# Ultrasound in Ophthalmologic Diagnosis

# Ultrasound in Ophthalmologic Diagnosis

## A Practical Guide

Rudolf Guthoff

With a contribution on physical principles by Johann M. Thijssen
Translated by F. C. Blodi
Foreword by Robert Machemer

204 illustrations, 29 tables



1991
Georg Thieme Verlag
Stuttgart · New York

Thieme Medical Publishers, Inc.
New York

Prof. Rudolf Guthoff, M.D.
University Hospital, Eppendorf
Eye Clinic
Martinistrasse 52
2000 Hamburg 20
West Germany

*Library of Congress Cataloging-in-Publication Data*

*Guthoff, Rudolf:*
Ultrasound in ophthalmologic diagnosis: a practical guide / Rudolf Guthoff; with a contribution on physical principles by Johann M. Thijssen; foreword by Robert Machemer, p. cm.
Includes bibliographical references an index.
ISBN 3-13-755901-4. – ISBN 0-86577-378-5
1. Eye-Ultrasonic imaging, I. Thijssen, J. M. II. Title. [DNLM; 1. Eye Diseases-diagnosis. 2. Ultrasonic Diagnosis. 141 G984u]
RE79.U4G87 1991
817.7.07543 – dc20
DNLM/DLC
for Library of Congress

Cover drawing: Renate Stockinger

**Important Note:** Medicine is an ever-changing science. Research and clinical experience are continually broadening our knowledge, in particular our knowledge of proper treatment and drug therapy. Insofar as this book mentions any dosage or application, readers may rest assured that the authors, editors and publishers have made every effort to ensure that such references are strictly in accordance with the **state of knowledge at the time of production of the book.** Nevertheless, every user is requested to examine carefully the manufacturer's leaflets accompanying each drug to check on his own responsibility whether the dosage schedules recommended therein or the contraindications stated by the manufacturers differ from the statements made in the present book. Such examination is particularly important with drugs that are either rarely used or have been newly released on the market.

This book is an authorized, expanded and revised translation from the 1st German edition, published and copyrighted 1988 by Ferdinand Enke Verlag, Stuttgart, Germany. Title of the German edition: Ultraschall in der ophthalmologischen Diagnostik. Ein Leitfaden für die Praxis. (Bücherei des Augenarztes, 116).


Thieme Medical Publishers, Inc., 381 Park Avenue South, New York, N.Y. 10016

Typesetting by Gulde-Druck GmbH, Tübingen
Printed in Germany by Gulde-Druck GmbH, Tübingen

ISBN 3-13-755901-4 (GTV, Stuttgart)
ISBN 0-86577-378-5 (TMP, New York)

1 2 3 4 5 6

# Foreword

Ultrasonography has become an essential part of the diagnostic armamentarium of the ophthalmologist. This is especially true for those interested in disease of the posterior segment of the eye. Despite the superb precision of A-scan ultrasonography, it has always been easier for the nonspecialist to read B-scan pictures.

The present monograph provides an excellent introduction to the theoretical background of ultrasonography and a superb atlas of the most commonly found clinical entities. Excellent schematic drawings explain the important features of the ultrasonogram at a glance. This is a book that I hope will find its way into many offices and serve as a quick guide to diagnosis.

October, 1990
*Robert Machemer, M.D.*
*Helena Rubinstein Foundation Professor of Ophthalmology Duke University Medical Center*

# Preface

"Measure whatever can be measured, and what cannot be measured, make measurable." Galileo Galilei

"What cannot be made measurable..?" Herbert Pietschmann

The pioneer work in the area of ophthalmic echography was already performed before 1960. This work fertilized other areas of ultrasound use. Nevertheless, ophthalmology was neglected for a long time when new machines were developed. A highly developed diagnostic tool evolved which was mainly based on the A-mode. Ossoinig, in particular, described this under the general concept of "standardized echography." For a few years ophthalmologic machines have been available which use digital processing, thereby producing temporal and spatial high-resolution echograms. This easily interpretable method of presentation facilitates learning the first steps of making an ultrasound diagnosis. At the same time we do not have to abandon quantifying the ultrasound signal with the simultaneously stored A-mode echogram. Dr. J. M. Thijssen has worked for twenty years on the physical principles of diagnostic echography in ophthalmology; his chapter on this topic contributes to this book greatly.

This monograph attempts to delineate the possibilities of echography in our specialty, while putting the cross-section echogram at the center of our considerations. By comparing the echogram with histopathologic sections, we try to demonstrate the limits of ultrasound diagnosis. Physical limitations prevent us from attempting to obtain a "tissue differentiation" in the true pathologic anatomical sense. Photomicrographs taken in loupe magnification will help us to correlate the substrate of the echogram – the acoustic interfaces of the tissues – with the resulting echographic pattern. Computerized B-scan guided ultrasound Doppler equipment has only recently been introduced into ophthalmology, and has opened up remarkable new perspectives. Examples of color-coded Doppler examinations are given for the differential diagnosis of intraocular tumors and the differentiation of ocular and orbital vascular diseases. In this way we attempt to determine the position of ultrasound diagnosis in the clinical decision-making process, therby facilitating the learning process for the neophyte.

I would like to thank here numerous consultants and assistants: the Chairman of the Department, Prof. Draeger, for the critical review of the manuscript; Prof. Naumann, for his editorial contribution. I am indebted to Mr. Helmdach for his instructive sketches; to the photo laboratory of the eye clinic, especially to Mrs. Bauer for photographic services; and to Mrs. Sebestyen for her extensive secretarial help. I would like to thank Dr. Beckenkamp and Prof. von Domarus for letting me use histopathologic illustrations, which they also interpreted. I am grateful to Dr. Helmke and Dr. Winkler for their close collaboration in preparing the Duplex and color-coded Doppler examinations.

I have to thank all my colleagues in the Eye Clinic, Radiology Clinic, Oral Surgery and Ear, Nose and Throat Clinic for referring patients and for stimulating discussions.

I am especially indebted to Dr. W. Schroeder, my friend and colleague, who introduced me to ophthalmologic ultrasound diagnosis. Lastly, I am indebted to Prof. Blodi, who translated the original German edition with great skill.

Hamburg, October 1990 *Rudolf Guthoff*

# Contents

# 1 Principles

## 1.1 History of Ultrasound Diagnosis

R. Guthoff and J. M. Thijssen

Toward the end of the last century it was found that acoustic energy also existed outside of the limits perceived by the human ear. This was a scientifically fruitful time during which radio waves, radioactivity and Roentgen rays were discovered. However, only a few scientists concerned themselves with ultrasound. In 1793 the Italian scholar Spallanzani (Figs. 1.**1** and 1.**2**) discovered that bats could fly in a completely darkened surrounding. If the animals' heads were covered by hoods, they could not avoid obstacles when flying, even when the hoods were transparent. Spallanzani modified this experiments in order to prove that a type of hearing helps the animals in orientation. Rather than using hoods, he placed wax spherules into the animals' auditory canals; this also eliminated their faculty of orientation. He postulated: "The uncanny faculty of bats to orient themselves when flying in darkness is connected with hearing."

Spallanzanis contemporaries thought the concept that bats could "see with their ears" was absurd. Scientists ridiculed the so-called Spallanzani bat problem. Finally, in 1940 Griffin and Galambos proved the connection. Bats and some water mammals have the capability to emit ultrasound impulses and then recognize and evaluate their echoes; this actually represents the principle of clinical ultrasound diagnosis.

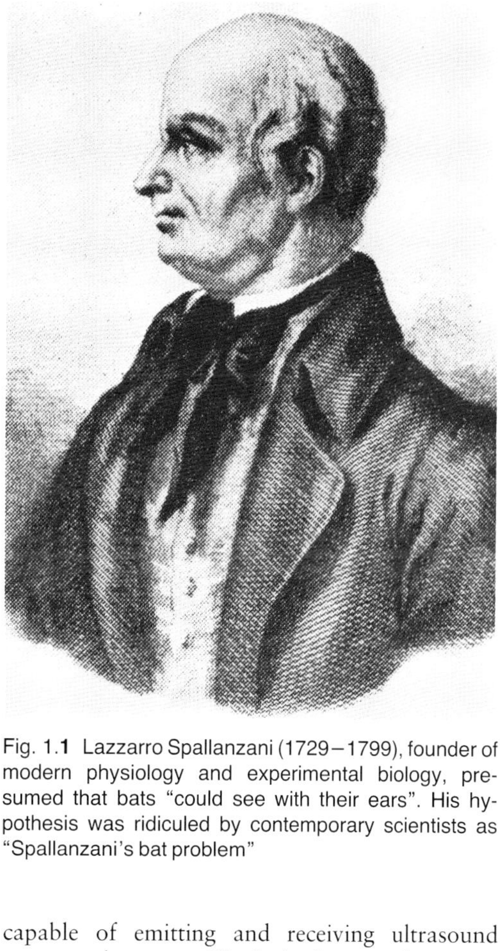

Fig. 1.**1** Lazzarro Spallanzani (1729–1799), founder of modern physiology and experimental biology, presumed that bats "could see with their ears". His hypothesis was ridiculed by contemporary scientists as "Spallanzani's bat problem"

It took a long time before the discovery of ultrasound energy was applied purposefully. The brothers Curie described in 1880 the piezo-electric effect. They discovered that by mechanically pressing on a tourmaline crystal, a difference in electric potential is created between opposing surfaces. On the other hand, an electric current will deform the shape of the crystal.

During World War I, the French physicist, Paul Langevin, used an underwater orientation device which, on the basis of the piezo-electric effect, was capable of emitting and receiving ultrasound waves under water. His device became the principle for the sonar system which was important during World War II.

The invention of the so-called "reflectoscope" by Firestone (1942) was the most significant advance for ultrasound diagnosis. This instrument is used for testing different kinds of material without damaging the material itself. With a similar device, Ludwig (1949) succeeded in detecting gallstones in patients. The first publication on ophthalmologic

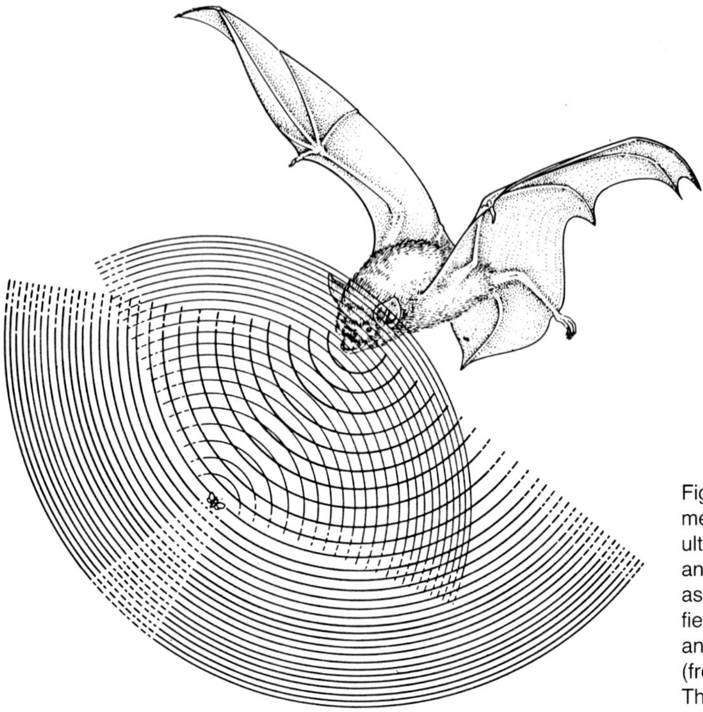

Fig. 1.2 Schematic illustration of methods used by bats for orientation by ultrasound. Sounds emitted by these animals will be reflected from obstacles as long as they lie within the ultrasound field. The echo is used for orientation and for estimating the speed of flight (from R. Ekkert: Tierphysiologie. Thieme, Stuttgart 1986)

ultrasound diagnosis appeared in 1956 and was published by G.H. Mundt and W.F. Hughes (1956). They succeeded in localizing intraocular tumors with a certain degree of reliability. In 1957 Oksala and Lethinen published a series of fundamental papers on the ophthalmologic A-mode diagnostic method. This method was further developed, especially in Europe (Buschmann, Ossoinig), and was complemented by the diagnosis of orbital processes and by biometry (Gernet). Around the same time G. Baum and J. Greenwood introduced their two-dimensional B-mode to ophthalmology. They stated that their apparatus simulates a slit lamp, except that a pulsed ultrasound beam is substituted for the light beam. It projected light-modulated points on a screen, thereby obtaining acoustic tissue sections. They succeeded already in recognizing retinal detachment, hemorrhages and even orbital pathologic changes. This technique required a complicated water bath coupling between the eye and the transducer. Bronson (1972) developed a hand-held contact B-mode transducer. This led to a rapid dissemination of echographic diagnostic methods in ophthalmology. In 1964 Buschmann founded in Berlin the Societas Internationalis Pro Diagnostica Ultrasonica in Ophthalmologia (SIDUO), which is the oldest medical specialty society for ultrasound diagnosis. Its meetings are held at two-year intervals and attended by interested ophthalmologists and basic scientists.

## 1.2 Physical Principles with Special Consideration of Ophthalmologic Problems

J. M. Thijssen

### 1.2.1 Characteristics of Ultrasound

Ultrasound is sound with a frequency beyond the range of human hearing (20 000 Hz). The frequency expresses the number of cycles per second. The unit hertz (Hz) is based on Heinrich Hertz, a German physicist.

Sound represents mechanical waves, i.e., a periodic movement of mass. This differentiates ultrasound diagnosis from other imaging modalities, which all use electromagnetic waves. This means that echograms provide entirely different information about the examined tissues.

We distinguish longitudinal and transversal waves. Figure 1.**3** is an example of a transversal wave. The excursion runs here vertical to the direction of the sound beam. The temporal distance between two points of identical position, e.g., the peak of the wave, is called a period (T). Frequency is the reciprocal of this value. The spatial distance corresponding to one period defines the wavelength. If we know the speed of propagation (c), we can calculate the wavelength:

$\lambda = c \times T$ (m).

In a similar way we define and calculate the wavelengths of longitudinal waves, to which ultrasound belongs. In liquids and gases only longitudinal waves occur. As Fig. 1.**4** shows schematically, ultrasound is produced by a transducer. A ceramic plate (K), serves as a piezo-electric element which is coupled to thin conductor layers (L). On the front surface is a protective layer (S) and on the back surface, a piece of damping material (D). The latter is installed to dissipate energy from the excursions of the ceramic plate after the electric impulse, thereby shortening the duration of the emitted ultrasound signal.

The periodic densifications and rarefactions of the ceramic plate are transmitted as a longitudinal wave (Fig. 1.**5**) to the patient's body. That means that a pressure wave extends in the tissue. Local pressure changes (P) periodically densify and rarefy the tissue. The molecules are pushed to and

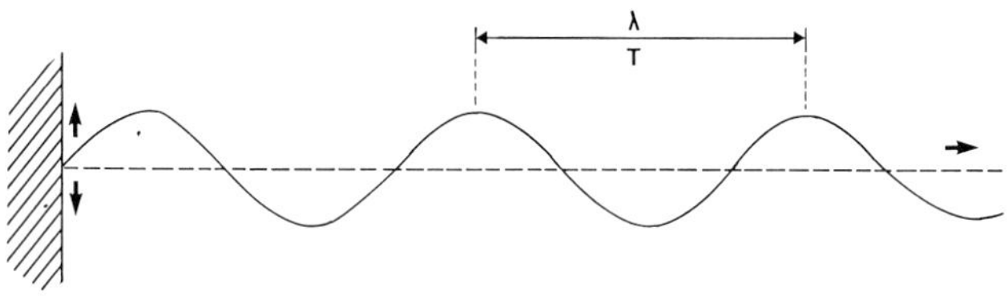


Fig. 1.**3** Example of a sinusoidal wave. Period time T and wavelength lambda

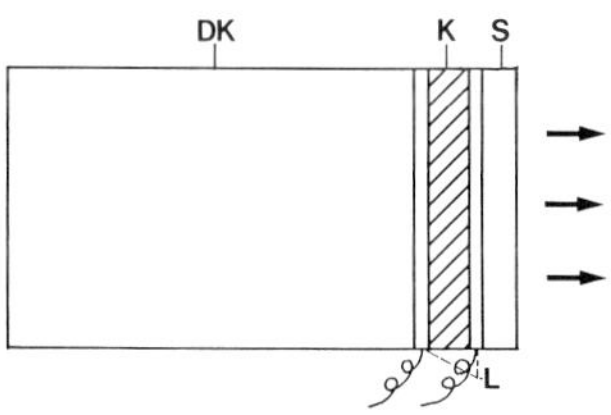


Fig. 1.**4** Structure of a transducer (DK = dampening body, L = conductor layers, K = piezo-electric ceramic, S = protective layer)

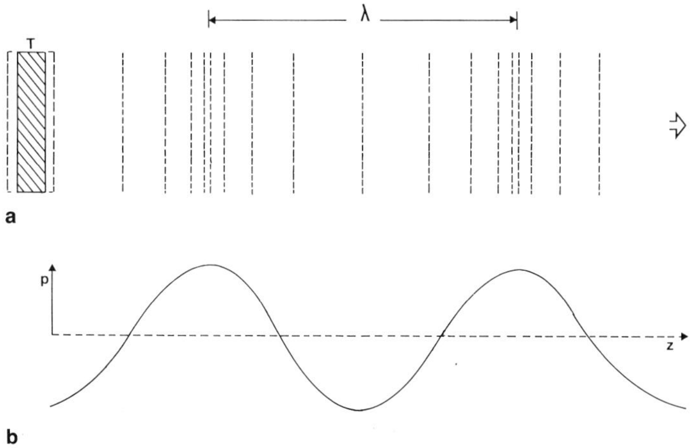


Fig. 1.**5 a, b**
**a** Longitudinal compression wave (T = transducer).
**b** Temporal course of sound pressure (lambda = wavelength, p = sound pressure, z = depth)

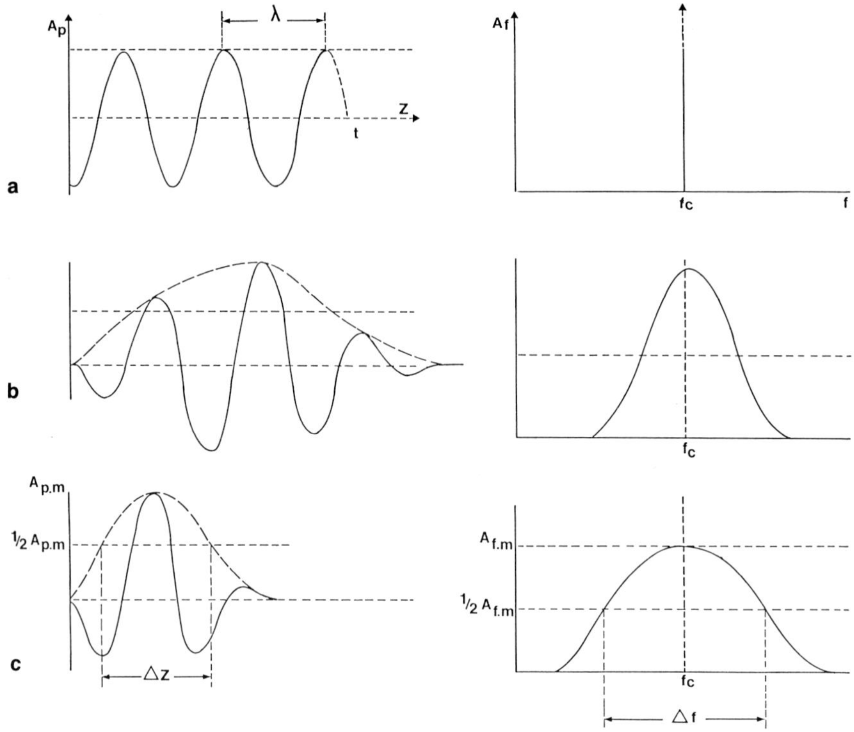


Fig. 1.**6a–c** Correlation between impulse duration and spectrum
**a** On the left: continuous wave, dashed line; the envelope, $A_p$ = pressure amplitude, t = time. On the right: spectrum, $A_f$ = pressure amplitude in the domain of frequency, f = frequency, $f_c$ = central frequency commensurate with the wavelength
**b** On the left: pulsed wave (4 periods). On the right: the corresponding spectrum
**c** On the left: pulsed wave (2 periods). Half-width value delta z. On the right: spectrum, half-width value delta f

fro. These motions extend into the direction of the ultrasound. Their magnitude lies considerably beneath the wavelength of ultrasound.

The wavelength can be calculated from the frequency of the ultrasound and the speed of sound: $\lambda = c/f$ (m).

**Example:**

The speed of ultrasound in tissue is about 1500 m/s. The diagnostic frequency lies above 1 MHz (= 1 megahertz = 1 million hertz). This means for a transducer of 10 MHz:
$\lambda = 1500/10^7 \text{(m)} = 1.5 \times 10^6/10^7 \text{(mm)} = 1.5/10 = 0.15$ (mm).

The calculation has been simplified by transposing 1500 m/s into 1.5 mm/μs (1μs = 1 microsecond) and $10^7$ Hz into 10 megahertz. In this way we always work with units of millimeters and MHz in ultrasound diagnosis.

Wavelength is an important quality characteristic of any ultrasound device. If we place an alternate current over the electric conductor layers of the ceramic plate, the plate will show continuous vibrations and will emit a continuous acoustic wave (Fig. 1.**6a**, left). This constant wave can be characterized by its amplitude and its wavelength in tissue. In a frequency spectrum of this wave (Fig. 1.**6**, right), only one frequency ($f_c$) will be present, which has an infinitely high amplitude ($A_f$). In diagnostic echography we use continuous waves only to measure blood flow (see Sect. 1.2.5, Doppler effect).

For the pulse-echo technique we use short pulses as shown in Figs. 1.6**b** and **c**. The corresponding frequency spectra are drawn on the right side of the figure. They show that a short pulse duration is necessarily connected with a wide frequency spectrum.

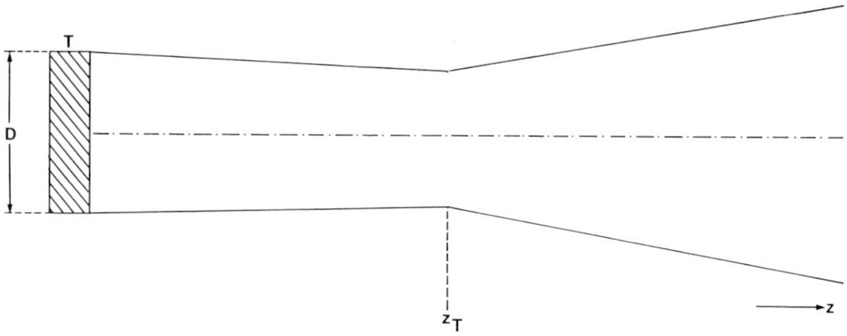


Fig. 1.7 Schematic sketch of a sound field from a flat transducer. D = diameter, $z_T$ = transition distance (transition from near to far field)

The duration of the pulse and the width of the spectrum are characterized by their half-width values (Fig. 1.6). In the time diagram of ultrasound pressure, the envelope, a curve necessary for the determination of half-width values, is represented by a dashed line.

From the definition we can deduce that for a higher frequency, the duration of the pulse – if the number of oscillations remains the same – becomes shorter, which implies that the depth resolution of the instrument increases. In other words: in order to elicit the same number of oscillations during an impulse, a shorter period of time is necessary and therefore the following holds true: the shorter the wavelength, the greater the resolution power.

**Example:**

The impulse in Fig. 1.6c has a half-width value of about 1 period. The depth resolution therefore corresponds to one wavelength.

Transducer: 8 MHz

Speed of sound: 1.5 mm/μs

$\lambda = c/f \approx 0.2$ mm.

The impulse in Fig. 1.6b, on the other hand, has a half-width value of about 2 periods, i.e., the value 2. For a transducer of 8 MHz, this means a depth resolution of 0.4 mm. This value applies to most ophthalmologic A-mode machines.

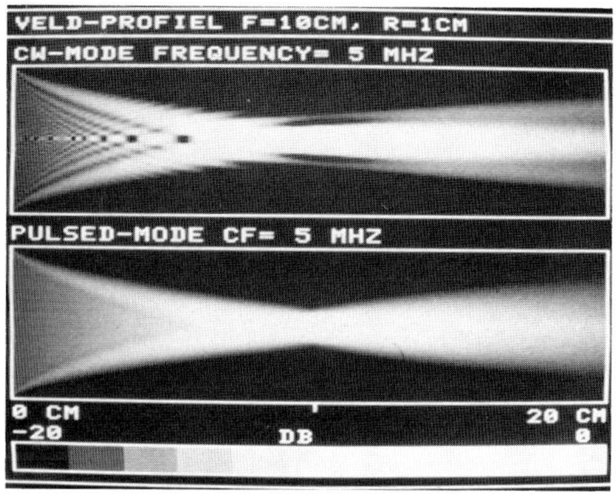


a

b

Fig. 1.8 a, b Calculated cross-sections of the sound field.

**a** Continuous wave. The interference in the near field and the lateral lobes is well visible.

**b** Pulsed mode, nearly no interferences (after Verhoef, Cloostermans, Thijssen 1984)

### 1.2.2 Sound Field Extent

The sound field produced by a transducer in a homogenous medium, e.g., water, is shown schematically in Fig. 1.7. Physically, this field can be compared with a laser beam or a Fraunhofer field which appears when light exits through a small shutter opening. The transducer is, like a laser device, a source of coherent waves; thus we must distinguish a **near field** from a **far field**. In optics this corresponds to the Fresnel and the Fraunhofer regions. The transition distance ($z_t$), where one region changes into the other, can be described by the calculation:

$z_T = D^2/4\lambda = D^2f/4c$ (mm).

**Example:**

Transducer diameter D = 5 mm

Frequency f = 8 MHz

Sound velocity c = 1.5 mm/s

$z_T = 33.3$ mm.

Fig. 1.7 shows that the near field has a cylindrical shape, whereas the far field diverges while it expands. Figure 1.8 shows cross sections through the axis of a sound field. The upper picture was calculated for a continuous wave transmission. It clearly shows the numerous interference patterns in the near field. Diffraction of the waves at the edge of the transducer causes the side lobes, which branch from the main lobe of the sound beam.

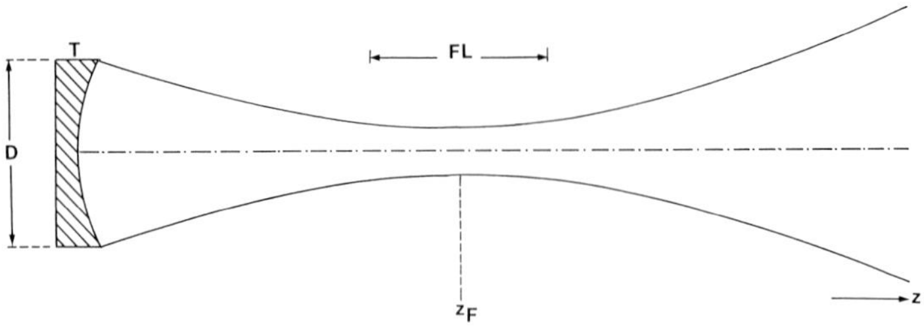


Fig. 1.**9** Schematic drawing of the sound field of a focused transducer. FL = focal length, $z_f$ = focal distance

a
b
c

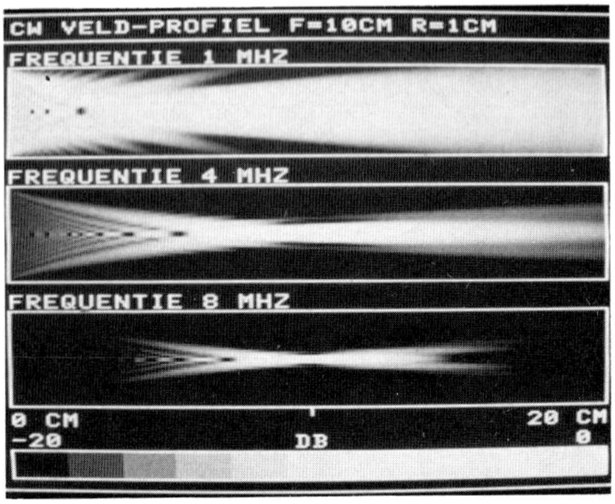


Fig. 1.**10a–c** The effect of frequency on the cross-section of the sound field in the focus (continuous waves), focal distance 10 cm
**a** 1 MHz, practically no focusing
**b** 4 MHz, focus well visible
**c** 8 MHz, diminution of the diameter in the focus

With the pulsed mode of operation, the sound beam is not so complicated (Fig. 1.**8b**). There is less danger of overlooking small structures lying in the region of sound field minima, the so-called "acoustic holes".

The relatively large diameter of the sound field limits the lateral resolution in the area of the main lobe also. Acoustic lenses bonded to the transducer will focus the beam in the near field. Figure 1.**9** shows that such a transducer can be characterized by its focal distance ($z_F$). The relation of focal distance and transducer diameter (D) is a measure for the strength of focusing.

The focal diameter ($x_F$) can be calculated in the following way:
$x_F = 2.44\ \lambda F/D = 2.44\ cF/fD$ (mm).
**Example:**
Sound velocity: c = 1.5 mm/s
Transducer-focus distance: F = 25 mm
Transducer frequency: f = 10 MHz
Transducer diameter: D = 5 mm
$x_F = 1.8$ mm.

The lateral resolution of an ultrasound device is often characterized by the **half-width value of the sound field** in the focus. Figure 1.**10** illustrates how focusing depends on the frequency. The sound beam cross sections were calculated for the given frequencies. This shows that both lateral resolution as well as depth resolution increase with high frequencies.

A characteristic of focusing is the length of the focus (FL). It is defined as the distance between the two sound beam diameters which are twice as large as the focal diameter (Fig. 1.**9**).

### 1.2.3 The Interactions of Ultrasound and Tissue

These interactions are summarized in Fig. 1.**11**. Snellen's laws apply here for reflection and refraction as they do for light.
Reflection:
1. $\Theta_1 = \Theta_1'$.
Refraction:
2. $\dfrac{\text{sine}\ \Theta_1}{c_1} = \dfrac{\text{sine}\ \Theta_2}{c_2}$

**Example:**
Sound velocity in aqueous: 1530 m/s
Sound velocity in the lens: 1640 m/s
$\Theta_1 = 30°$
$\Theta_2 = 32°$.

The acoustic impedance (Z) determines the reflected (r) and the transmitted (t) amplitude of sound when the beam is perpendicular to the interface (Fig. 1.**12**).

This relationship is described by the following formulas, i.e., the fraction of sound reflected:

$$r = \frac{Z_2 - Z_1}{Z_2 + Z_1} \times 100\% \text{ and } t = 1 - r.$$

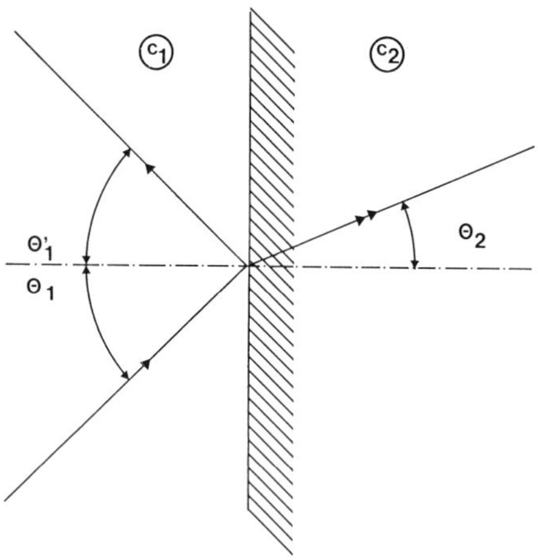


a

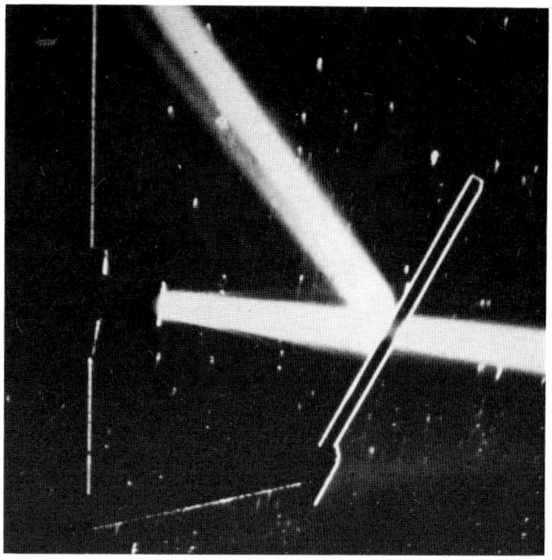

b

Fig. 1.**11 a, b** Snell's laws of reflection and refraction
**a** Schematic drawing ($c_1$ larger than $c_2$)

**b** Schlieren image (turned 90° to the left). The refraction on the anterior and posterior surface of the reflector is visible as a parallel displacement of the sound beam

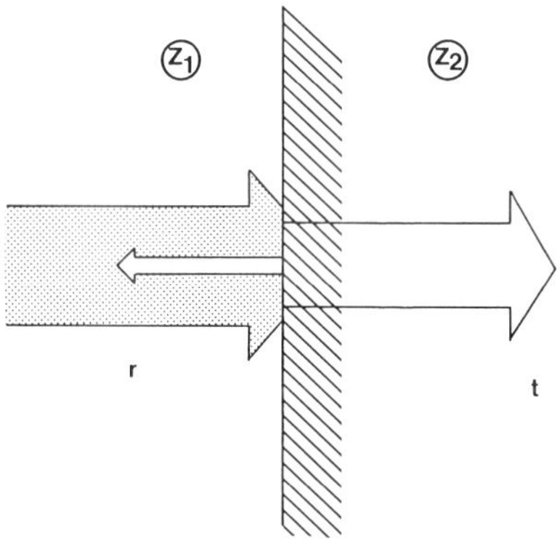


Fig. 1.**12** Determining the amount of reflection (r) and of transmission (t) when the angle of incidence is 90°

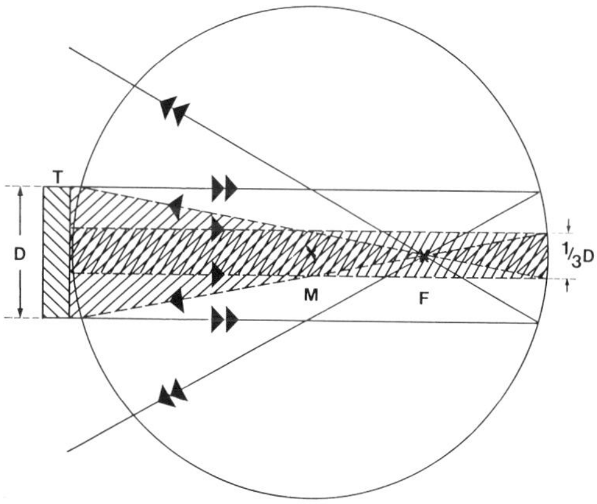


Fig. 1.**13** Reflection from a spherical surface (e.g., the ocular fundus). Focus of the concave mirror (F), center (M). After reflection the diameter of the field is exactly three times larger, i.e., the effective diameter of the sound field is one-third of the original diameter (after Thijssen: Echo-ophthalmography: Physical principles and diagnostic value. In: H. E. Henkes (editor), Doc. Ophthalmologica Proc. Ser. Vol. 3, Junk, Den Haag 1973, p. 273)

Acoustic impedance is defined as
$Z = \varrho c$
with $\varrho$ = thickness of the mass
c = sound velocity.

**Example:**
Sound velocity as in the previous example: 1500 m/s
Density of aqueous: $10^3$ kg/m$^3$
Density of the lens: $1.07 \times 10^3$ kg/m$^3$
r = 7%.

When a sound beam impacts a surface obliquely, the amount of reflected sound is lower the more the angle deviates from the vertical direction.

Ultrasound reflection influences the imaging of the **shape of the eyeball**. We see in Fig. 1.**13** that the spherical shape of the eyeball wall creates a focal point for the reflected ultrasound. This point lies at a distance of one-half the radius of curvature in

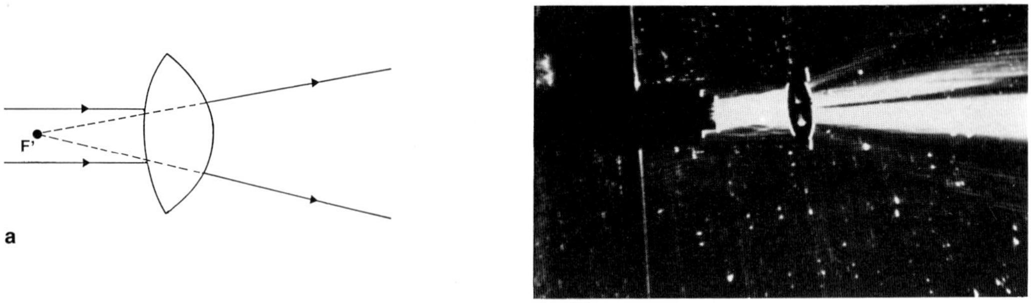


Fig. 1.**14** a, b Biconcave acoustic lens when the sound velocity in the lens is greater than in the surrounding media

**a** Schematic drawing, focus (F′)
**b** Schlieren image of the effect by the lens

front of the posterior pole. Because of this phenomenon, only about one-third of the diameter of the sound field can be received by the transducer to the formation of the image. For the same reasons, increased curvature of the retina in the fovea leads thereby contributing, to a considerable widening of the sound field after reflection. Thus, the intensity of the echo from the fovea is too low to allow exact imaging in this sector.

The lens presents another intraocular structure which, on the basis of the laws of refraction, will influence the ultrasound. The sound velocity in the aqueous and in the vitreous is slower than in the lens. Therefore, the biconvex shape of the lens will diverge the ultrasound (Fig. 1.**14**), in contrast to the behavior of light rays. The focal distance of the lens equals −55 mm.

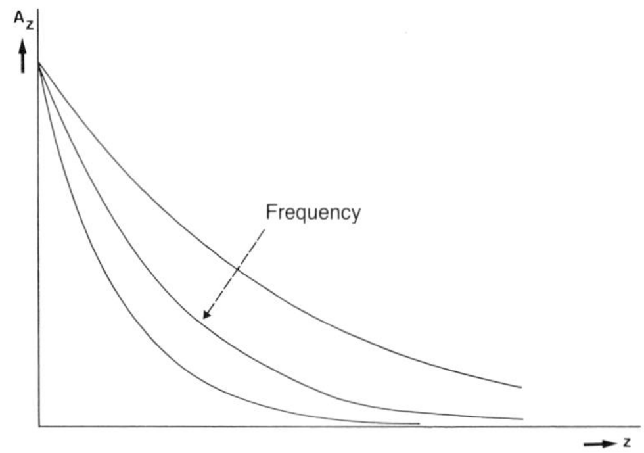


Fig. 1.**15** Sound attenuation; the exponential curves represent sound pressure as it decreases in the tissue. The attenuation is greater the higher the frequency (i. e., also: decreasing depth penetration)

### 1.2.4 Attenuation and Scattering of the Sound Waves

Attenuation of sound is based on two tissue effects: absorption and scattering. Absorption is the transformation of sound energy into heat. This process occurs at the molecular level and consists of relaxation oscillations of organic macromolecules. Scattering is a reflection in all directions which occurs from small structures, e. g., the walls of capillaries, connective tissue septa or cell membranes. The scattered sound energy is thereby eliminated from the sound field and only a small fraction will be received by the transducer as a tissue echo. Both of these mechanisms attenuate the ultrasound pulse as well as the reflected ultrasound signal. This attenuation increases exponentially with tissue depth and linearly with the frequency (Fig. 1.**15**). On the other hand, axial resolution increases when a higher frequency is employed; therefore, choosing a certain frequency for echographic examination will always represent a compromise between the desired depth of penetration and the possible resolution.

The attenuation (in cm) and the amount of reflection are denoted in **decibels**:

$dB = 20 \log_{10} (p_2/p_1)$,

whereby $p_2/p_1$ expresses the relation between the sound pressure in the media 1 and 2 (reflection) or in the depths 1 and 2 (attenuation).

**Example:**

| | | | | | | | | |
|---|---|---|---|---|---|---|---|---|
| $p_1/p_2$ = | 1 | 2 | 3 | 10 | 100 | ½ | ⅓ | |
| dB = | 0 | 6 | 10 | 20 | 40 | −6 | −10 | etc. |

The sound attenuation in the aqueous and in the vitreous is negligible. In the lens it is 20 times as high; this is one of the reasons why the sound waves should not have to traverse the lens when

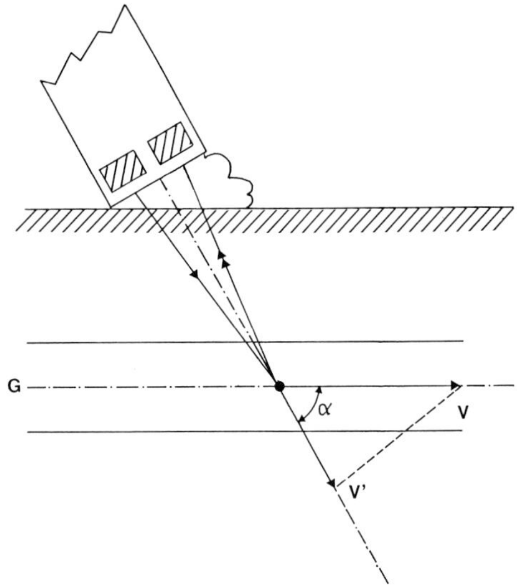


Fig. 1.**16** Measuring conditions for determining blood flow velocity by the Doppler effect. G = vessel, v = blood flow velocity, emitter and receiver transducers

pathologic changes in the posterior segment of the eye are diagnosed.

### 1.2.5 The Doppler Effect

Up to now we have assumed that the reflecting interfaces are stable compared to the generation and detection of the ultrasound. If the generator and/or the receiver moves with a relative velocity (v), the reflected waves will undergo a frequency shift (Delta f) compared to the emitted frequency. For this purpose, in ultrasound diagnosis we use a single transducer with two ceramic plates (Fig. 1.**16**). One element emits a continuous wave of ultrasound (CW-Doppler), while the other receives the reflected signals.

In this way we can measure the shift in frequency caused by the intravascular blood particles which act as scattering reflectors. The Doppler effect can be described by the following equation:

$$f = -2vf/c = \frac{-2v'f\cos\alpha}{c},$$

with f = frequency, v = blood flow velocity, c = sound velocity, $\alpha$ = angle between axis of sound beam and direction of movement (Fig. 1.**16**).

The equation shows that in order to determine blood flow velocity exactly, we have to know the angle "alpha". In practice we can omit exactly measuring this angle if it lies between 0 and 30° because only the cosine is considered in the calculation. By frequency demodulation, Doppler shifts can be made audible over a loudspeaker. With modern pulse-echo Doppler (pulsed-Doppler) devices, we are able to determine the velocity of blood flow in an area selected in a real-time B-mode echogram. These techniques are at present only of experimental interest for ophthalmology.

## 1.3. Dosimetry

As far as we know today, diagnostic ultrasound devices do not cause any tissue damage. Nevertheless, a brief description of the relevant dosimetric quantities may be indicated. We also have to consider the time during which ultrasound is applied, i.e., the length of the examination, because there may be a summation of injurious effects in the tissues.

The energy is defined as the product of sound power (P) and exposure time (t).
E = Pt (Joule, J).

Sound power is therefore energy per time unit. The formula is: P = E/t (J/s = Watt, W).

Measuring the sound power is done in a water bath with a material that completely absorbs the ultrasound. In this way we can measure the force exerted on this material. It increases proportionately to the sound power.

In order to measure biological damage, we calculate the power per unit area (intensity, I):
I = P/D ($W/cm^2$) (D = cross section of the ultrasound beam).

The intensity can also be determined by pressure measurements, for this purpose, a hydrophone is used. In the focus of the sound field the intensity can be derived from the sound pressure p. The following formula applies:
$I = p^2/Z$ ($W/cm^2$) (Z = acoustic impedance).

The transformation of ultrasound energy into heat causes a local rise in temperature. This leads to a heat conduction in the tissue and counteracts the heat convection via the vascular system. The extent of possible thermal damage is therefore not determined by the impulse intensity, but by the spatial peak temporal average intensity (Ispta). According to the recommendations of the American Institute for Ultrasound in Medicine, this value should, in diagnostic ultrasound, **not** exceed 100 $mW/cm^2$.

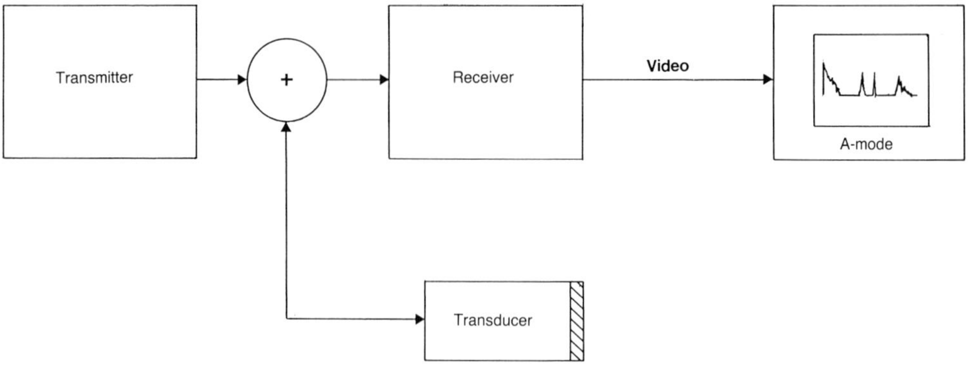


Fig. 1.**17** Schematic sketch of an A-mode instrument. The transducer is connected with the transmitter and the receiver. A-echogram = time pattern of the echo amplitudes

## 1.4 Ultrasonic Instruments

### 1.4.1 The A-Mode Technique

The A-mode system derives its name from "amplitude". This is an amplitude modulation. The A echogram is one-dimensional, i.e., it indicates – with known sound velocity – exactly the location of a reflecting interface within the organs insonified by the ultrasound.

Figure 1.**17** depicts such as instrument in a schematic way. An electronic transmitter generates periodically (1000 ×/second) a short impulse with high amplitude (200 V). This electrical pulse is transmitted to the transducer which then emits a short ultrasound pulse. The signals reflected from the tissues will deform the piezo-electric element. This produces an electric signal (rf-signal) which is registered by the receiver. Figure 1.**17** shows that the receiver is connected to the transducer and to the pulser. The electric pulse produces at the same time a saturation of the receiver, causing a "dead zone" at the left in the A-mode display.

The receiver consists of an adjustable radio frequency amplifier (dB-control), a demodulator and a filter. The function of a demodulator is explained in Fig. 1.**18**: the rf-oscillations are nearly completely eliminated and each echo signal is represented as a separate spike. Additional filters smooth the ripples of the now rectified video signals. Figure 1.**19** shows the influence of the filters.

It may be mentioned that filtering of the signals will unavoidably lessen the steep increase of the individual spikes and therefore reduce the theoretically possible exactness of depth measurements (see Sect. 1.5). The video signal is then led into the vertical deviation system of the oscilloscope while the horizontal deviation is synchronized with the transmitted pulse. The first signal which is due to this pulse is presented as a spike of maximal height and definite width (Fig. 1.**18**), i.e., the dead zone. The covering layer of the transducer (protective layer or acoustic lens) will also lead to a temporal delay between the emission of ultrasound waves and their entrance into tissues. This so-called **"null point error"** depends upon the apparatus used and should be known for the individual case. For this reason, distance measurements with direct contact of the transducer on the eye are not necessarily absolutely correct.

#### Amplification Characteristics of Ultrasound Devices

The total amplification of A-mode equipment may be linear, logarithmic or S-shaped (Fig. 1.**20a**). In **linear** amplification the height of the spike on the screen is proportional to the amplitude of the received echo (Fig. 1.**20a**), at least below a certain maximal value. Higher amplitudes will always be displayed as maximal spikes (saturation of the amplifier). **Logarithmic** amplification (dotted line in Fig. 1.**20a**) leads only at higher echo amplitudes to saturation, so that the dynamic range of an amplifier can be increased. The relations are presented in Figure 1.**20b** in a semilogarithmic form. It should be noted that the logarithmic amplification now yields a straight line. Ossoinig (1971) introduced as an alternative the **S-shaped** amplification mode to ophthalmology (Fig. 1.**20b**). Its advantage is an optimal display of tissue echos, i.e., between

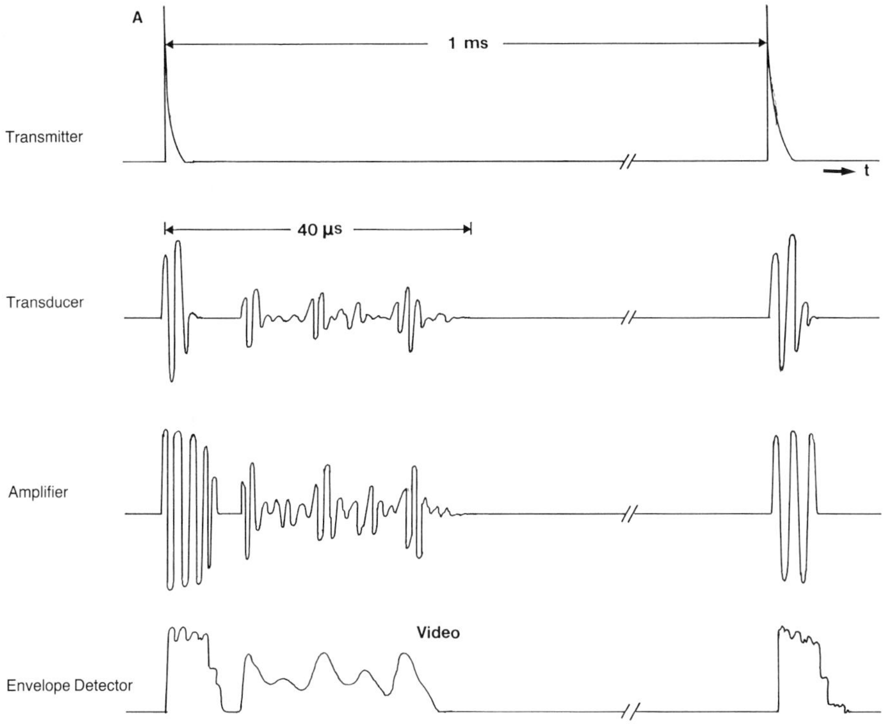


Fig. 1.**18** Time pattern of signal processing in an A-mode instrument. Time distance of the emitted pulses: 1 ms (see text) Amplifier and demodulator are in the receiver (Fig. 1.**17**)

a

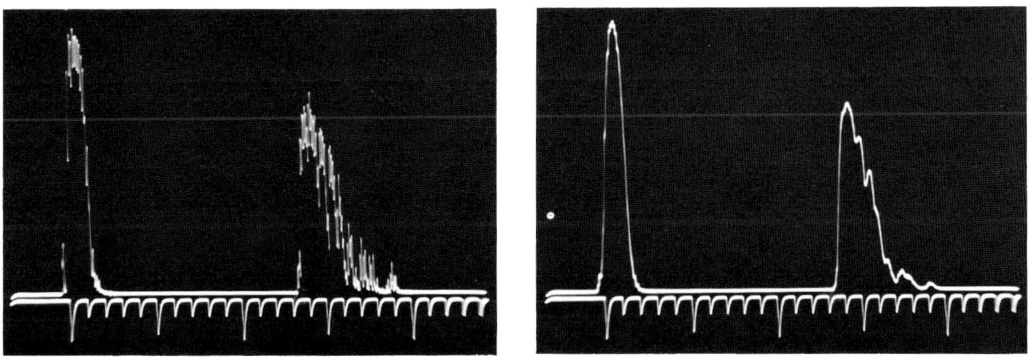

b

Fig. 1.**19a, b** Effects of less (**a**) and more (**b**) deep filtering of the echo signal (video) after demodulation

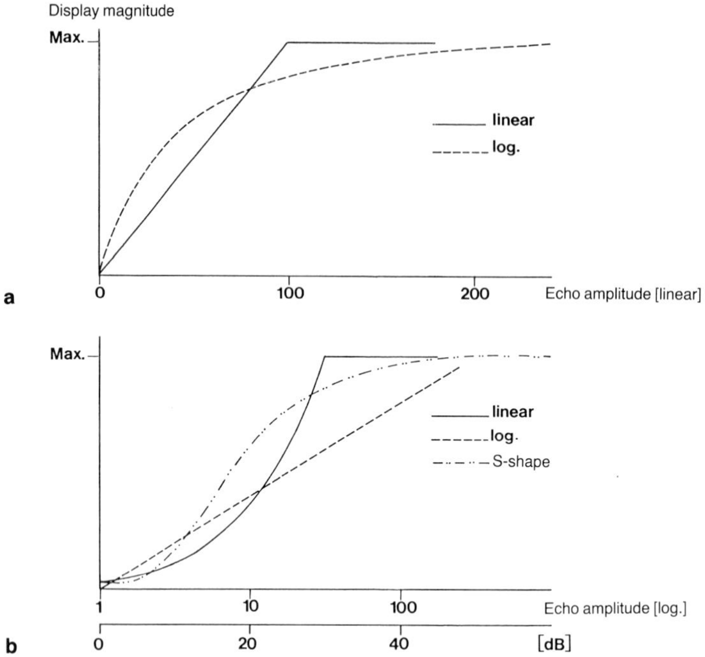


Fig. 1.**20** **a, b** Characteristic curves for various amplifications: the amplitude of the image on the A-mode screen (ordinate) and of the echos (abscissa)
**a** Linear representation, tangent of linear representation = amplification
**b** Logarithmic representation on the abscissa. S-shaped amplification added. Dynamic range = range of echo amplitudes up to saturation (in dB)

10 and 30 dB in Fig. 1.**20b**. This method is considered most valuable for tissue differentiation. Linear amplification modes are used in some biometry devices.

Figure 1.**21** shows tissue echograms obtained with a logarithmic or an S-shaped mode under various amplifications. The advantage of the logarithmic mode is obvious: the attenuation of the sound in tissues, i.e., the decay of amplitude heights commensurate with tissue depth (the angle kappa of Ossoinig), does not depend upon the setting of the amplifier (cf. Fig. 1.**21a** vs. **b**, left, and **c** left). The amount of reflection for individual structures can be determined in dB directly on the screen because the amplitude of the echogram is proportional to the logarithmic value of the height of the echo signal. The advantage of the S-shaped amplification is a somewhat enhanced opportunity to differentiate echo amplitudes within a middle range of reflections. A disadvantage is that the angle kappa depends upon the setting of the amplifier (cf. Fig. 1.**21a** vs. **b**, right, and **c**, right).

Exact **calibration** of the machine is necessary to make tissue differentiations possible. For this purpose, reflectors made of contact lens material (Trier 1977, Haigis 1980, Buschmann 1977) and a solid tissue model of a synthetic rubber with microbeads (Till 1976) have been recommended.

The total sensitivity of the instrument depends upon the transducer, the amplifier and the oscilloscope display. For calibration purposes we determine the amount of amplification which generates a certain echo level on the screen under well-defined conditions. A prerequisite is a reliably calibrated amplification control (dB-control). In practice it is recommended that the calibration level be based upon a definite total sensitivity. Ossoinig coined the term "tissue sensitivity" for this type of calibration. For biometric purposes, it is reasonable to decrease the amplification by about 15 dB. This amount of amplification is also called measuring sensitivity.

### Possibilities of Calibrating an Apparatus

The Hema-W-38 reflector (1, 2, 6) consists of a soft contact lens material with a water content of 38%. The amount of reflection of this material is quite high compared with that of biological structures. The difference from total (i.e., 100%) reflection is −16.5 dB. We achieve the tissue sensitivity recommended by Ossoinig if we set the decibel regulator 58 dB above the standard echo of the Hema reflector.

The tissue model of Till (1976) is composed of silicone and vulcanized microbeads (producer:

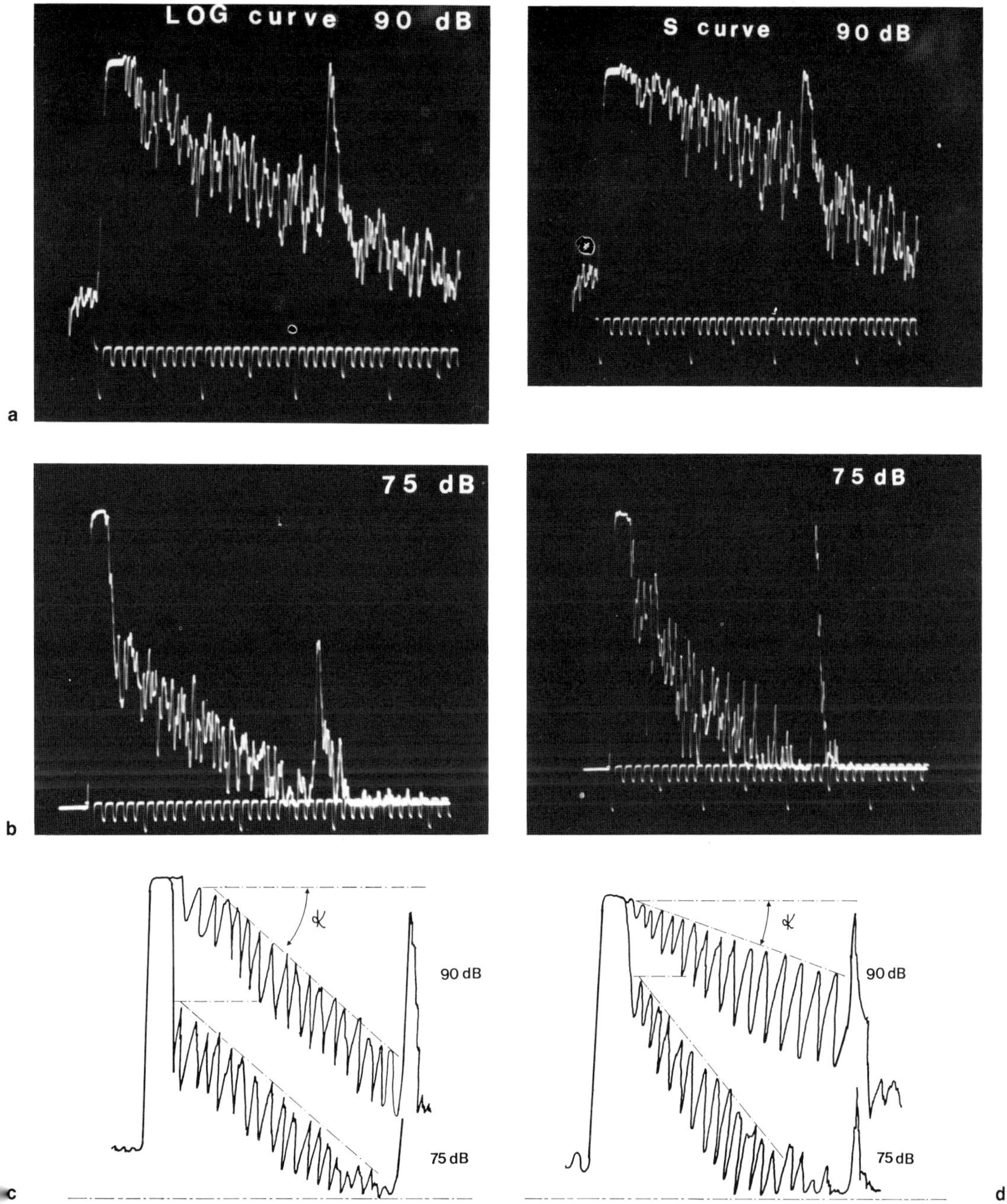


Fig. 1.**21 a–d** The consequences of logarithmic and S-shaped amplification for imaging tissue echograms
**a** Logarithmic amplification (40 dB dynamics): parallel displacement of the echo pattern, angle kappa (degree of attenuation) is independent of the amplification or the amount of reflection. The amount of reflection is the initial height of the spikes. Tissue model of Till, Triscan (Biophysique Medical)
**b** S-shaped amplification (33 dB dynamics): the angle kappa depends upon the height of imaging. Wide dynamic imaging spectrum for echos of average amount of reflection
**c, d** Schematic sketches of the imaging shown in **a** and **b**

Eisenbamberger, St. Pölten, Austria), e.g., glass pearls. We attempt to find an amplification which produces a typical, easily reproducible echogram pattern. This pattern is illustrated in Figs. 1.**21a** and **b**. The amplitude of the spikes decreases continuously between the initial peak and the reflection at the metal bottom of the test tube. When setting for tissue sensitivity, the dB-control is set in such a way that the model pattern lies symmetrically between 100 and 0% of the amplitude.

Modern A-mode instruments make it possible to **"freeze" the echogram**. Electronically, this technique is based on digital data storage. Its principle is shown in Fig. 1.**22**: at regular intervals the amplitude pattern is read, i.e., a sample is taken, and changed into digital information. The frequency of sampling per time unit determines the precision with which the original, analog, signal is stored. The (technical) precision of measuring with such an analog-to-digital converter (ADC) is explained in the following example.

**Example:**

Sampling frequency $f_m = 20$ MHz

Sampling time $\triangle t = 1/f_m = 50 \times 10^{-3}$ µs

Sampling depth extension $\triangle z = \frac{1}{2} \times c \times \triangle t = \frac{1}{2} \times 1.5 \times 5- \times 10^{-3} = 0.0375$ mm $= 37.5$ µm.

## 1.4.2 The B-Mode Technique

In the B-mode technique (time-brightness method) the echos are displayed as light dots of varying brightness (B = brightness). In addition to this brightness modulation, there is an electromagnetic coupling between the transducer position and the image screen. In this way a two-dimensional section through the tissue is obtained. The B-mode or "B-mode echogram" allows good evaluation of anatomical relationships. It is, however, more dif-

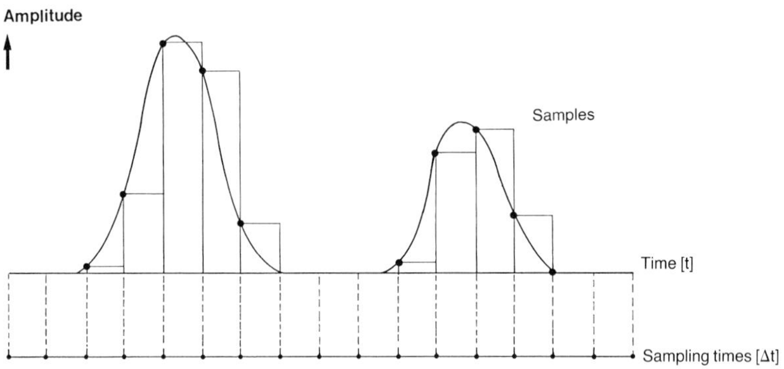


Fig. 1.**22** Digital representation of the echo pattern. For each sample the amplitude is stored electronically as a binary digit. The sampling frequency is the recriprocal of the interval period

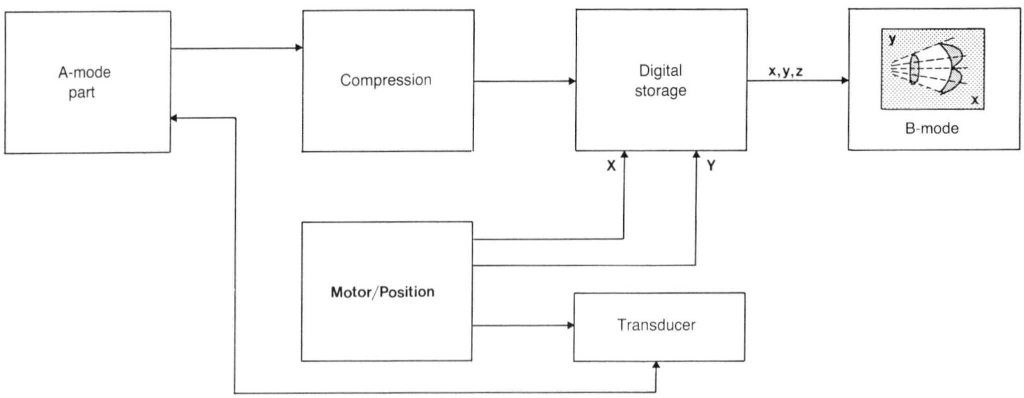


Fig. 1.**23** Schematic presentation of a B-mode instrument. Trasmitter-receiver in the A-mode part. Compression of the amplitude dynamics depends upon the extent of digitalization (number of bits). Motor drive and position coding system of the transducer (sector scanning) Digital storage of the echo and position informations. Readout on a B-mode screen

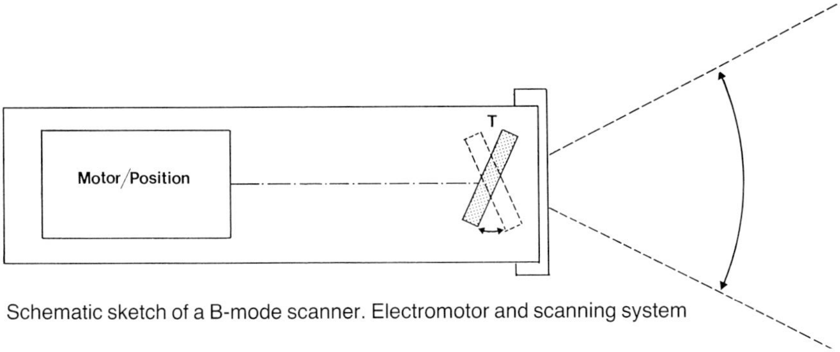


Fig. 1.**24** Schematic sketch of a B-mode scanner. Electromotor and scanning system

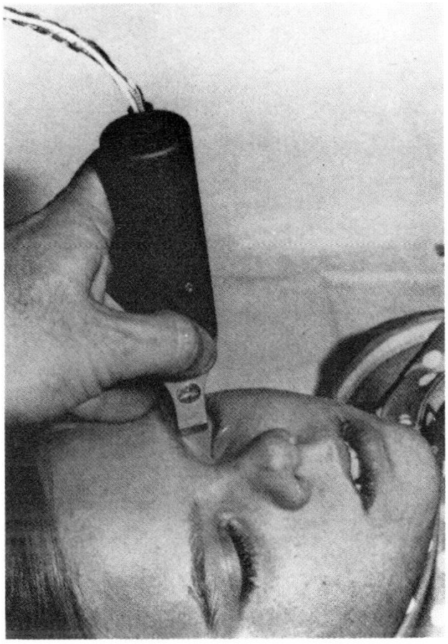

Fig. 1.**25** The Bronson scanner (1972)

ficult to judge the amplitudes of individual signals because the differentiation of a gray scale by the human visual system is limited. This can be more easily achieved by the A-mode.

Figure 1.**23** illustrated schematically a B-mode instrument. Principally, we need an A-mode part (Fig. 1.**17**) which receives, amplifies and rectifies the echogram. The transducer contained in the scanner is moved automatically and governed by an electromotor (Figs. 1.**24** and 1.**25**). The position of the transducer is registered electromechanically.

Modern instruments also contain a system for digital storage of the position signals (X/Y). By using these signals a video signal (Z) is generated which allows direct display on a television monitor, or storage on videotape. Figure 1.**26** shows a vector scan schematically. By using digital storing a post-processing is possible. Figure 1.**27** shows a modern ophthalmologic A- and B-mode apparatus.

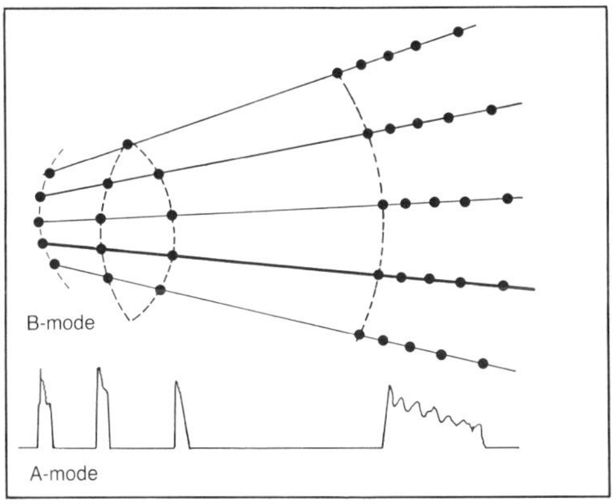


a

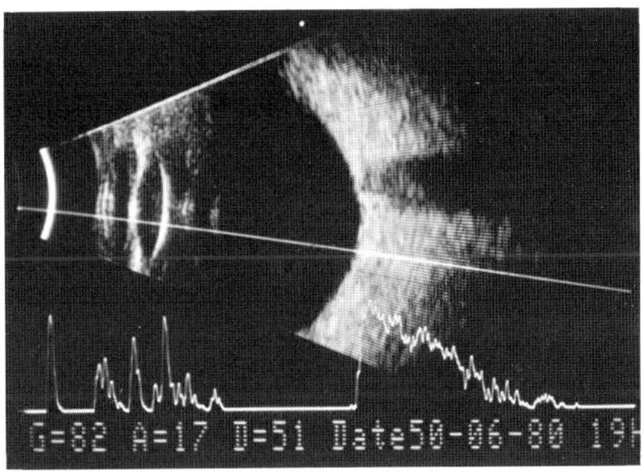


b

Fig. 1.**26a, b** B-mode display
**a** Schematically: The amplitudes are coded according to brightness and sectorial cross section. Vector selection of a line and A-mode display

**b** Example of a B-mode display (Ophthascan, Biophysique Medical)

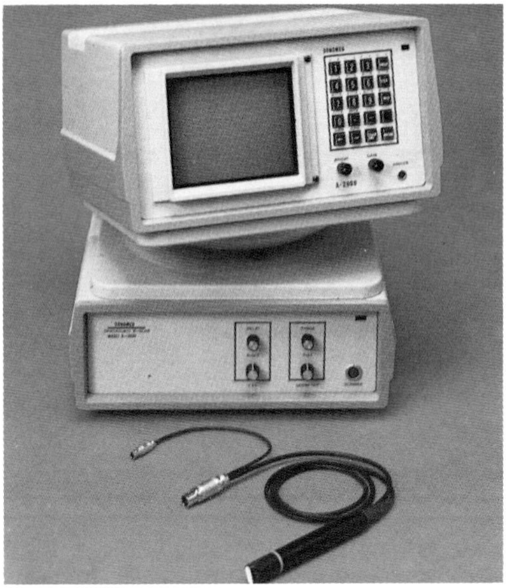

Fig. 1.**27** Example of a modern A- and B-mode instrument (Sonomed)

### 1.4.3 Biometric Instruments

The ultrasonic measuring devices in ophthalmology consist of an A-mode part and an electronic clock. The simplest instrument contains a time scale which is simultaneously presented with the A-mode echogram. Modern instruments allow a digital evaluation of the dimensions of the individual components of the eye.

This possibility is explained in Fig. 1.**28**. During the examination the signals of the cornea (H), the lens (L) and the retina (R) are identified by the examiner or by the device and are delineated by measuring windows. An electronic system automatically measures the sound transmission time between the individual marks (measuring times), provided a certain amplitude threshold has been exceeded. The time intervals calculated in this way are then recalculated to distances considering the velocity of sound in various eye media. Many instruments feed the measured values to a small computer which, while taking into account, the refractive power of the cornea and the expected postopera-

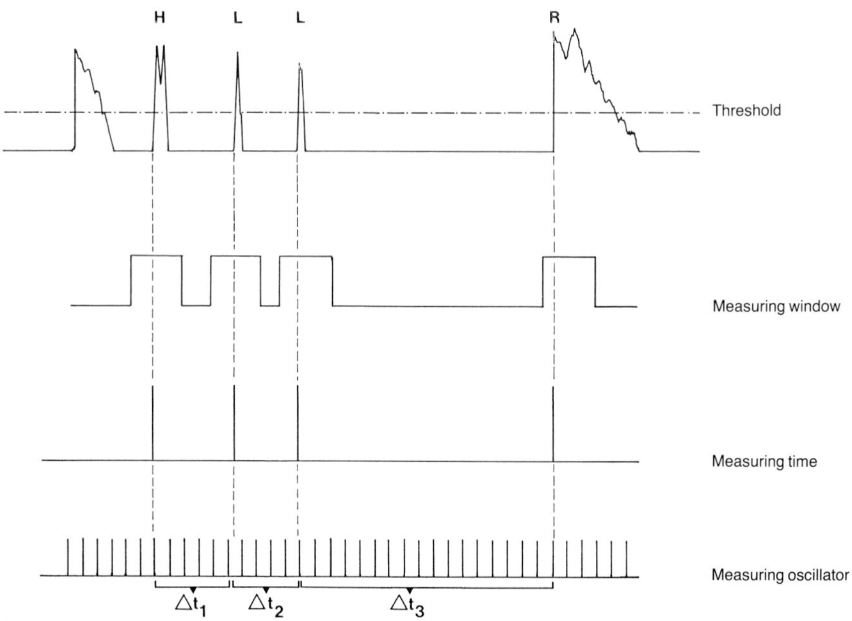


Fig. 1.**28** Time pattern of electronic ultrasound biometry. The rise times of the amplitudes within the measuring windows are determined by a measuring oscillator. The amplitude threshold prevents measuring weak reflections

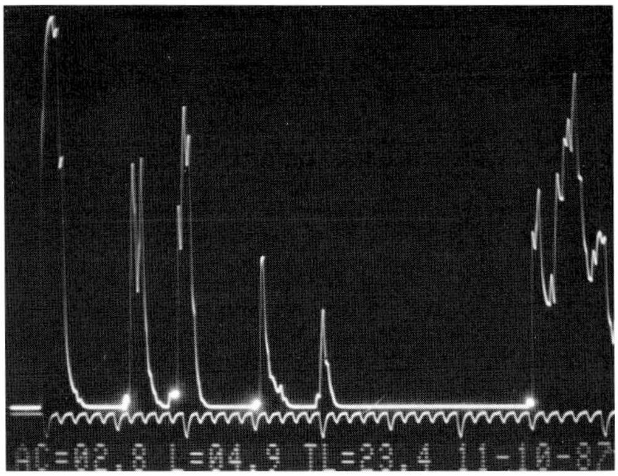

Fig. 1.**29** Biometrical measurements after digital storage of the A-mode images. Measuring points (adjustable) are shown by increased brightness

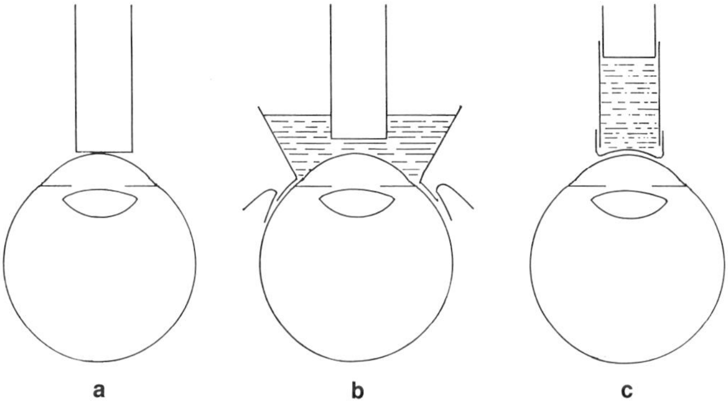


Fig. 1.**30 a–c** Techniques of biometry
**a** Direct coupling
**b** Measurement with an open corneal shell
**c** Measurement with a closed water-containing stand-off chamber

tive depth of the anterior chamber, will recommend the dioptric power of the intraocular lens to be implanted. The accuracy of these machines depends upon the frequency of the measuring oscillator or on the sampling frequency of the AD converter. With an oscillator frequency of 20 MHz, we achieve a measuring precision of about 0.1 mm.

In modern biometric instruments the echograms are evaluated in freeze frame (Fig. 1.**29**). The measuring precision of such machines is related to the sampling frequency (Fig. 1.**28**) and lies around 0.2 mm. In principle, biometric machines should be **calibrated at regular intervals**. For this purpose, we need electronic clocks (echo simulators) or exactly ground, plane-parallel plastic or metallic blocks.

The sound velocity in the lens is 7% greater than in the aqueous or vitreous. Many of the commercially available ultrasound biometric devices correct this fact automatically by implementing a single sound velocity for axial length measurements. We can expect more precise results if we measure and calculate the dimensions of the eye media separately.

The sound velocity in the aqueous and in the vitreous is 1532 m/s; in the lens, 1642 m/s. Taking into account the dimensions of the media, a mean sound velocity for the schematic eye is calculated to be 1550 m/s.

For measuring the **axial length of the globe**, we use high-frequency transducers (10–15 MHz), the sound field of which is focused on the ocular fundus. The acoustic coupling (Fig. 1.**30**) is here achieved by direct contact between the transducer and the cornea (A); via a corneal shell filled with fluid (B); or using a closed, water-filled container (C). In principle the immersion method (B) should be preferred, though in the meantime systems for contact coupling have been perfected and are commercially available.

Lately, **ultrasound devices** have been designed **to measure the thickness of the cornea** (pachymetry), a prerequisite for refractive corneal surgery. In principle they are constructed similar to the above-described biometric instruments. However, we usually use higher ultrasound frequencies for this purpose.

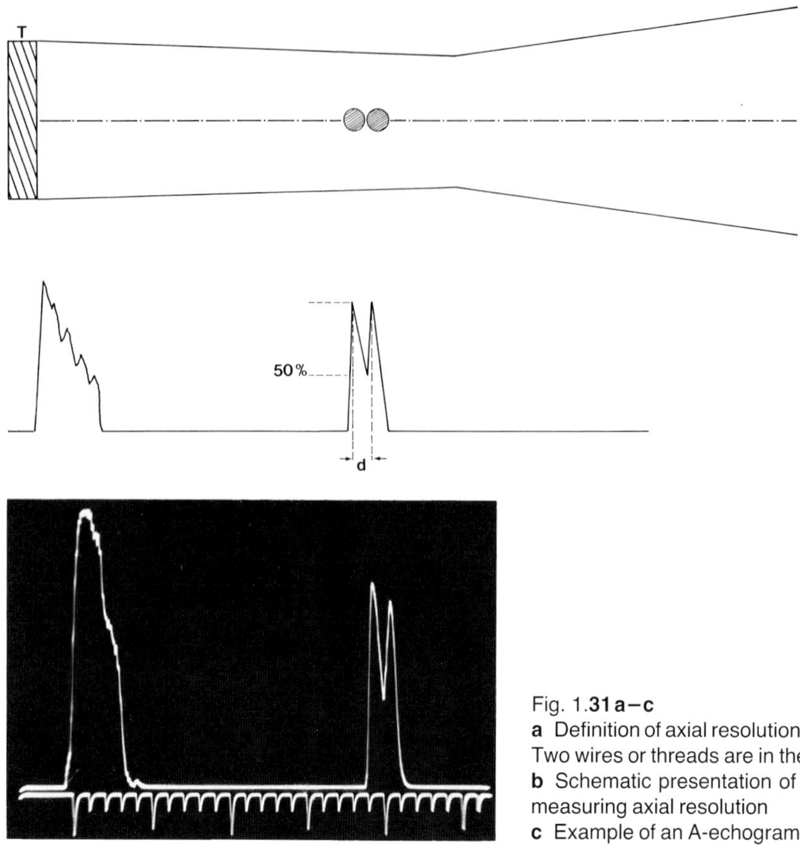


Fig. 1.**31 a–c**
**a** Definition of axial resolution of an A-mode instrument. Two wires or threads are in the near field
**b** Schematic presentation of the A-mode image when measuring axial resolution
**c** Example of an A-echogram

## 1.5 Technical Limits and Artifacts

### 1.5.1 Resolution

In Sect. 1.2 we have already considered the relationship between impulse duration and resolution power of an ultrasound device. The axial resolution of an A-mode apparatus (Fig. 1.**31 a**) is defined as the distance between two reflectors whose echo spike amplitudes differ by 50% (Fig. 1.**31**). This definition is not generally applicable for devices with a nonlinear amplification mode. For an unequivocal measurement of amplification modes, we use special flat reflectors of glass or the water-containing contact lens material Hema W-38. This technique of measuring is illustrated in Figure 1.**32**. We can measure the axial resolution power of an A-mode signal by comparing the width of a predetermined echo spike with that of an echo amplified by 6 dB with respect to the first one.

We use a wire target to determine the axial and lateral resolution power of a **B-mode system** (Fig. 1.**33 a–e**). Because of the focused sound beams in the B-system, the distance of the test reflectors from the transducer surface plays an essential role. The measurements should be taken at the focal distance. Figure 1.**33** explains how this is done. The commercially available devices have a lateral resolution power of 2 mm and an axial resolution of 0.3 mm.

### 1.5.2 Precision of Measurements

All instruments use filters which alter the course and amplitude of the individual echo spikes in order to display smooth and unequivocal spikes on the screen (Fig. 1.**19**). Only that part of the signal which exceeds a certain threshold will be displayed. This will delay the rise of the signal spike depending upon the amplification or the reflectivity

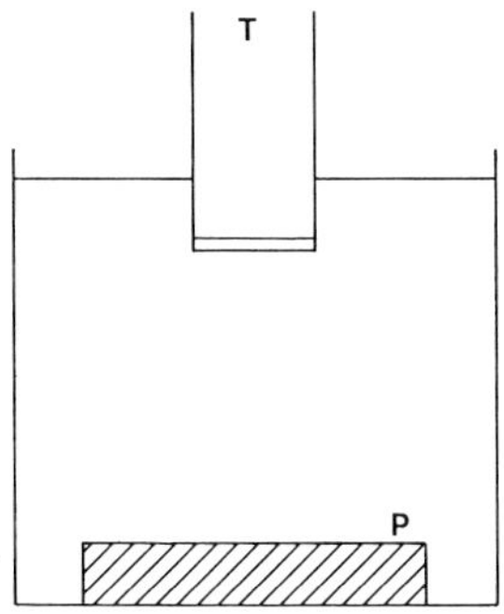


a

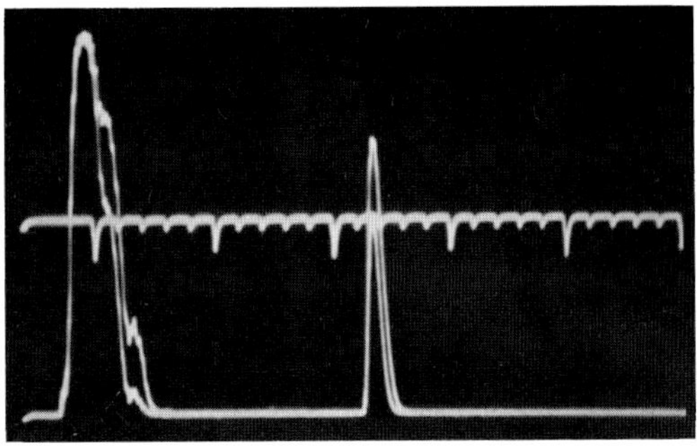

b

Fig. 1.**32a, b** Measuring axial resolution: half-width value of an echo spike
**a** Schematic sketch of the measurement: reflection on a plate (P)
**b** A-mode echogram of the measurement: the echo spike lies just at the height of the measuring line higher spike: after increasing the amplification by 6 dB (2 ×). Resolution = width of the echo at the measuring line

level. Figure 1.**34** demonstrates how high this error of measurement can be.

The following considerations are important for clinical practice: A dense nuclear cataract may lead to a considerable sound absorption; this may occasionally suppress the retinal signal, and only the more intensively reflecting choroid, or even sclera, will be displayed; this spike can then be erroneously interpreted as the posterior border of the vitreous. Thus, for biometry we recommend focused transducers, the focus of which lies at the posterior pole of the globe.

### 1.5.3 Multiple Reflections

Strong reflections may produce two types of multiple reflections. The first example is concerned with repeated reflections between a strong reflector and the transducer (Fig. 1.**35**). This occurs, for instance, when sound waves strike the lens in a perpendicular direction. We see multiple echoes in the vitreous when there is direct contact between the transducer and the cornea, as well as when a water-filled closed plastic stand-off is used. Multiple echoes may also appear within a regularly shaped structure, e.g., the lens, or within bird shots (Fig. 1.**36a**). The sound velocity is usually higher in these structures than in the less dense surroundings (e.g., the vitreous). The repeatedly imaged distances (d) within these structures therefore appear imaged shorter than the actual dimensions (Fig. 1.**36a** bottom).

These multiple echoes may appear over a larger distance when the ultrasound is "caught" within a structure, e.g. in bird shots (Fig. 1.**36b**). Such an artifact is therefore most helpful in detecting a foreign body in the orbit. If the foreign body has an irregular shape, then the production of multiple reflections depends mainly on the angle of incidence of the sound. In some cases it is reasonable to select a lower amplification so that the foreign body can be detected because of its relatively high degree of reflectivity.

### 1.5.4. Shadow Formation

A shadow is defined as a change in sound intensity produced by a definite structure, i.e., a change in the amount of reflection behind that structure. Increased reflection appears behind a relatively weakly reflecting or attenuating structure, e.g., a cyst in the orbital adipose tissue. The apparent reflectivity may be decreased by a strong attenuation or strengly reflecting structure. Examples are intraocular tumors (Fig. 1.**37a, b**) and a foreign body. This artifact therefore can also be used to localize intraocular foreign bodies.

### 1.5.5 Distortion

The first part in the echogram corresponds to the area which is closest to the transducer. The near field of the sound beam has a relatively wide lateral extension and therefore, when concave structures, e.g., the retina, are sector scanned, the image appears more concave than it really is (Fig. 1.**38**). Convex structures, on the other hand, are imaged too flat or as a plane. This distortion also occurs when the sound beam does not transverse the

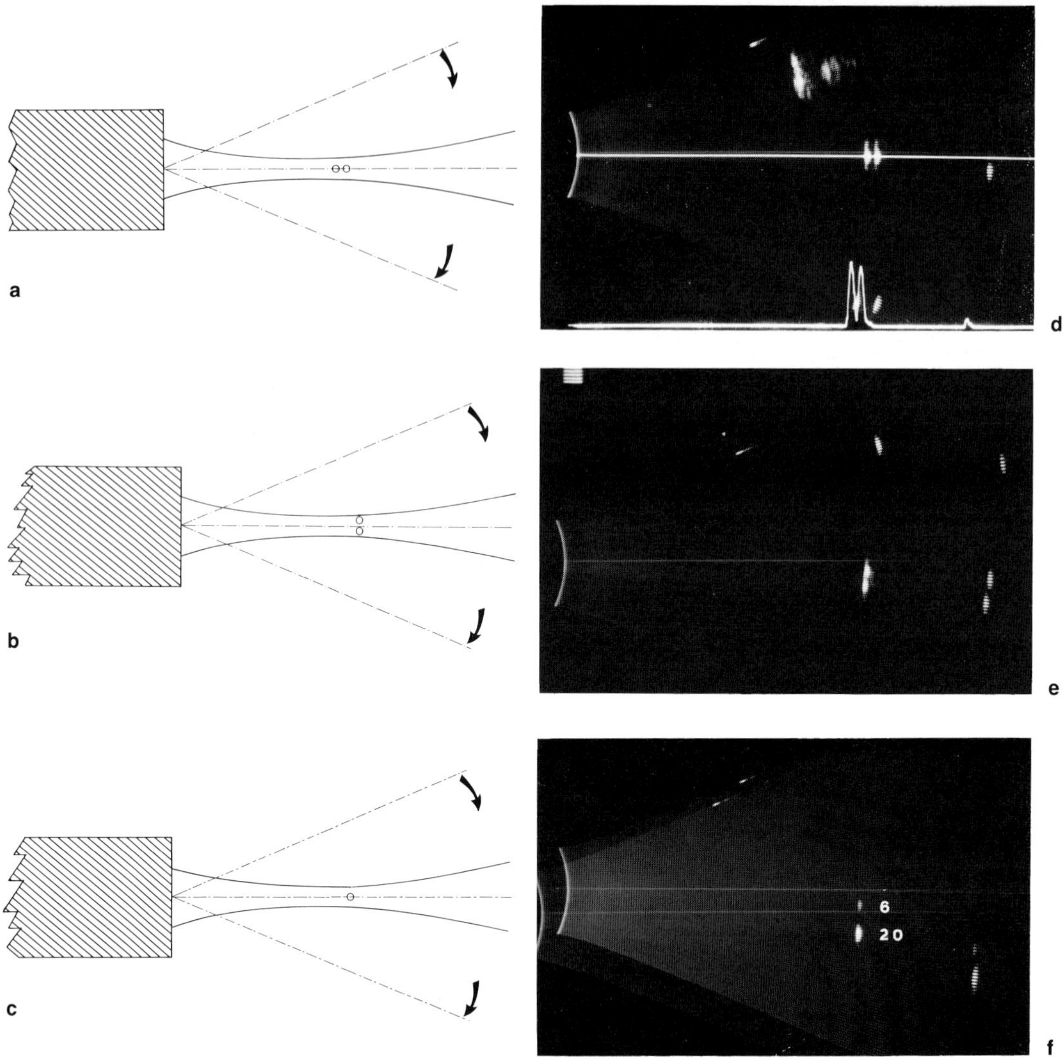


Fig. 1.**33a–f** Axial and lateral resolution of a B-mode instrument. On the left: schematic illustration of the measuring procedure. On the right: photos of the B-mode image of a wire model
**a** Axial resolution, A- and B-echogram 20 dB above the perception threshold; distance between the wires 1 mm
**b** Lateral resolution, B-mode echogram 20 dB above threshold; distance between wires 1 mm
**c** Axial and lateral resolution, B-mode echogram of a single wire, 6 dB and 20 dB above threshold
**d, e, f** Corresponding photos

lens (i.e., not a central transducer coupling) (Fig. 1.**38b)**).

Another distortion is produced by the strong curvature of the lens periphery (Fig. 1.**39**). The negative (i.e., outward-directed) refraction leads to an apparent shortening of the eye. This has to be differentiated from the above-described type of distortion, because the imaged retina will by further deviation of the sound beam be apparently displaced backward.

A marked change in sound velocity will also lead to a distortion. We have mentioned this case before, when discussing multiple reflections.

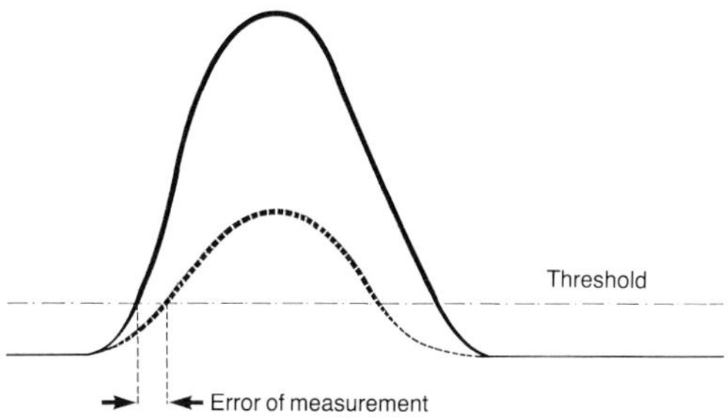


a

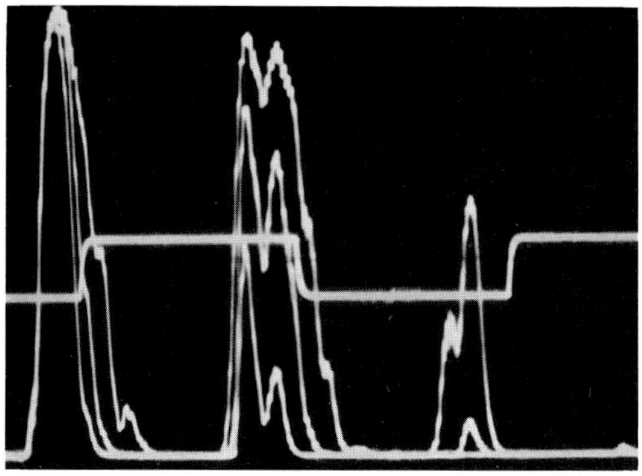

b

Fig. 1.**34a, b** Influence of amplification or of the amount of reflection on the precision of measurements
**a** Delay of the spike rise, depending upon the height of the amplitude, by the imaging threshold of the echo instrument
**b** Example of the amplification influence: overlapping echograms, photographed with 6 dB steps of amplification

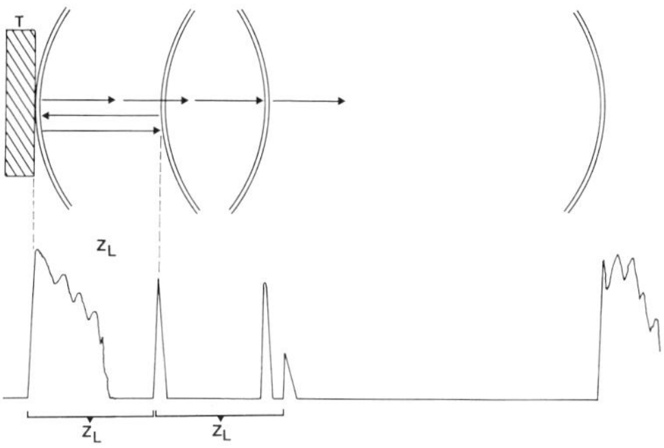


a

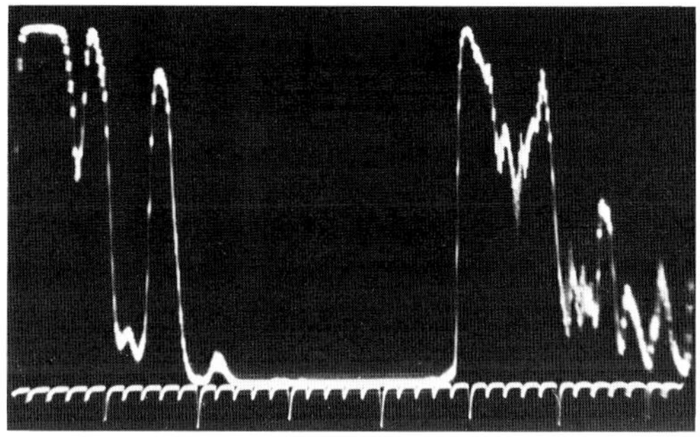

b

Fig. 1.**35a, b** Multiple echo artifacts of the first kind: reflections between reflector and transducer
**a** Schematic sketch
**b** Example: multiple echo from the lens

Furthermore, a markedly calcified cataractous lens will also possess an increased sound velocity; the resulting apparent shortening of the eye may easily be confused with a pathologic process in the macula (Fig. 1.**40**). It is therefore most important not to direct the sound beam through the lens when establishing an ultrasound diagnosis. During the examination the transducer should always be applied to the conjunctiva and never to the cornea.

Another reason for artifacts caused by change in sound velocity are implants, e.g., silicone oil in the vitreous. Figure 1.**41** (top) shows the A-mode echogram of a patient with unilateral vitreous replacement. If we examine such a patient for the first time, the result may be surprising: the operated eye appears to be 30% longer than the healthy one. The solution of the problem is simple: the sound velocity in silicone oil is only about two-thirds of the velocity in the vitreous (i.e., only two-thirds of the sound velocity for which the ultrasound machine has been calibrated). For this reason, the actual size of the eye is only two-thirds of the imaged size, as will become evident from the A-mode image of the fellow eye in Fig. 1.**41** (bottom).

## 1.6 Tissue Differentiation

Ophthalmologists have known for a long time that it is possible to differentiate tissues with the help of A- and B-mode echograms. The following tissue properties can be differentiated sonographically:

- **Kinetic** (dynamic) characteristics, e.g., motility and mobility of intraocular structures, e.g., aftermovements,

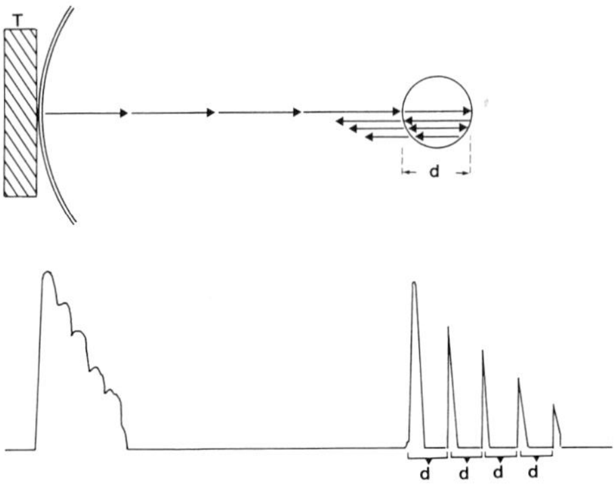


a

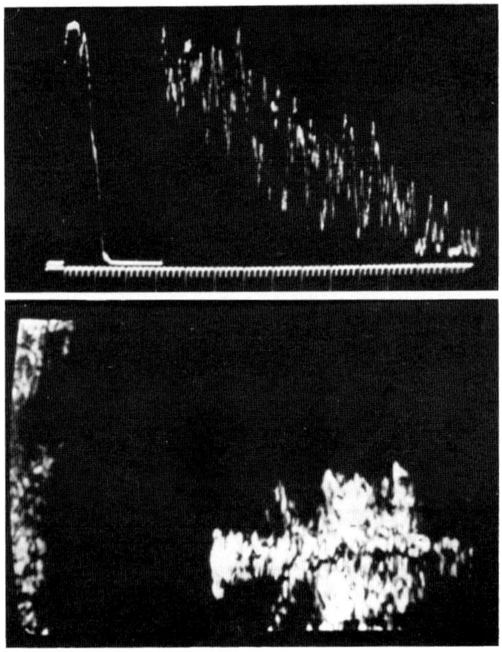

b

Fig. 1.**36** **a, b** Multiple echo artifacts of the second kind: reflections within a structure (e.g., foreign body)
**a** Schematic sketch
**b** A- and B-echogram of a bird shot

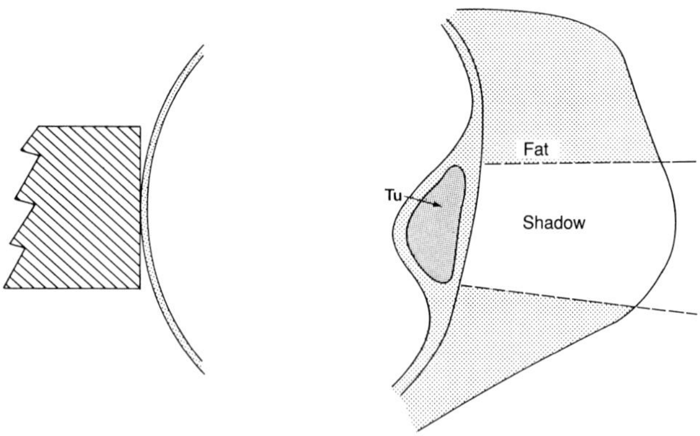


a

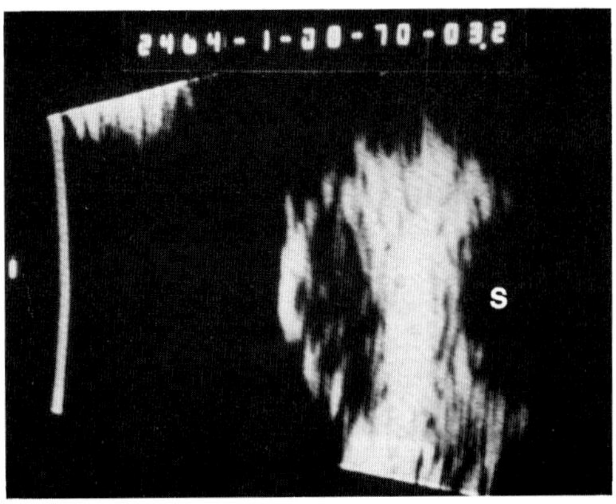


b

Fig. 1.**37** **a, b** Shadow formation produced by marked attenuation or by a strong amount of reflection from one structure
**a** Schematic sketch of an intraocular tumor
**b** Shadow formation in the orbital fat (S)

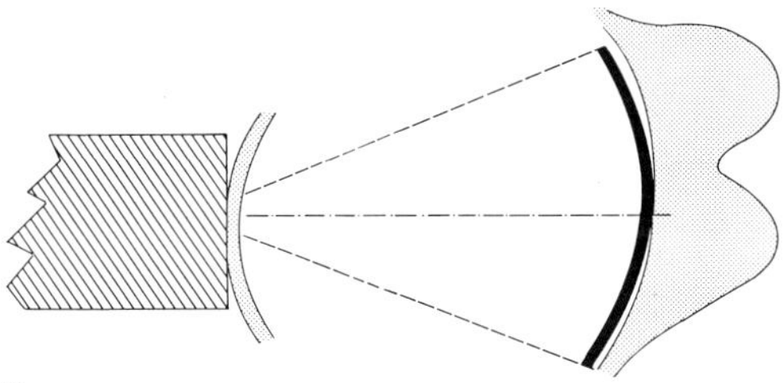

a

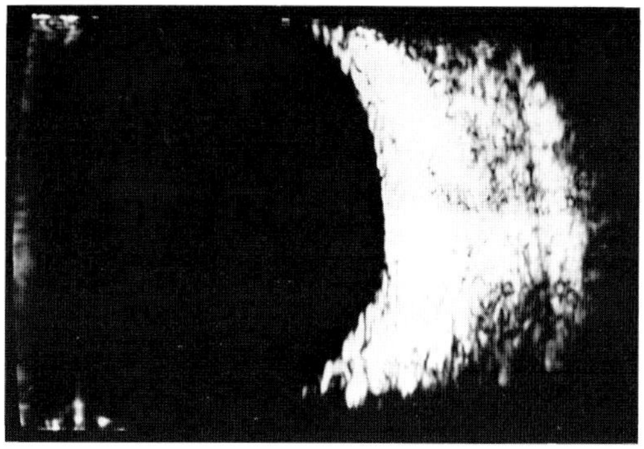

b

Fig. 1.**38** **a, b** Distortion produced by the sector scanning of the B image: exaggerated curvature (concave)

**a** Schematic drawing of the distortion in a central beam
**b** Example for a peripheral light beam

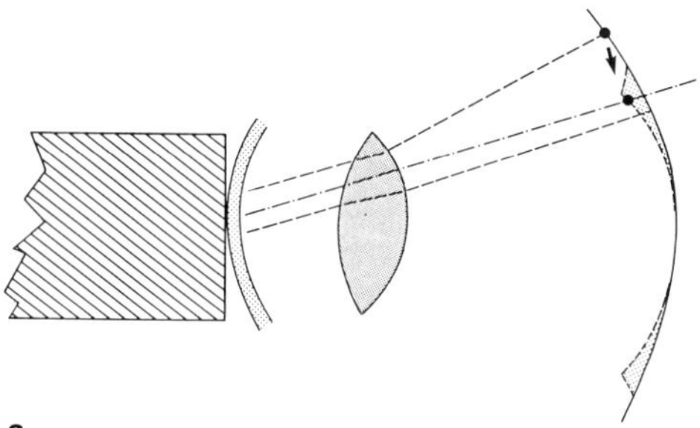

a

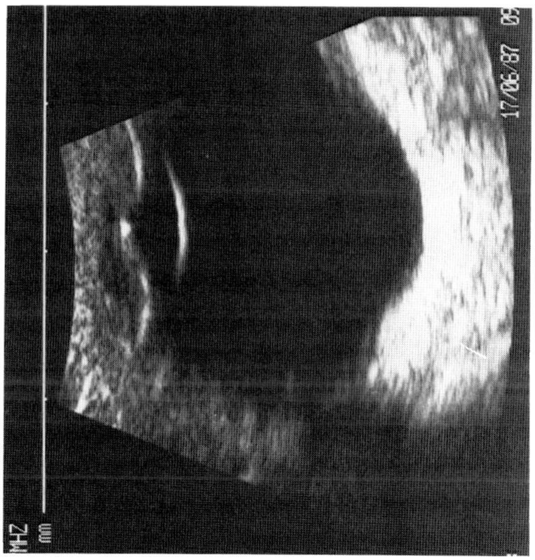


b

Fig. 1.**39** **a, b** Distortion produced by the strong refraction of the lens periphery

**a** Schematic drawing of this distortion: the peripheral retina is imaged more centrally
**b** B-echogram of this type of distortion

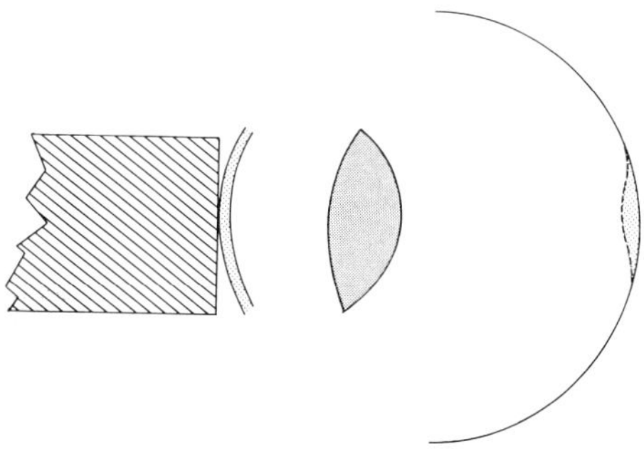

Fig. 1.**40** Distortion produced by the high sound velocity and densification within a cataractous lens; schematic sketch seems to demonstrate a pathologic process in the macula

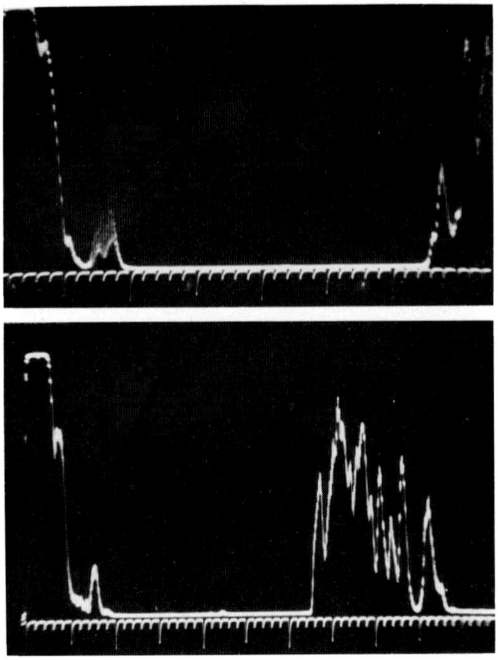

a

b

Fig. 1.**41** **a, b** Distortion of the A-mode echogram by silicone oil replacement of the vitreous body
**a** Eye with silicone oil
**b** The normal fellow eye

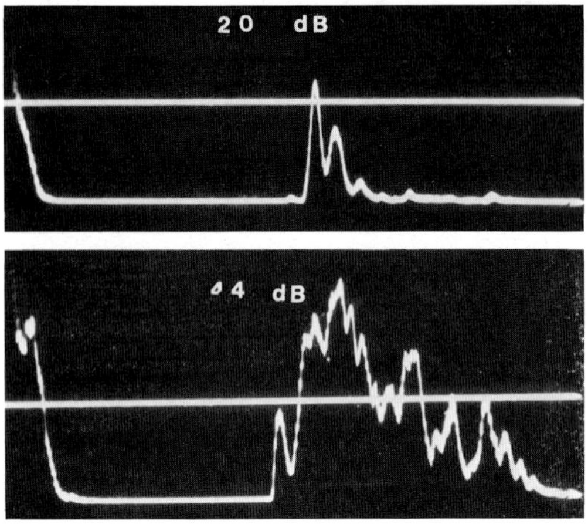


a

b

Fig. 1.**42** **a, b** Quantitative echography of relative amounts of reflection
**a** Scleral spike reaching the measuring line, amplification 20 dB
**b** Echo of a vitreous membrane at this amplitude, amplification 44 dB, i.e., difference of 24 dB. The diagnosis therefore is: vitreous membrane

- anatomic characteristics, like the delineation and shape of various tissues, e.g., the mushroom shape of a choroidal melanoma, the choroidal excavation behind a melanoma or the spherical shape of a choroidal detachment;
- quantitative characteristics, e.g., relative strength of reflection, sound attenuation or shadow formation.

As mentioned above, ultrasound machines with a logarithmic total amplification make a direct visual evaluation of the amount of reflectivity level possible, if the total sensitivity of the machine is calibrated on a model. When using an instrument with S-shaped amplification, the amplifier has to be set in such a way that a certain echo will reach a predetermined amplitude (e.g., 50% of the A-mode echogram) for measuring the amount of reflection. The corresponding amplification is measured in decibels and is carefully maintained for all examinations.

Another possibility is the so-called **"relative reflectivity"** (dB-difference) measurement, in which the echo to be measured is compared with a scleral echo. By changing the amplification, the two echoes are then sequentially brought down to half the maximum display (Fig. 1.**42**). The difference in dB of the amplifier control settings indicates the relative reflectivity of this structure. This method is often used to differentiate intraocular membranes.

A new development in the area of tissue differentiation is the mathematical analysis of radio frequency signals, the so-called **"acoustic spectography"**. Using a powerful computer system, this method gives quantitative data on the frequency-dependent attenuation and scattering of ultrasound in tissues. In a few centers this method is already used for the differential diagnosis of tumors and for follow-up examinations after radiation therapy.

# 2 Examination Techniques

## 2.1 The Evaluation of Echographic Findings

It is the aim of a diagnostic method to describe the findings and to characterize them as precisely as possible. The expertise of the examiner, his general clinical experience and the methods he uses influence these findings in a nonquantifiable way. They especially influence the evaluation of the findings.

Statements on the diagnostic value or the accuracy of a specific examination method appear frequently in the literature, but are difficult to compare. When using a method routinely it is important to know its technical and physical **limits**.

> It is absolutely necessary to separate the **objective findings** from the **interpretations** of the results, which will necessarily also be influenced by other clinical parameters.

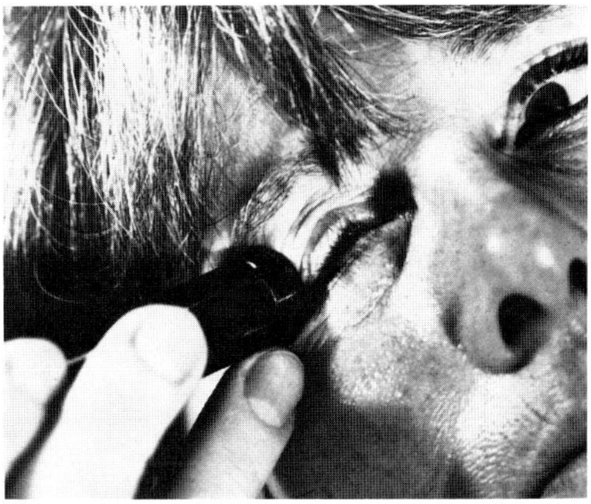

Fig. 2.**1** The B-mode transducer is applied to the closed lids with the help of a coupling substance (e.g., methylcellulose solution). In order to facilitate exact gaze excursions, it is advisable to cover the nonexamined eye of the patient only partly

## 2.2 Recommendations for a Rational Sequence of Examinations

### The Examination Procedure

The echographic examination of the eye and the orbit can be performed in a facile way if the patient lies flat or sits in an examining chair that can be tilted backward. Infants and children are best examined in their mother's arms.

The high frequency of the ultrasound cannot be transmitted through air; therefore, a gel-like contact substance, e.g., 2% methylcellulose solution, has to be applied to the transducer or to the patient's skin. Sterility should not be a problem if commercially available gels are used. The transducer is cleaned by wiping with a disinfectant, whereby the number of microorganisms can be kept low. If sterile conditions have to be maintained (e.g., when examining during a surgical intervention), a sterile plastic finger cot or a surgical glove can be pulled over the transducer. In order to reduce impedance differences between the membranes, it is necessary to apply a drop of the methylcellulose solution on the transducer to guarantee direct coupling. In the area of the exit window of the ultrasound, the plastic finger cot should be in direct contact with the transducer cover.

Examining through the closed lid does not appreciably weaken the sound energy. This allows a wide radius of rotation when turning the transducer. In order to facilitate quantitated gaze movements, the nonexamined eye should be only partly coverd (Fig. 2.**1**).

Direct contact of the transducer with the globe is only necessary for special A-mode techniques. In this way the less well-defined sound attenuation by the lids can be avoided when using quantitative examination techniques (e.g., "quantitative echography" (Fig. 2.**2**).

One problem for biometric measurements of the axial length is the coupling pressure, which neces-

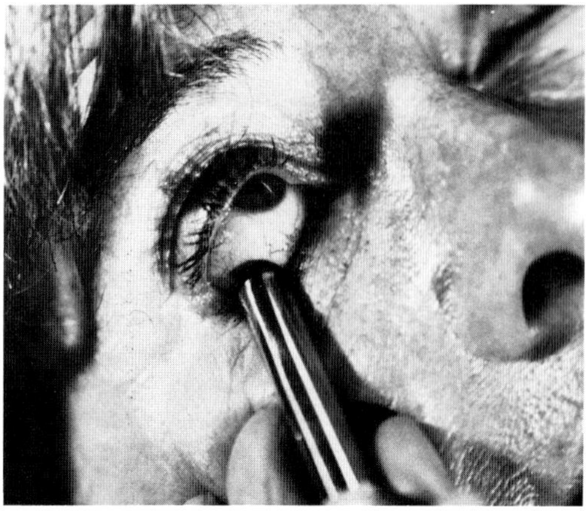

Fig. 2.2 It is advisable to place the transducer for quantitative A-mode echography directly on the anesthetized conjunctiva

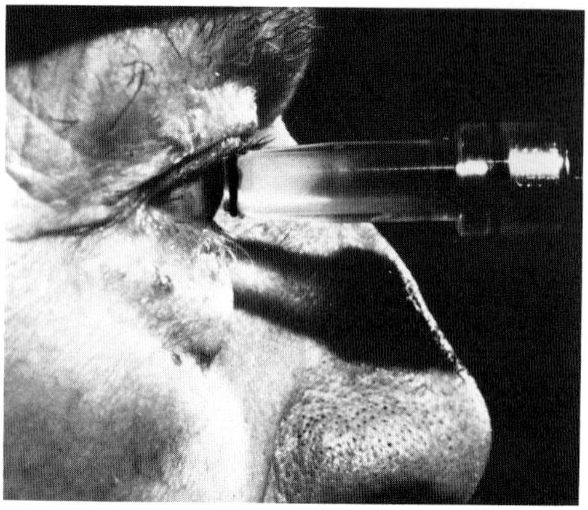

Fig. 2.4 Contact method to measure the axial length by using a tonometer suspension to hold the transducer

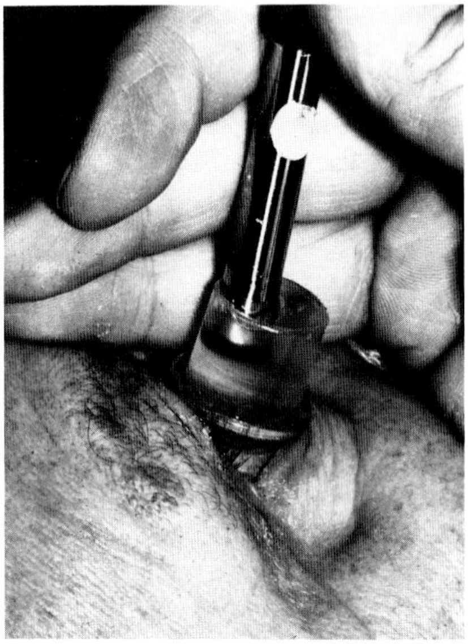

Fig. 2.3 In order to measure the axial length of the eyeball without distorting the globe, a water-containing stand-off in the form of a funnel is placed against the lids (immersion method)

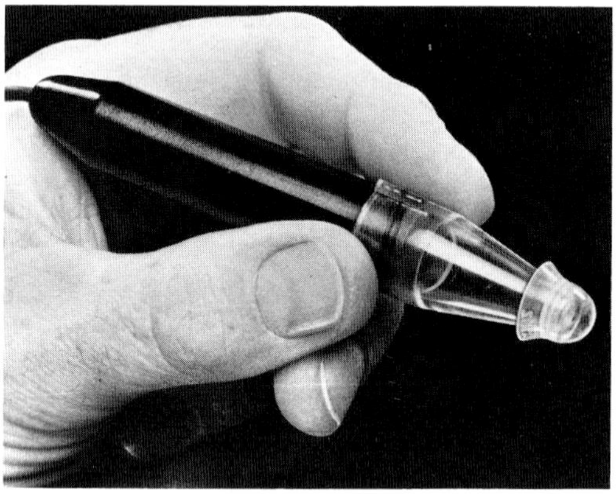

Fig. 2.5 Flexible water-filled stand-off for a hand-held biometry transducer

sarily leads to a minimal deformation of the globe. The following solutions are possible:

1. A closed water container in the shape of a funnel held in front of the lids allows measurements without deforming the globe in any way, the so-called immersion procedure (Fig. 2.3).

2. Using a special holder for the transducer (e.g., a tonometer suspension) guarantees minimal and constant coupling pressure when the patient is in a sitting position (Fig. 2.4).

3. A flexible, integrated, water-filled stand-off will cause only a negligible deformation of the cornea (Fig. 2.5).

Experiments have shown (Guthoff 1988) that the coupling pressure and the intraocular pressure influence the measurements. The resulting differences in measuring the axial length can be compensated for in clinical practice by following the above-mentioned recommendations. The procedures are of equal value (Shammas 1984, Schelenz et al. 1988).

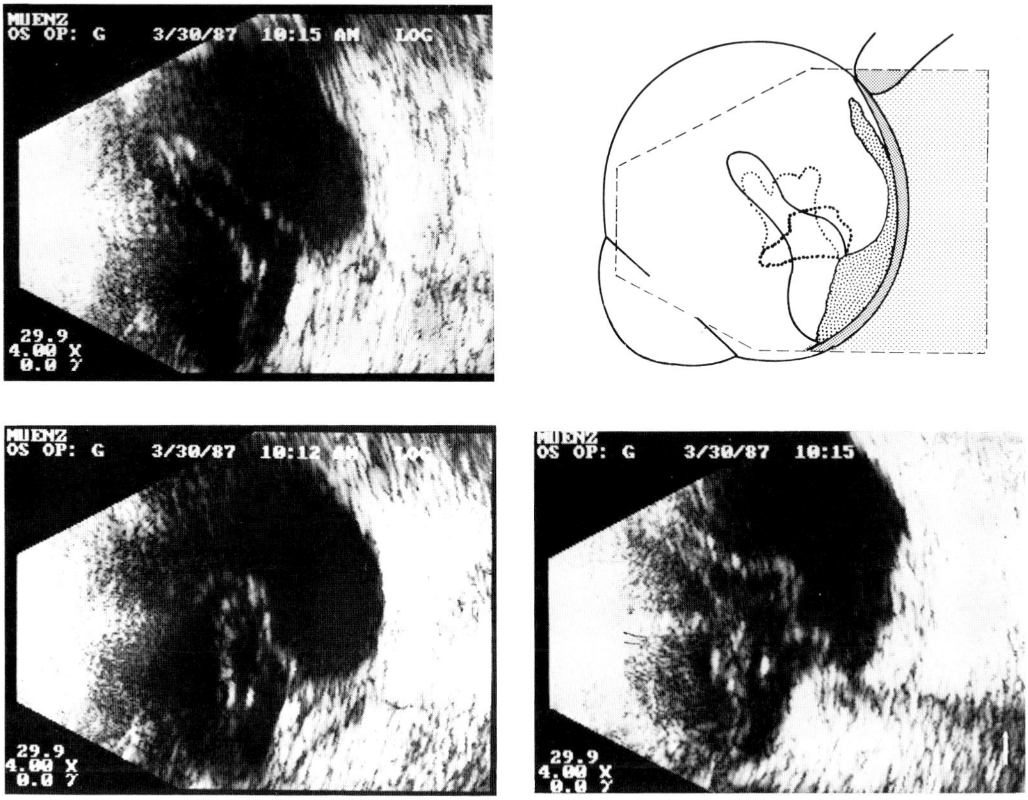


a b c d

Fig. 2.**6a–d** Various stages of aftermovements of a vitreous membrane adherent to the area of the exoplant. In the schematic drawing the various cross sections are projected above each other

#### Principles of Obtaining the Optimal Ultrasonogram

During the entire examination, we should pay attention so that:

1. the examined structure is in the middle of the scanned sector; and
2. acoustic interfaces are at a right angle to the propagation direction of the ultrasound.

These postulates can be fulfilled by corresponding changes in the patient's gaze and by the appropriate movements of the transducer (kinetic echography). It is absolutely necessary to follow these rules if we want to quantify signal intensities (quantitative echography) (see Sect. 2.5).

#### Spontaneous Motions as a Diagnostic Sign

Already after a few examinations, the echographic neophyte will realize that diagnosis can only be made during the examination procedure. He will be impressed by the extent of intraocular movements, e.g., of floating vitreous opacities (Fig. 2.**6**). The type of **aftermovements** of the vitreous induced by changes in the patient's gaze also provides valuable information.

Some pathologic processes will produce echographically demonstrable movements which are extremely important for the diagnosis. Among these are arteriovenous fistules of the orbit or the effect of blood flow within highly vascularized melanomas. It is also important to examine all normal anatomical structures from different directions so that we get a clear picture of the extent of a pathologic process.

**Identical** examination parameters are difficult to reproduce during an examination – and even more so during a follow-up examination. We have discussed in Sect. 1.2 the importance of calibrating and standardizing the instrument. The variables induced by the examiner represent an uncertainty factor which cannot be quantified. The ultrasound reflected by the tissues is influenced by the angle

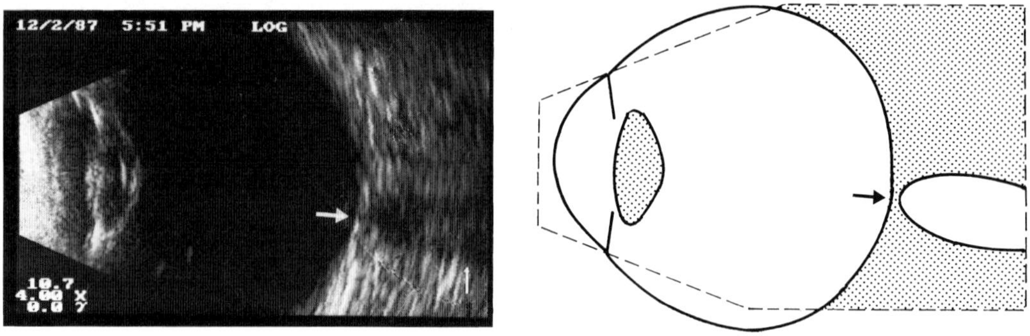


a b

Fig. 2.7 **a, b**
**a** Cross sectional echogram through a normal globe; the arrow marks the entrance of the optic nerve
**b** Schematic drawing

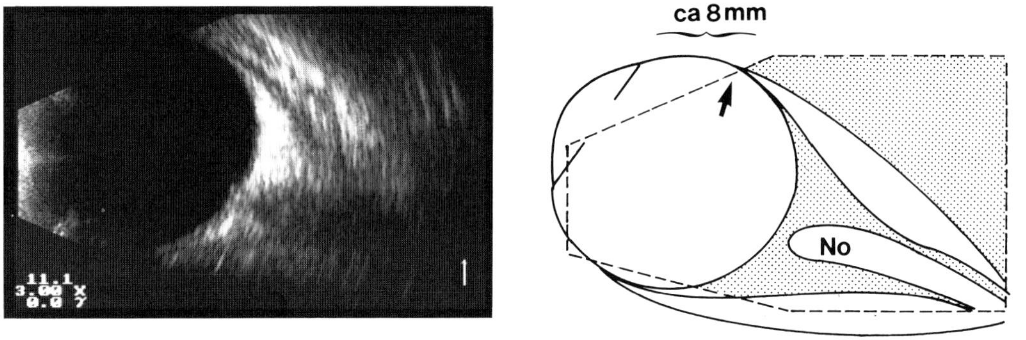


a b

Fig. 2.**8 a, b** Image of the globe and the orbit. The insertions of the recti muscles (arrow) projected onto the ocular coats provide some orientation. Distance of muscle insertion to limbus is about 8 mm; NO = optic nerve

under which the transducer is applied, by the location of the scanning plane, by the position of the globe and, not least of all, the pressure with which the transducer is applied.

#### The "Critical Moment" Decides

In X-rays and in magnetic resonance imaging we project the soft tissues onto skeletal structures which are imaged simultaneously. This allows an unequivocal topographic orientation. Echographic techniques imaging soft tissue only, however, need "landmarks" for orientation. Such landmarks are the entrance of the optic nerve into the globe (Fig. 2.**7**) or the insertions of the extraocular muscles (Fig. 2.**8**).

**Amplification control** plays an important role in gaining orientation in the area to be examined. Absorption of ultrasound energy in the tissue depends upon the specific sound running time. It is therefore impossible to display with equal quality in acoustic cross section structures lying at different distances from the transducer.

In the B-mode echogram, quality of imaging is identical with creating "a pretty image" in which the crucial structures can be well recognized. It is therefore not only necessary to shift our attention to various structures, but also to adjust amplification so that we always obtain an optimal setting of the apparatus.

No examination should be terminated before all echographically visible structures, from the ciliary body to the orbital soft tissues, have been evaluated. Anybody who is well versed in the method will take no more than a few minutes for this type of screening.

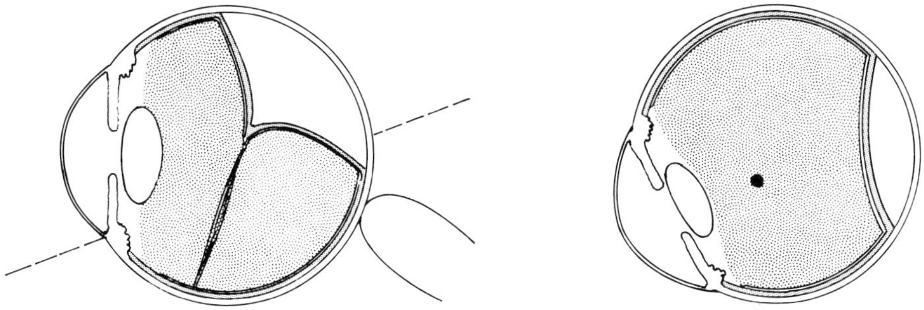

a b

Fig. 2.**9a–d**
**a, b** Schematic drawing of traction detachment in two planes at 90° to each other. Only examination from different directions enables us to differentiate strands and membranes
**c, d** See color plates

#### The Three-Dimensional Image

The introduction of rapid scanning contact B-mode devices with high resolution power have made the results of our examinations much more vivid. However, constructing a three-dimensional image from individual acoustic sections may occasionally represent difficulties (Fig. 2.**9**). Bronson (1976) refers in this connection to the surprising cross sectional images which can be obtained when examining a wine bottle (Fig. 2.**10**).

The currently available instruments suggest a course of examination which, independent of the problem at hand, consists of four steps:

1. finding the known anatomical landmarks with the help of contact B-scan technique;
2. determining the location of pathologic findings with special consideration of the motility of pathologic structures;
3. giving a detailed description of the pathologic findings on the basis of its reflection properties considering quantitative echography (comparison with standards) and estimating the sound attenuation;
4. including all available clinical information for final evaluation.

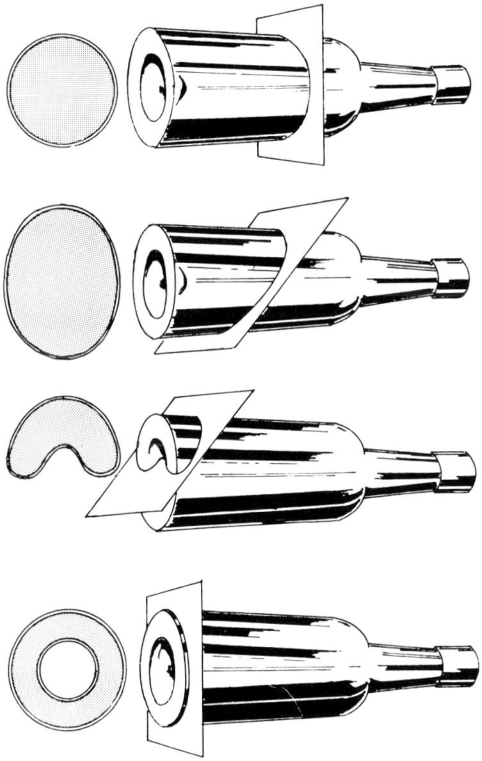

Fig. 2.**10** Bronson (1976) has pointed out the surprising sectional images which we obtain when examining a wine bottle echographically

#### The Integration of B-Mode Doppler Instruments (Duplex Scanner) into Ophthalmologic Diagnosis

The routine A- and B-mode techniques have matured; the possibilities and limitations of these methods are known. Only during the last years have we been able to use the Doppler effect of frequency shifts to evaluate and measure movements within a tissue and flow conditions within vessels. These frequency shifts can be observed in tissue volumes of less than 10 $mm^2$; they therefore represent additional information about the circulation in small tissue areas. So far there is no instrument available which is designed specifically for use in ophthalmology. On the basis of interesting results in cardiology and pediatrics (Winkler and Helmke 1988), it seems worthwhile to use similar instruments in ophthalmology (Guthoff et al. 1989, Berger et al. 1989). With this examination method small tissue areas can be investigated in cross sectional echograms and tested for a frequency shift. By color coding a large ultrasonic cross section, all areas in which a frequency shift occurs can be made conspicuous by a specific color (Figs. 2.**9c–d**; 4.**80c–d**). The first results were reported and summarized in 1989 (Guthoff et al.).

## 2.3 Documentation of Echographic Findings

Imaging the results of an echographic diagnostic examination on a cathode ray tube is a dynamic process and is best documented by videotape. We have to keep in mind that even a continuous documentation of the echographic examination is actually only a memory support or a visual aid for teaching sessions. It is hardly possible to make a delayed diagnosis as we know it from ordinary plain X-ray pictures or from digitally stored examination results in radiology. The selection of the information to be documented is essentially decided by the examiner's procedure.

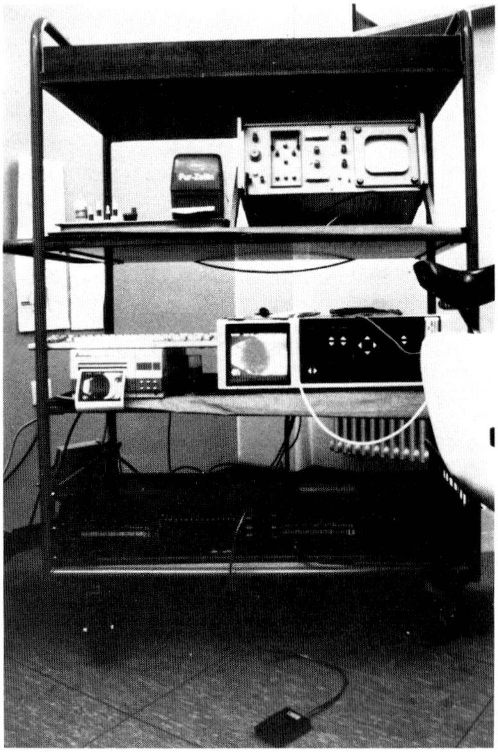

Fig. 2.**11** Ultrasound examination unit
Above: Device for analog A-mode diagnosis
Center: Digitalized A/B display system with video
Below: Video recorder

It has been proven sufficient to obtain representative cross sectional echograms, occasionally complemented by A-mode pictures with defined amplification settings. Most commercially available instruments have a window for videotaping and videoprinting, thereby allowing a simple and quite economical documentation, compared to Polaroid photos (Fig. 2.**11**).

Unfortunately, we have to forego part of the gray scale in the digitally stored B-echograms. This disadvantage could be compensated by the expensive method of using a sophisticated camera or the negatives of small images. Most of the illustrations used in this book are reproduced from videoprints. The originals are printed as so-called "hard copies" on thermal paper by a video imprinter directly coupled to the digital ultrasound machine.

## 2.4 Ultrasound Biometry

In order to measure biological structures with ultrasound some prerequisites are absolutely necessary:

1. The sound velocity has to be known.
2. It must be possible to correlate exactly acoustic interfaces with anatomical structures.

The **propagation velocity** of ultrasound used for diagnostic purposes is at 37° C
for aqueous and vitreous 1532 m/s
for the lens 1641 m/s
for the cornea 1639 m/s.

For ultrasonographic measuring techniques the globe represents a collective of spherical interfaces. Their centers of curvature all lie on the optical axis of the eye. This arrangement explains why only this direction of examination will lead to maximal echoes from acoustic interfaces. Any deviation of the transducer from the optical axis reduces the spike amplitudes, because under these circumstances only one of the interfaces will be maximally imaged (Fig. 2.**12**).

The prerequisite for an exact ultrasonic biometry is

therefore a careful positioning of the transducer, which has to be adjusted. This position has to be maintained until all interfaces involved produce an echo of maximal amplitude.

Most of the commercially available instruments for ultrasound biometry are equipped with an electronic pattern-recognition devivce which facilitates routine examinations. Many authors (Gernet 1966, 1973, Lepper 1984, Strobel et al. 1978) have pointed out that it may be erroneous to accept uncritically measurements obtained by such a method. The device recognizes and stores not anatomical structures, but signal patterns. Therefore, a retinal detachment involving the posterior pole may mimic normal coats of the eyeball and lead to serious diagnostic errors.

The cornea and the posterior ocular wall are the only structures of the eye which can also be measured by ultrasound outside the optical axis. Both are delineated by concentric surfaces so that it suffices to obtain a maximal signal intensity (maximal amplitude) in order to determine when we are dealing with a vertical acoustic section (Lepper et al. 1984). Thickness measurements in a clear cornea can be obtained with optical instruments (Taeger 1952). During the last years a few automat-

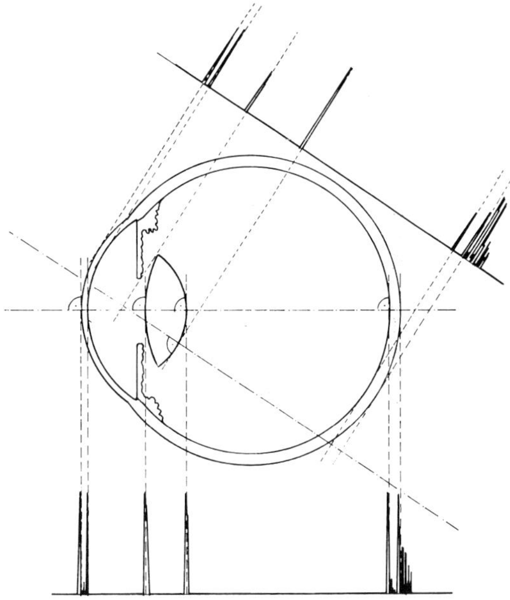

Fig. 2.**12** Schematic drawing of A-mode echograms obtained with axial and paraxial biometric measurements. Maximal signal spikes of all involved interfaces can be obtained only when the examination is performed in the optical axis

a

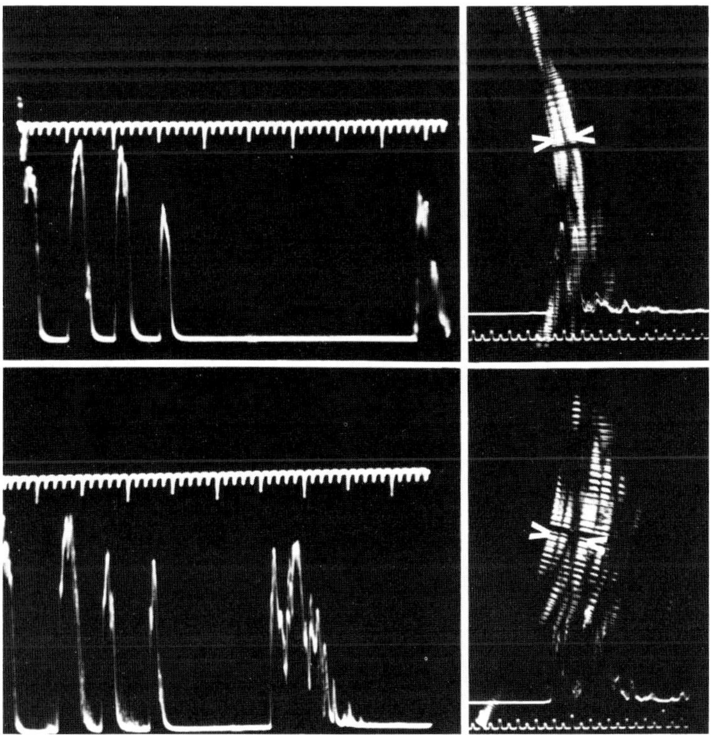

b

Fig. 2.**13a, b** A- and B-mode echogram of a myopic and of a hyperopic eye

**a** An axial length of 30.2 mm corresponds to a thickness of the ocular coats of 0.93 mm

**b** With an axial length of 18.4 mm the thickness of the ocular coats doubles to about 2 mm

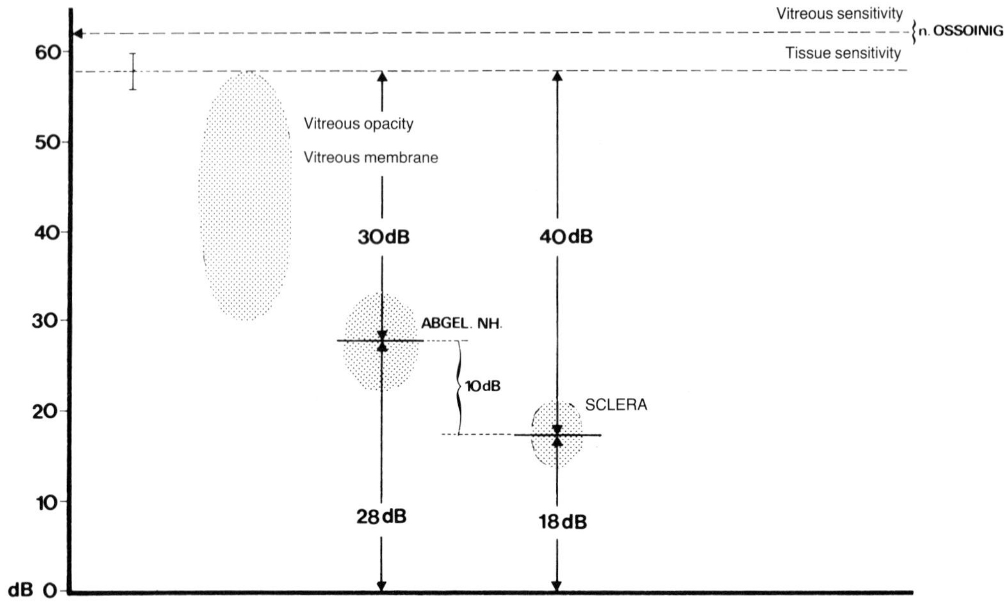


Fig. 2.**14** Published results of quantitative echography differentiating between retina, sclera and vitreous opacities, according to the tissue sensitivity method of Ossoinig (above) and the Hema-Reflector W 38 of Buschmann and Haigis (below)

ic ultrasound biometric devices for the use in corneal refractive surgery have become commercially available; they also provide quite precise measurements.

These instruments enable us, for instance, to determine corneal thickness as a function of endothelial damage following various techniques of cataract extraction (Jaffe et al. 1987). These instruments have not yet been accepted for routine clinical diagnostic purposes.

### The Thickness of the Ocular Wall

In 1965 Nover and Grote reported on the first attempts to measure the thickness of the ocular wall at the posterior pole by using ultrasound. The teams around Coleman, Purnell and Trier (Coleman 1971, Purnell et al., Lepper 1978) succeeded in measuring the thickness of the retina and the choroid, as well as in registering choroidal pulses. This was achieved by using special laboratory instruments.

It is also possible to estimate the thickness of the ocular wall with commercially available diagnostic devices. Figure 2.**13** demonstrates biometric findings in eyes with different axial length. By echographically measuring the thickness of the ocular walls, we can calculate their volume. A statistical comparison of these volumes between myopic and hyperopic eyes has established these volumes to be approximately 1.6 ccm; they are independent of the length of the ocular axis. This applies to the ocular wall posterior to the equator. In vitro it is possible to correlate individual layers of the ocular wall to definite spikes. However, this was not possible in clinical practice, though the same machines were used.

## 2.5 Principles of Quantitative A-Mode Echography

It is the aim of quantitative echography (Buschmann 1972, Ossoinig 1972, Trier 1977) to measure the reflection properties of membranes accurately. Usually the following question is asked:

In the case of an acoustic interface, are we dealing with the retina or with another membrane?

In order to perform quantitative echography, we need an exactly calibrated decibel control in the instrument (see Sect. 1.4.1) (Buschmann et al. 1989). We attempt to adjust the transducer in such a way that the structure in question displays the highest possible spike on the screen. It is sometimes necessary to reduce the sensitivity of the amplifier so that we can exactly determine the maximal amplitude and remain beneath an overload of the amplifier. Once the optimal direction for the examination has been found, we reduce the amplifier sensitivity so that the pathologic echo will just reach a horizontal measuring line projected onto the screen. In this way spikes are determined (the lowest setting of the amplifier should be regarded as decisive) which can then be compared with a standard. Two methods have been recommended in the literature:

1. **normal sclera (Ossoinig 1971);**
2. **a standard obtained under certain well-defined conditions from a test reflector** (Haigis et al. 1980, Buschmann et al. 1989) (Sect. 1.4.1).

**Regarding 1.** Some authors found on systematic examination relatively large individual variations of scleral reflectivity (Buschmann et al. 1981). According to our experience, this measuring method is suitable for clinical routine examinations.
**Regarding 2.** The W-38 reflector (Haigis et al. 1980) consists of the contact lens material Hema and represents a physically well-defined and useful standard. Basic changes in the amplifier characteristics and in the decibel control quality may develop. Therefore, occasional checking of these instrument parameters is indispensable.

Figure 2.**14** graphically shows the published results in the acoustic differences between retina, sclera and a test reflector.

# 3 The Echographically Demonstrable Ocular Anatomical Structures

When using contact B-mode instruments for examining the anterior segment, we have to keep in mind that these focused transistors will reach good imaging properties only at a distance of 5–8 mm from the transducer surface. During contact coupling over closed lids the anterior segment lies in the area of the poorly resolved near field. There are two possibilities of solving this problem:

1. using a water bath between transducer and lids; for this purpose a water-filled fingercot is suitable (Fig. 3.**1**);
2. using the vitreous space as an internal coupling device (Fig. 3.**2**).

The latter possibility is less expensive, but satisfactory results can only be obtained if there is at least a slight exophthalmus and the globe can be sufficiently ab- and adducted. Lid edema of any etiology may also be used for coupling (Fig. 3.**4**).

## 3.1 Cornea

The cornea is characterized echographically by two acoustic interfaces. For exact thickness measurements we need special A-mode devices. These are available for planning refractive corneal surgery (Lepper 1984).

Recent developments in diagnostic ultrasound (ultrasound biomicroscopy) make it possible to display images of cross sections with microscopic resolution (Pavlin et al. 1990). These devices are capable of producing images to a depth of 4 mm and an axial and lateral resolution approaching 200 μm. Corneal epithelium is displayed in front of the highly reflective Bowman's membrane (Fig. 3.**3a**). Signal height from the corneal stroma varies with the fluid content between the corneal lamellae.

## 3.2 Anterior Chamber

In a cross section the anterior chamber appears planoconvex. As mentioned in Sect. 2.4, we can obtain exact measurements echographically only in an axial direction. For this we need A-mode echography as we use it in axial biometry for calculating the strength of intraocular lens implants.

Chamber angle structures were first visualized with ultrasound biomicroscopy thechniques in eye

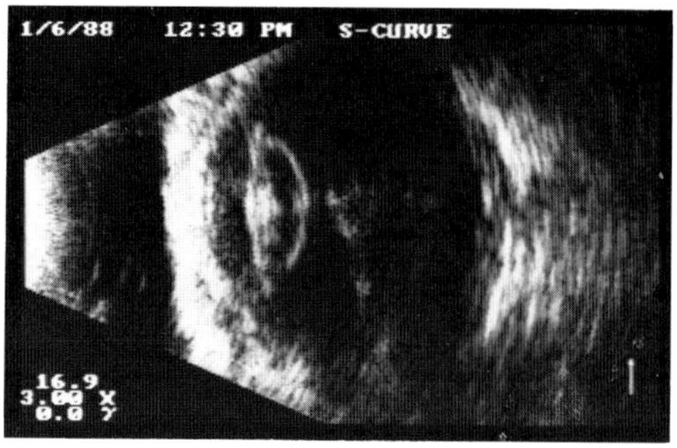


a

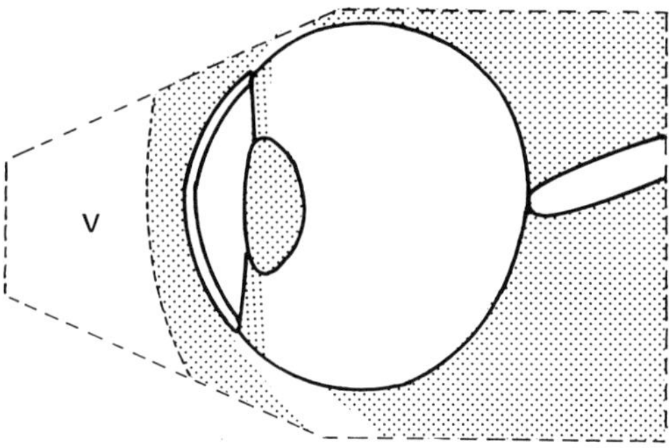


b

Fig. 3.**1 a–c**
**a** By using a stand-off (V), e. g., a water-filled finger cot, we can get optimal images from the anterior segment. The lens contour appears as a closed oval
**b** Schematic drawing

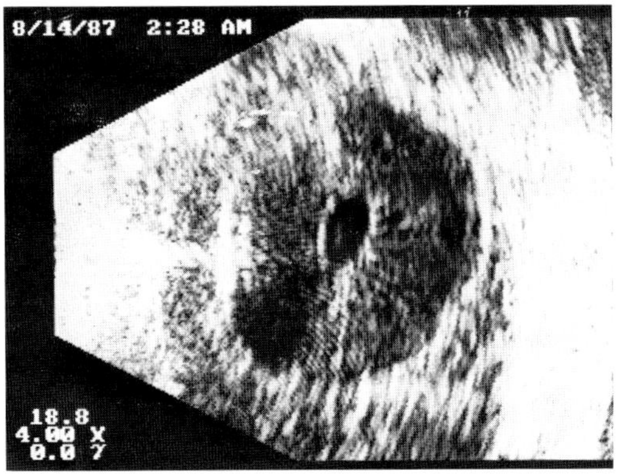


a

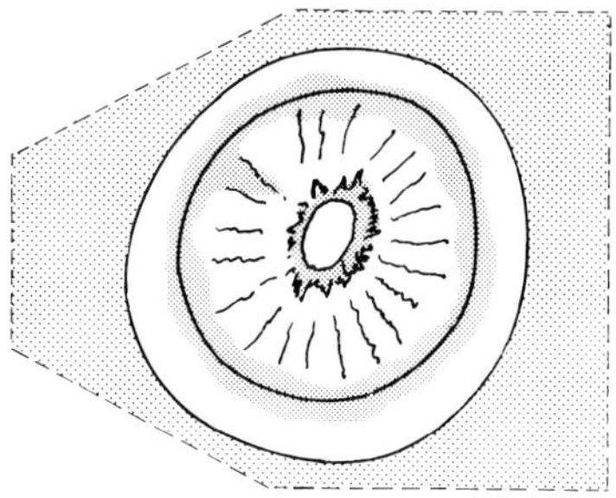

b

Fig. 3.**2** **a, b**

**a** Occasionally on maximal adduction, perhaps with the help of a long coupling, the iris diaphragm can be imaged in a frontal section. In this way it is possible to evaluate movements of the pupil even in eyes with dense corneal opacities

**b** Schematic illustration

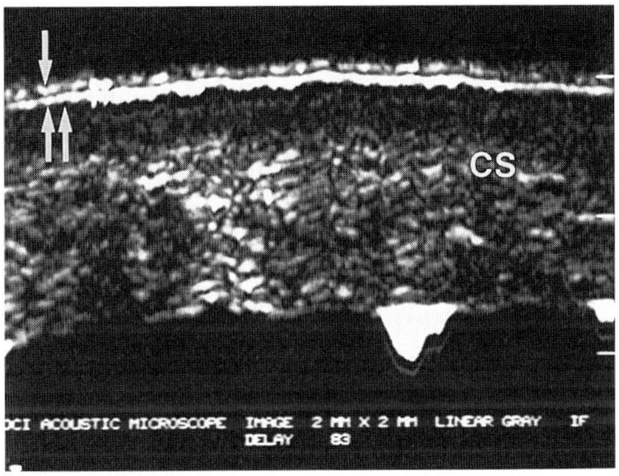


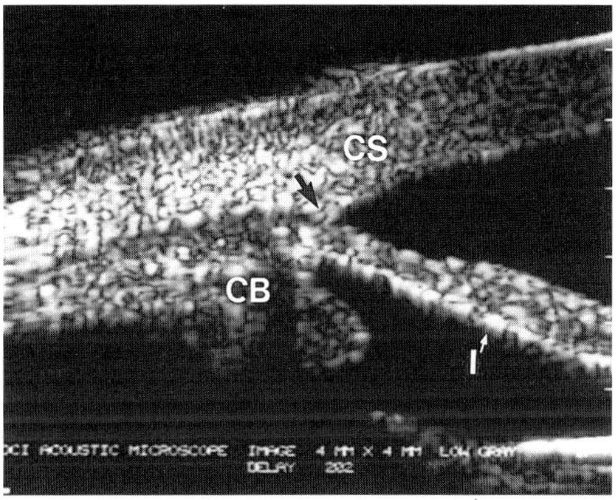


Fig. 3.**3** **a, b**

**a** Ultrasound biomicroscopic image of normal human cornea. Corneal epithelium (single arrow) is displayed in front of the highly reflective Bowman's membrane (double arrow). The signal height from the corneal stroma varies with the fluid content between the corneal lamellae

**b** Ultrasound biomicroscopic image of the angle structures seen from outside the intact globe (50 MHz). The corneo-scleral junction (CS) is defined by the different reflectivity of these two structures. The scleral spur (arrow) forms a distinct angle landmark. The ciliary body and ciliary processes (CB) are clearly imaged. The iris epithelium (I) forms a highly reflective layer at the posterior boundary of the iris (courtesy of Pavlin et al.).

bank eyes (Pavlin et al. 1990, 1), and recently in patients' eyes (Pavlin et al. 1990, 2). The scleral spur provides a landmark (Fig. 3.), ciliary body and ciliary processes are displayed separately and, the iris epithelium can be identified as a highly reflective layer at the posterior boundary of the iris.

## 3.3 Iris Diaphragm and Ciliary Body

Because of the limited lateral resolution power of the B-mode, the iris diaphragm cannot be satisfactorily imaged. It is occasionally possible to display the entire pupillary plane on frontal sections by using the soft lid tissue for coupling. Under these circumstances, we can also document a consensual pupillary reaction if optical evaluation is impossible (Fig. 3.**4**).

Due to its limited extent the ciliary body cannot be exactly localized. If it is imaged, we must first of all exclude a pathologic process.

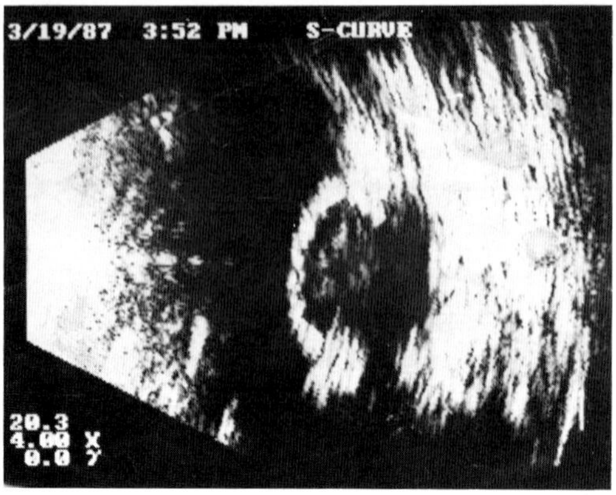


a

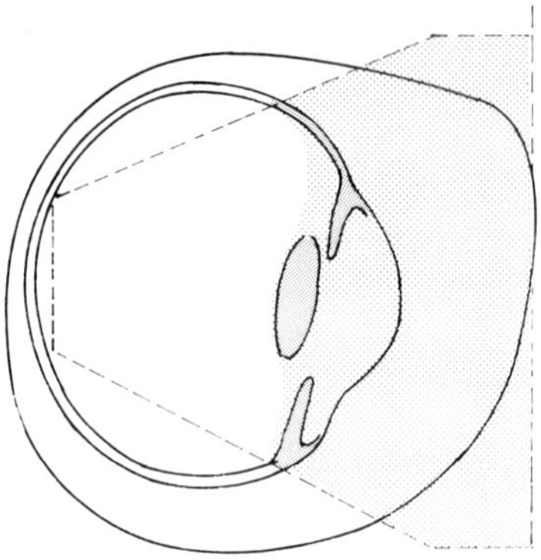

b

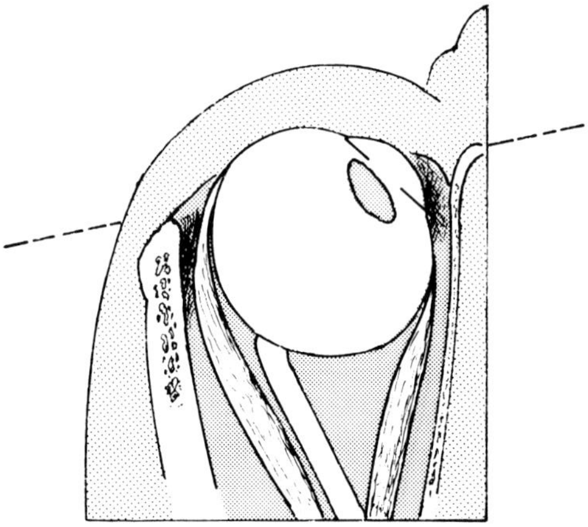

c

Fig. 3.**4a–c**
**a** Echogram at right angle to the plane of section shown in **c**. The vitreous body is used as an internal stand-off in order to demonstrate the anterior segment
**b** Schematic drawing
**c** Plane of section

## 3.4 The Lens

A clear lens is acoustically empty; in an axial cut it appears as an ellipsoid structure (Fig. 3.**1**). The lens contents accelerate the ultrasound and therefore the beam will diverge here (A-mode transducer), or the focal distance of the ultrasound waves will become longer (B-mode transducer) (see Sect. 1.5.5). In order to avoid disturbing artifacts, the ultrasound beam should not encompass the lens in its sound field during examination of the posterior segment of the eyeball.

## 3.5 The Vitreous

The vitreous space has a volume of about 5 ccm in an emmetropic globe and consists of more than 99% water. Its three-dimensional collagen framework is filled with hyalonuric acid molecules. The vitreous does not constitute an acoustic interface for diagnostic ultrasound and therefore does not give an acoustic signal.

The detached posterior vitreous membrane presents an interface which can be imaged by sufficiently high amplification (Fig. 3.**5**). This membrane is characterized on acoustic sections by a multicurved line with varying reflectivity. Well-imaged parts of the membrane alternate with areas where the continuity of the vitreous surface becomes only apparent during eye motions as an imaginary line between the condensations. In A-mode we see, under the same conditions (with maximal amplification), variable low spikes in the posterior segment. For the differential diagnosis it is important to pay special attention to the dynamics of aftermovements of the vitreous, which is only attached at the vitreous base. Figure 3.**6** attempts to demonstrate the movements of the vitreous framework in

a

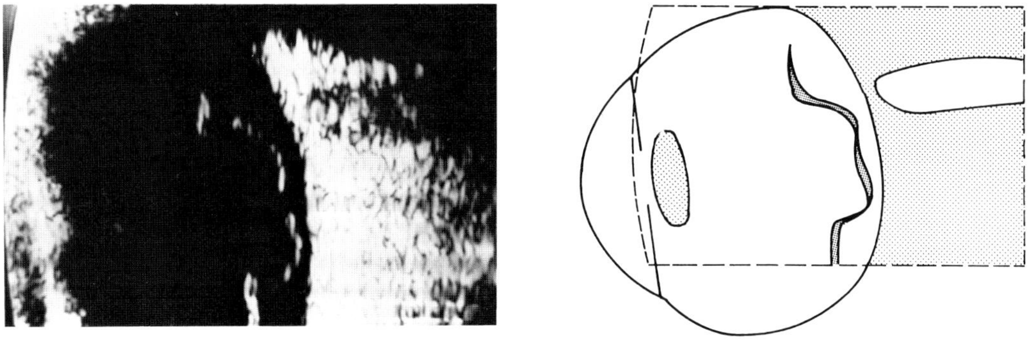

b

Fig. 3.**5a, b**
**a** The detached and slightly thickened posterior hyaloid membrane appears as a multicurved line not connected with the optic nerve head

**b** Schematic drawing

a b

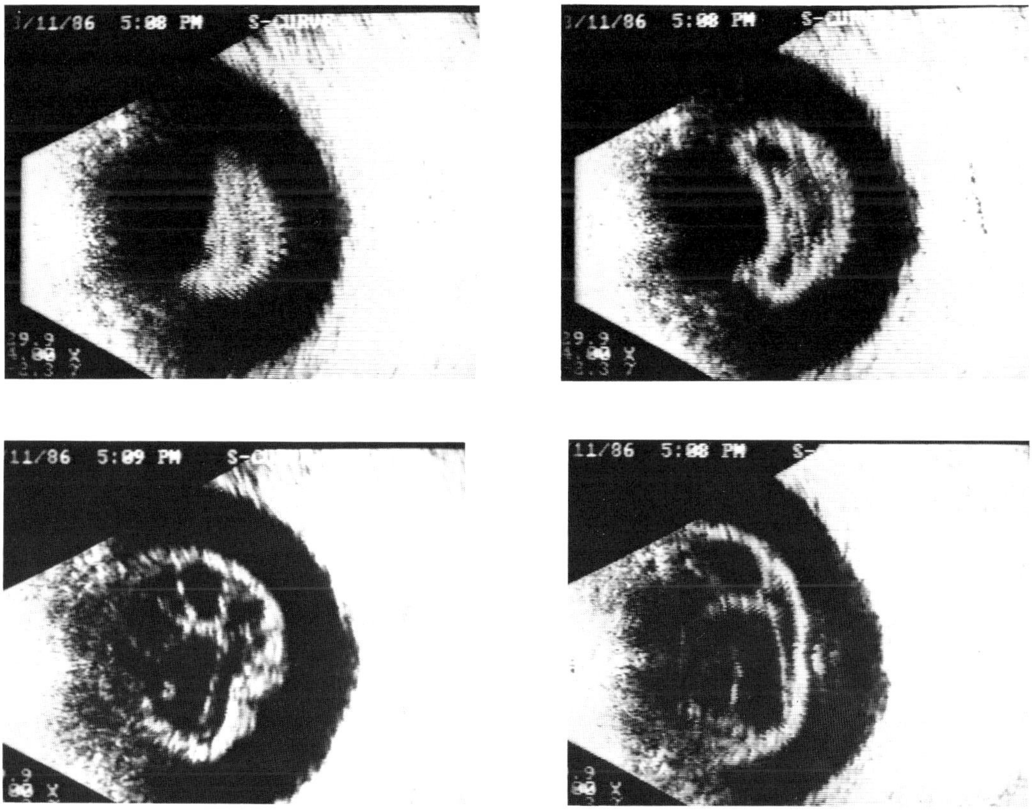


c d

Fig. 3.**6a–d** Sequential images during eye movement. The extensive dynamics of vitreous motions are here emphasized by the varying shape of the blood-covered vitreous framework

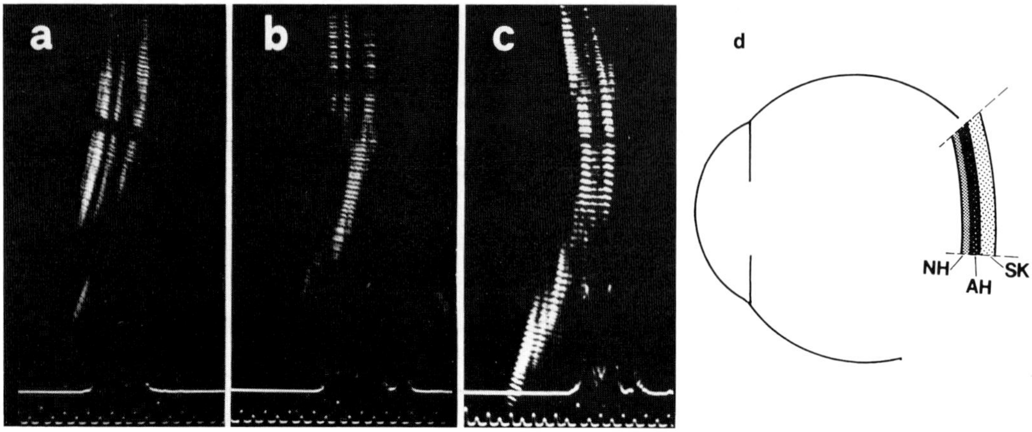


Fig. 3.7 **a–d** Demonstration of the individual layers of the ocular wall in vitro after layer-by-layer dissection of a pig eye
**a** Complete ocular wall
**b** Echogram after dissecting the retina
**c** Echogram after dissecting retina and choroid. In vivo, a reliable separate imaging of the various layers of the ocular wall cannot be obtained with commercially available instruments
**d** Schematic drawing (NH = retina, AH = choroid, SK = sclera)

various directions of gaze in a case of intraocular hemorrhage.

After only a short learning period, the examiner will soon be able to differentiate between after-movements of a taut vitreous membrane and free-floating opacities (see Sect. 4.2).

## 3.6 The Ocular Wall

The ocular wall is the most strongly reflecting structure in ophthalmology. Opinions differ concerning the normal variations of the reflectivity of this organ (Haigis et al. 1980, Ossoinig 1971, 1972). Many investigators (Till et al. 1972, Ossoinig 1972, Sampaolesi 1984) use the scleral echo for comparison when evaluating poorly defined membranes (see Fig. 2.**14**).

When attempting to **subdivide the ocular wall,** we reach the limits of our possibilities.

Instruments have been designed which are capable of differentiating even the individual retinal layers (Coleman 1971, Coleman et al. 1977, Lepper 1978). They are constructed for scientific purposes and will even demonstrate choroidal pulsation. Commercially available instruments will allow us to subdivide the ocular coats only under ideal experimental conditions (Fig. 3.**7**).

We can quite reliably determine the **thickness of the ocular wall** in the human eye (Guthoff et al. 1987, Nover et al. 1965) (Fig. 3.**8**) and can use these data for some differential diagnostic considerations (see Sect. 4.4.1). If we compare the thickness of the ocular wall in a high myope with a hyeropic eye, we find values of less than 1 mm in the myope and a thickness of up to 2.5 mm in highly hyperopic eyes. If we use these echographically determined measurements to calculate the volume of the ocular wall, we come to results which are interesting from a statistical point of view: independent of the axial length of the globe, the volume of the ocular wall at the posterior pole is about 1.6 ccm (Guthoff et al. 1987) (Fig. 3.**9**).

Echographically, we cannot decide whether the ocular coats are covered by retina or whether the retinal pigment epithelium lies bare and represents the inner border. Lepper et al. (1978) have tried to solve this problem by using frequency analyses and high-frequency transducers.

The **choroid** is in vivo 0.3–0.5 mm thick (Coleman 1971, Lepper 1978). Histologically, this organ is characterized by numerous blood vessels; there-

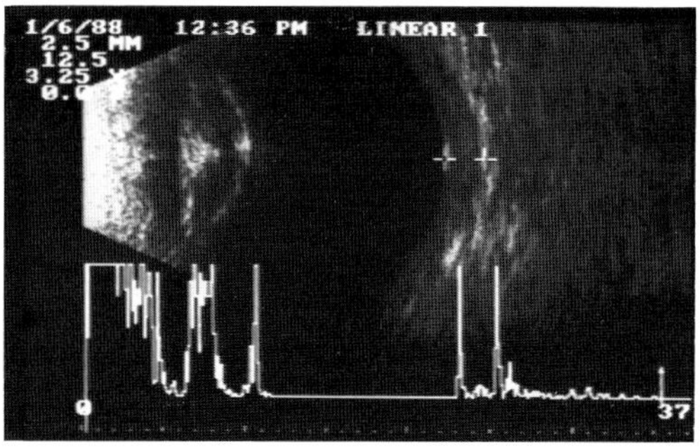


a

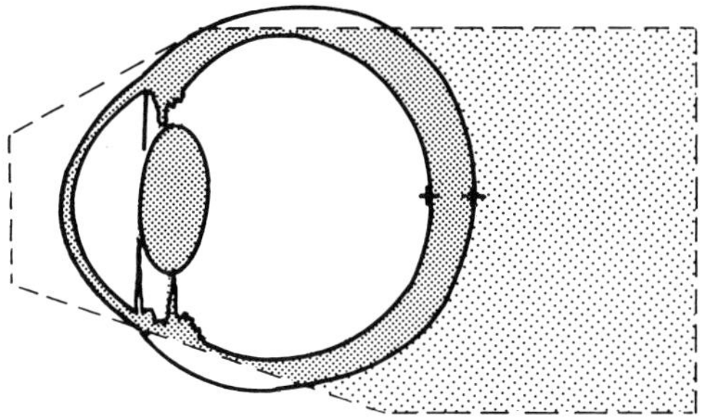

b

Fig. 3.**8 a, b**
**a** Ocular coats in an eye with an axial hyperopia of 10 diopters; axial length 20.2 mm. Using a linear amplification we obtain a sharp image of the retina and the scleral surface. Corresponding to the shortness of the hyperopic globe, we find a thickening of retina and choroid to a total of 2.5 mm
**b** Schematic drawing

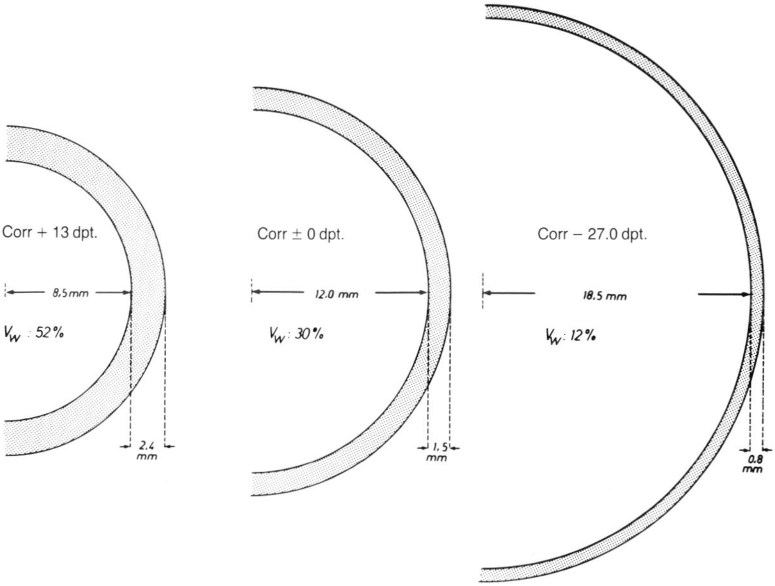


Fig. 3.**9** Schematic sketches of the posterior ocular wall in a hyperopic, emmetropic and myopic eye. The volume of the ocular wall behind the equator is constant and amounts to about 1.6 ccm. There is, therefore, a direct relationship between the axial length and the thickness of the ocular wall, which varies between about 2.4 and 0.8 mm

fore, we have to expect a strongly reflecting layer. An unequivocal imaging of this coat is, however, only possible under pathologic conditions (see Sect. 4.4.3). The suprachoroidal space is a tenuous layer of connective tissue in which the long ciliary vessels course. This potential space can be expanded by the accumulation of fluid as we see it in hemorrhagic or serous choroidal detachments.

The **sclera** is the strongest reflecting structure of the ocular coats. It is not possible to measure its thickness with commercially available instruments. A definite delineation toward the orbital fat is only feasible when pathologic alterations allow imaging of Tenon's space. According to histologic examinations, scleral thickness varies between 0.3 and 1.5 mm (Spalton et al. 1984).

# 4 Echographic Diagnosis of Intraocular Diseases

## 4.1 Anterior Segment

If corneal opacities make a visual examination of the interior of the eye impossible, we may obtain some information about the structure of the anterior segment by an ultrasound examination (Tejima et al. 1983, Le May 1978).

### 4.1.1 The Cornea

Damaged endothelial cell function may cause variations in **corneal thickness**. This may extend from 0.4 to 1.0 mm. In the infant eye, similar changes of the cornea may lead to a more pronounced increase of corneal thickness due to less developed axial stability (Fig. 4.**1**).

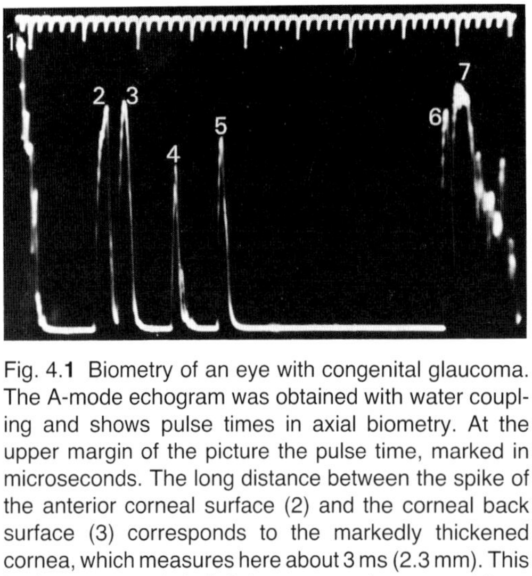


Fig. 4.**1** Biometry of an eye with congenital glaucoma. The A-mode echogram was obtained with water coupling and shows pulse times in axial biometry. At the upper margin of the picture the pulse time, marked in microseconds. The long distance between the spike of the anterior corneal surface (2) and the corneal back surface (3) corresponds to the markedly thickened cornea, which measures here about 3 ms (2.3 mm). This is due to an endothelial decompensation caused by a long-standing increased intraocular pressure
1 Emitted echo, 2 anterior corneal surface, 3 posterior corneal surface, 4 anterior lens surface, 5 posterior lens surface, 6 retinal surface, 7 scleral surface

### 4.1.2 The Anterior Chamber

Depending upon the **axial length of the globe**, the axial depth of the anterior chamber varies between 2.5 and 4.5 mm. François and Goes reported upon the correlation between the depth of the anterior chamber and the probability of developing an acute glaucomatous attack. Their review of the literature (François et al. 1981) is complemented by an extensive bibliography on biometry.

### 4.1.3 The Lens

The normal axial diameter of the lens lies between 3.5 and 4.5 mm (Jansson 1963). This diameter may increase up to 5.5 mm (Pallikaris et al. 1981), due mainly to a breakdown of the barrier represented by the anterior lens surface producing water clefts or an intumescent cataract. Pronounced optical heterogeneity usually also presents acoustic interfaces, so that opaque lens layers may become echographically visible (Fig. 4.**2**). Particularly brown nuclear opacities accelerate the sound velocity (Jansson et al. 1962, 1961). These changes induce biometric, but negligible, errors for the implantation of intraocular lenses. When examining infantile cataracts of uncertain etiology, the **retrolental space** should be especially carefully examined; otherwise, congenital anomalies, e.g., persistence and hyperplasia of the primary vitreous, could be overlooked (see Fig. 4.**35**).

Occasionally, we can also demonstrate intralenticular metallic foreign bodies by echography (Fig. 4.**3**). Calcifications of the lens nucleus may create images resembling those produced by foreign bodies (Fig. 4.**4**). Similar phenomena also appear on the surface of lens implants made of PMMA (Fig. 4.**5**) (Rochels et al. 1980, Scherer et al. 1982). Occasionally, we may be able to demonstrate a defect in the posterior lens capsule with prolapse of lens material into the vitreous after a perforating injury (Clemens et al. 1987).

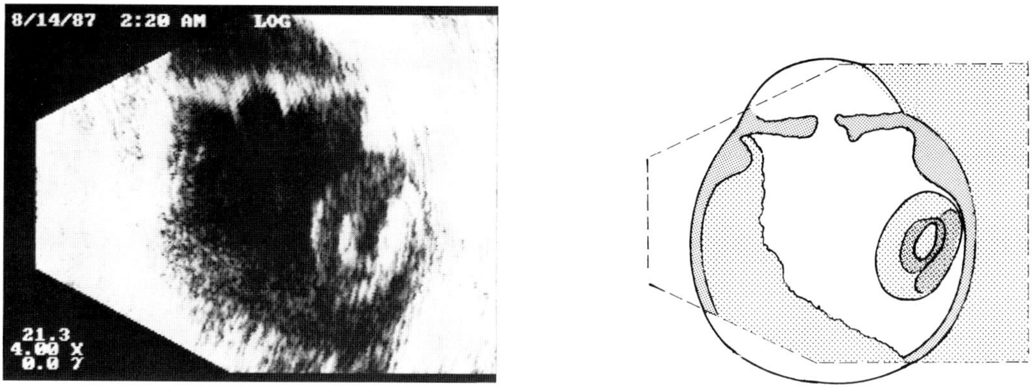


Fig. 4.**2 a, b**
**a** The opaque lens is luxated into the vitreous. Development of a cataract is usually associated with the formation of acoustic interfaces. In a completely opaque luxated lens we can differentiate the nucleus from the cortex in a cross section
**b** Schematic drawing

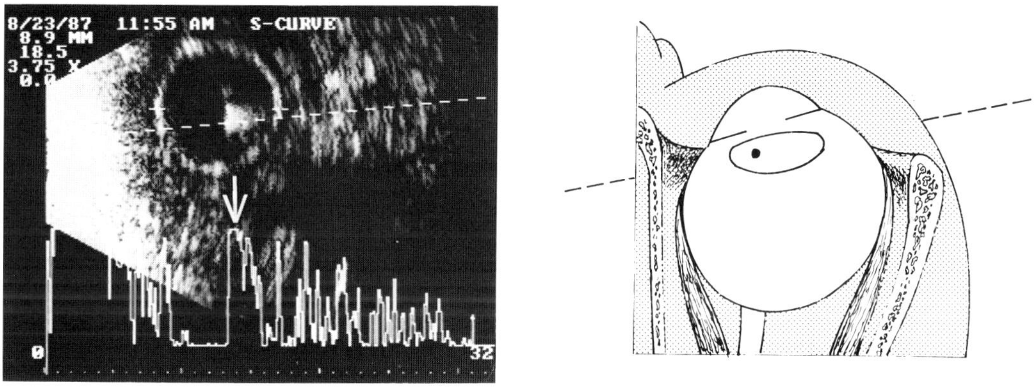


Fig. 4.**3 a, b**
**a** Intralenticular foreign body in a frontal examination (from temporal). The high reflectivity of the foreign body leads to a plateau formation in the A-mode echogram (white arrow). **b** Schematic drawing

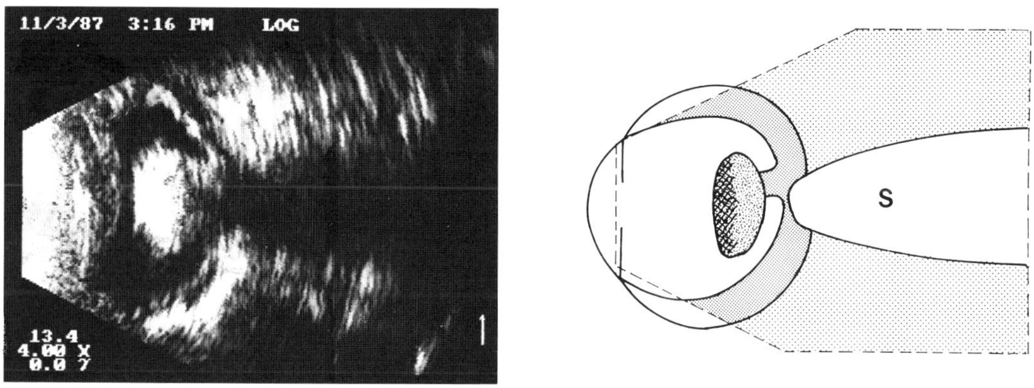


Fig. 4.**4 a, b**
**a** Calcified lens in a phthisical eye. Intralenticular calcifications lead to echos similar to those of an intraocular foreign body. Shadows obscure the images from the ocular coat and the orbital soft tissue
**b** Schematic drawing (S = sound shadow)

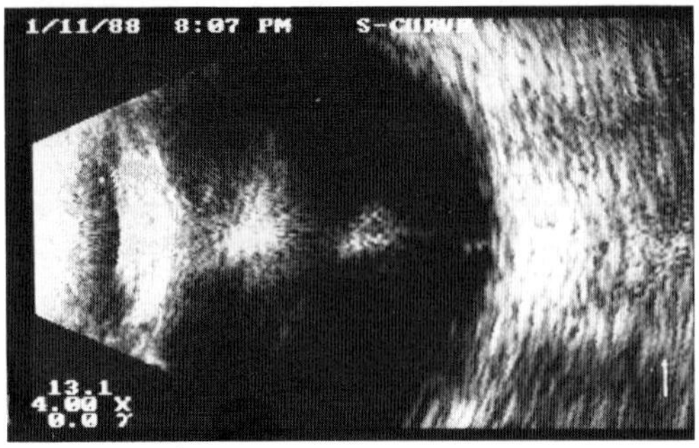


a

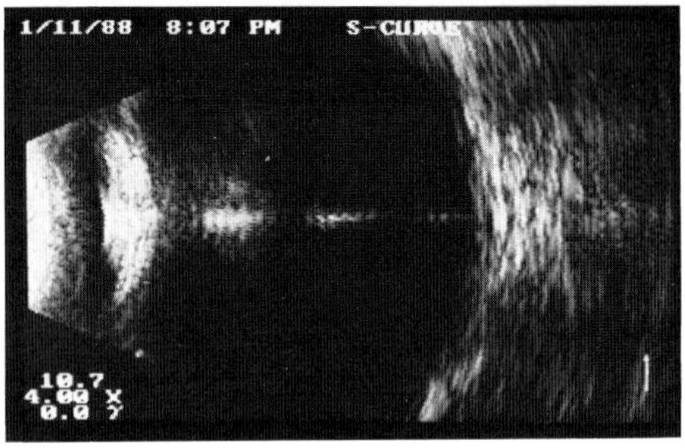


b

Fig. 4.**5 a, b** Echogram after the routine implantation of an intraocular PMMA lens. The intraocular PMMA lens produces artifacts, e.g., multiple echos and sound shadows. Only limited axial biometry is possible in pseudophakic eyes

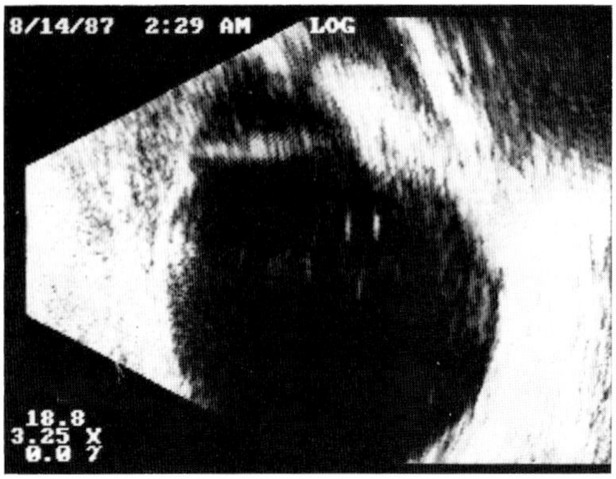


a

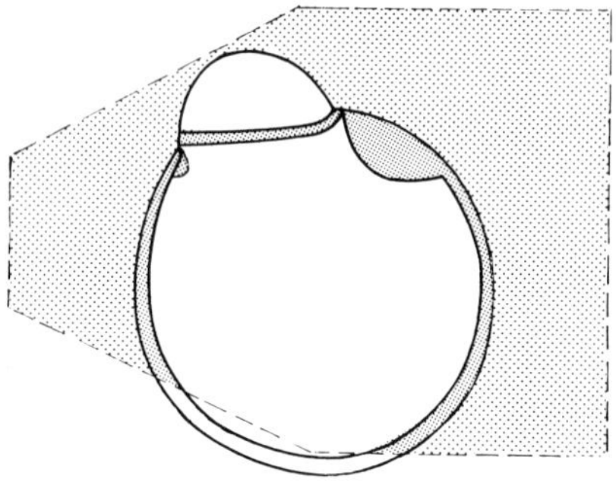

b

Fig. 4.**6 a, b**
**a** Solid space-occupying lesion in the ciliary body of a patient with Recklinghausen disease. Suspicion of a neurofibroma of the ciliary body
**b** Schematic drawing

### 4.1.4 The Ciliary Body

Increase in volume may make the ciliary body visible on echographic examination. This increase may caused by a tumor (Figs. 4.**6**, 4.**8**), or be posttraumatic (Fig. 4.**7**) or inflammatory. A differential diagnosis between a ring-shaped pseudogranulomatous cyclitis and a ring melanoma cannot be established echographically with the certainty necessary for a clinical decision. Figure 4.**8** shows the cross section of a ciliary body melanoma, the anterior surface of which touches the posterior lens surface.

### 4.1.5 Congenital Glaucoma

Congenital glaucoma is echographically characterized by a pathologic extension of the axial length (Buschmann et al. 1974, Sampaolesi 1969, 1981). As intraocular pressure measurements are here occasionally unreliable because of the influence of general anesthesia, ultrasound biometry becomes especially important for the diagnosis and follow-up of this disease.

Figure 4.**9** shows the growth curve of the eye during the first months of life as published by Sampaolesi. Once the intraocular pressure has been regulated, the growth of the globe becomes normal so that echographic follow-up examinations are indispensable in the postoperative period. It may be difficult to differentiate a mild type of hydrophthalmus from a rapidly progressing axial myopia (Bluth 1983, Gernet et al. 1969).

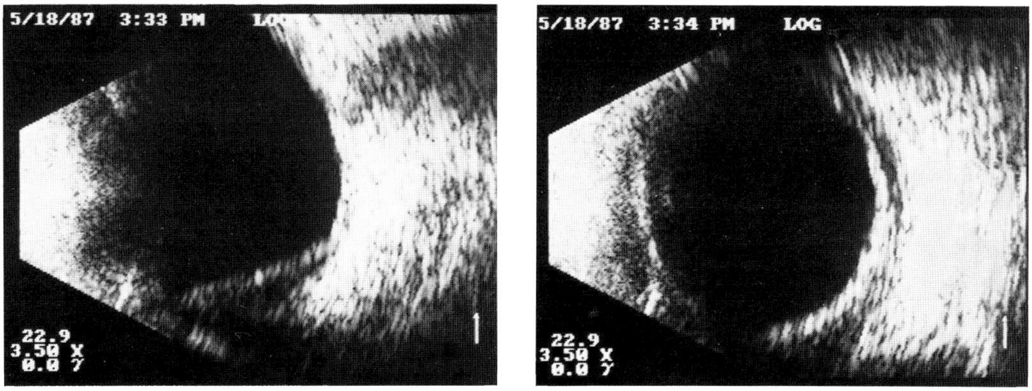


a b

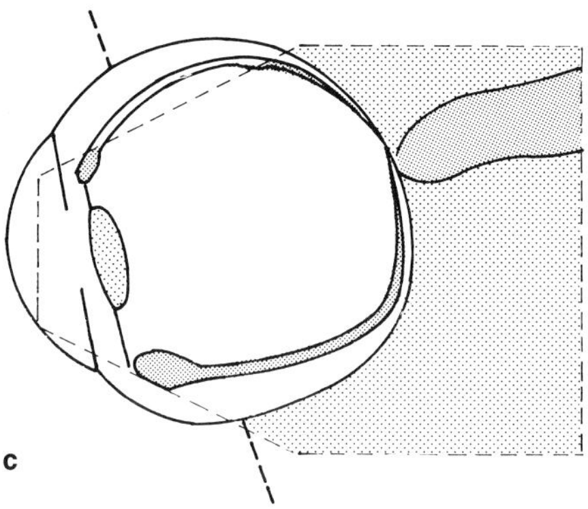

c

Fig. 4.7 **a–c**
**a, b** Perforating injury with regressing choroidal detachment. The area of the ciliary body is markedly involved
**c** Schematic drawing

## 4.2 The Vitreous

Echographic examination of pathologic changes in the vitreous will only be useful when the visualization of this organ is not good enough to allow a diagnosis. Echographic findings permit us to differentiate *dot-*, *strand-* and *membrane-like reflections*. Most important is the ultrasonic differentiation between membranous structures in the vitreous and a detached retina. Table 4.**1** summarizes the most frequent conditions associated with pathologic changes in the vitreous.

Table 4.1 **Clinical conditions with echographically demonstrable vitreous changes**

| |
|---|
| Changes in the shape of the globe |
| Vitreous opacities |
| Asteroid hyalosis |
| Synchisis scintillans |
| Acute posterior vitreous detachment |
| Vitreous hemorrhage |
| Uveitis (idiopathic) |
| Uveitis (infectious) |
| Intraocular foreign body |
| Persistence and hyperplasia of the primary vitreous (PHPV) |

### 4.2.1 Changes in the Shape of the Globe

#### Staphyloma

In cross section a staphyloma of the eyeball appears typically as an ectasia with a smaller radius of curvature than that of the globe (François et al. 1967, Makabe 1975) (Fig. 4.**10**). When the examination is performed in an oblique plane, the border between the normal ocular coats and the ectasia may appear under a more acute angle than is really the case. Scleral buckles lead to similar echograms (Fig. 4.**11**) (Rochels 1979). Koloszvary uses ultrasound biometry in the area of the staphyloma as an indication of his encircling operation for the treatment of progressive malignant myopia (personal communication). After an encircling detachment operation, the silicone explant will appear

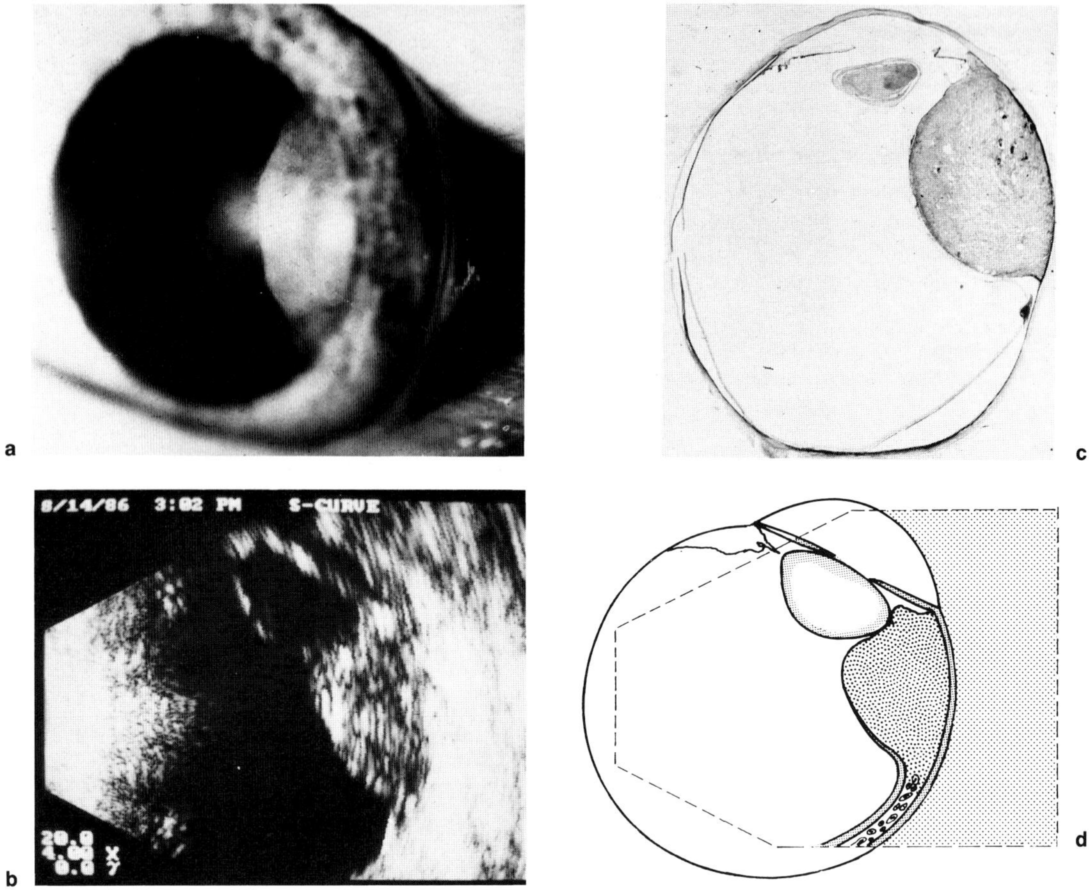


Fig. 4.**8a–d** A melanoma probably originating in the ciliary body
**a** Anterior segment with the tumor well visible on the nasal side
**b** Cross sectional echogram from the temporal side with maximal adduction of the globe shows the relation of the tumor to the lens
**c** Histologic section slightly outside the echographic imaging plane
**d** Schematic drawing

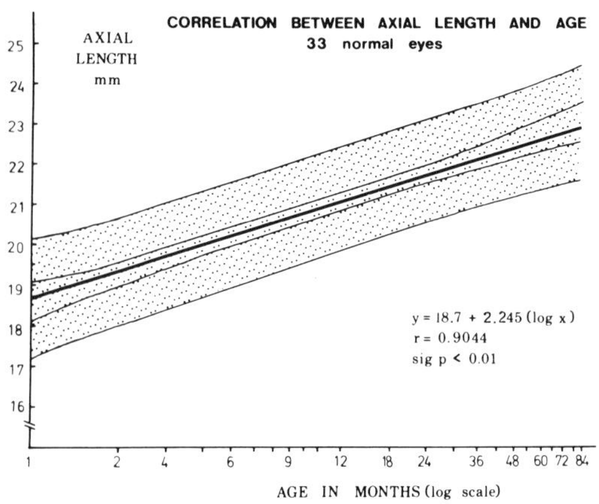


Fig. 4.**9** Correlation between axial length and age (after Sampaolesi (1981)

a

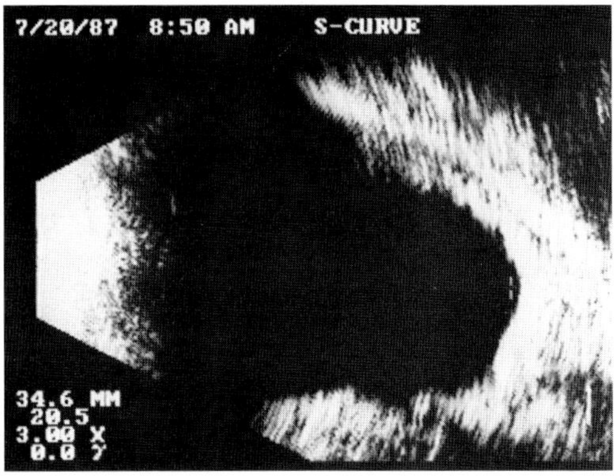


b

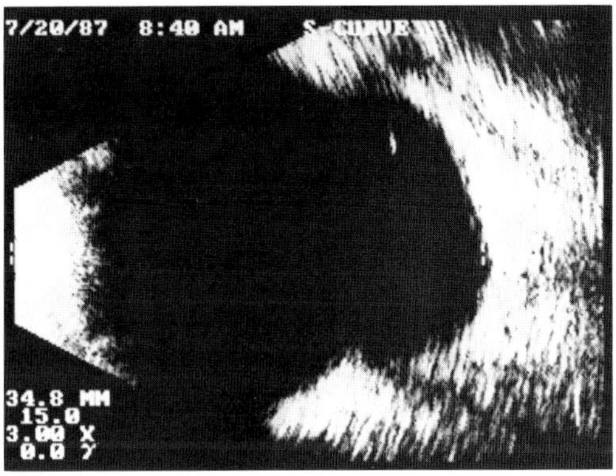


c

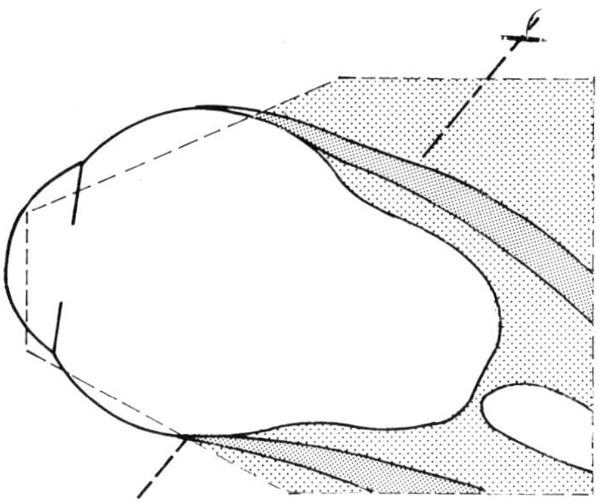

Fig. 4.**10a–c** Extensive staphyloma in a highly myopic eye (axial length 34.8 mm)
**a** In an axial section the eccentric entrance of the optic nerve can be seen
**b** The misshaped globe is especially well demonstrated on a sectional plane which lies outside the optical axis
**c** Schematic drawing

a

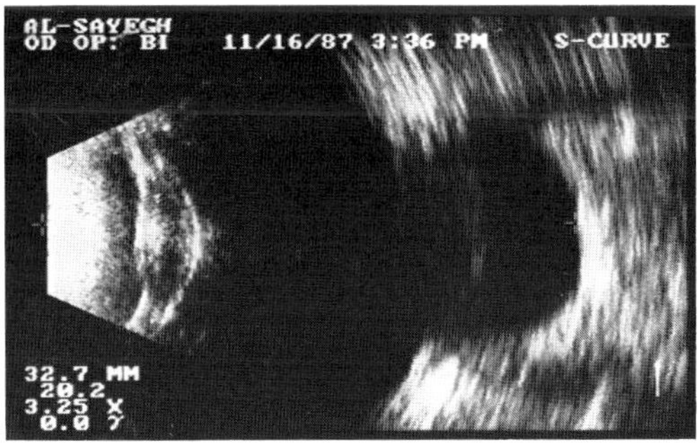


b

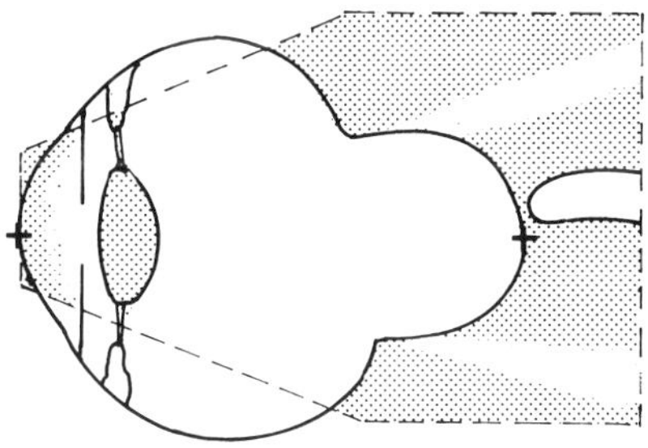

**+ 32,7 mm +**

Fig. 4.**11a, b**
**a** Scleral buckle in a highly myopic eye. Encircling retinal detachment operations may produce echographic cross sections similar to a staphyloma. If silicone rod was used, sound shadows will be produced as an extension of the scleral buckle. Distance between the electronic marker (+ +) 32.7 mm
**b** Schematic drawing

behind the deformed globe as a strongly reflecting and shadow-casting structure (Fig. 4.**12**) (Gerke 1979, Gernet 1965).

### Microphthalmus

Congenital microphthalmus frequently shows, in addition to the axial shortening, anomalies of other intraocular structures. We can occasionally prove the presence of a coloboma, which may involve the optic nerve head. In three of seven patients with congenital microphthalmus in our own material we found an isolated orbital cyst, which could be regarded as part of the globe, which was separated when the optic cup closed (Fig. 4.**13**).

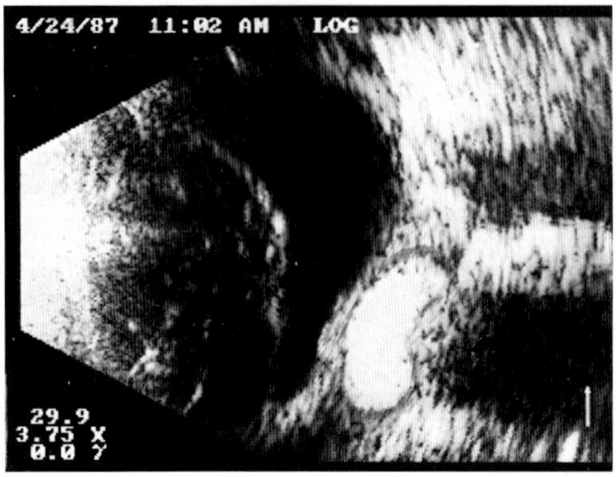


a

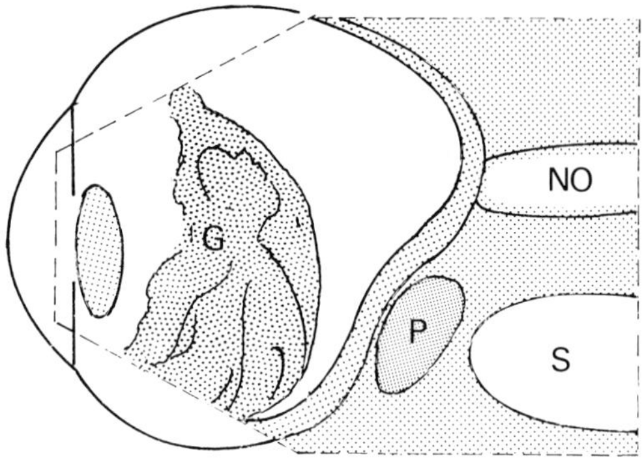


b

Fig. 4.**12** a, b
**a** Scleral buckle produced by a silicone sponge explant. After a scleral buckle, the deformity of the globe can be seen in an acoustic cross section. Silicone explants reflect the ultrasound nearly completely so that they can be compared with a foreign body. They also cast an acoustic shadow
**b** Schematic drawing (NO = optic nerve, P = explant, S = sound shadow, G = syneretic, densified vitreous)

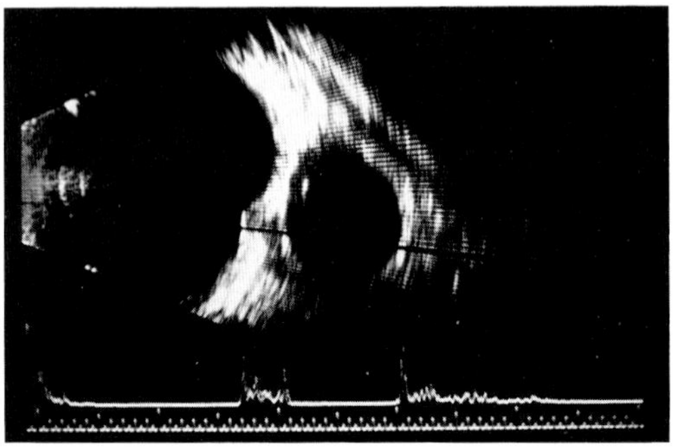

a

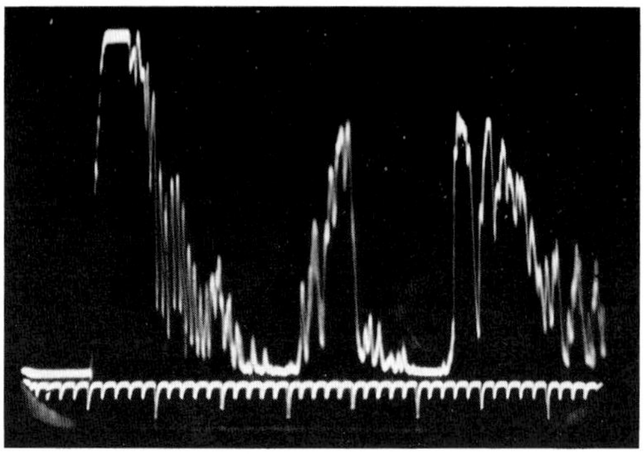

b

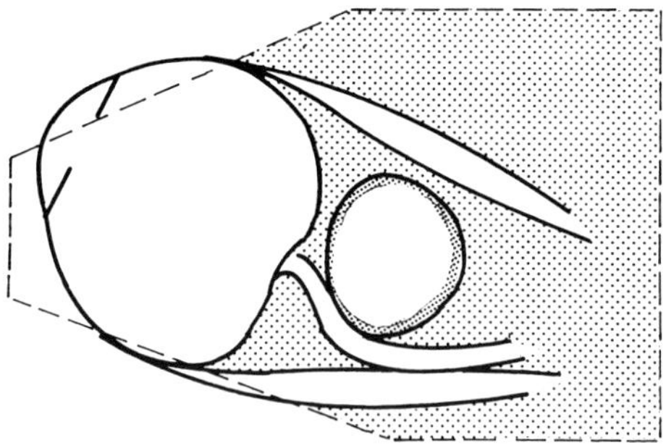

c

Fig. 4.**13** a–c
**a, b** Microphthalmus with orbital cyst. We occasionally find cystoid spaces within the muscle cone associated with microphthalmus, which are interpreted as »completely separated colobomas«
**c** Schematic drawing

### Phthisis

Severe atrophy of the globe may be associated with extreme hypotony. Echographically, phthisis is characterized by a thickening of the ocular coats. It is still not quite clear why this only rarely leads to a choroidal detachment; perhaps the latter is prevented by an atrophic choriocapillaris.

In contrast to severe axial hyperopia, here it is not possible to differentiate the various layers of the ocular coats. Occasionally, we see calcification or ossification (Fig. 4.**14**) which are probably due to degenerative processes and metaplasia of the retinal pigment epithelium. In advanced cases of phthisis, the sclera and choroid can represent 70%

a
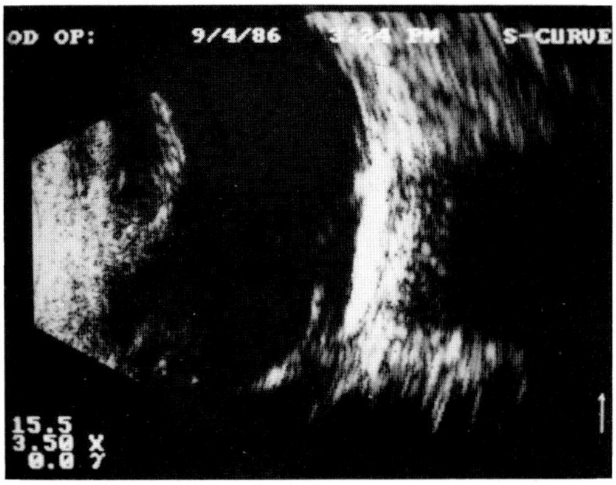


b
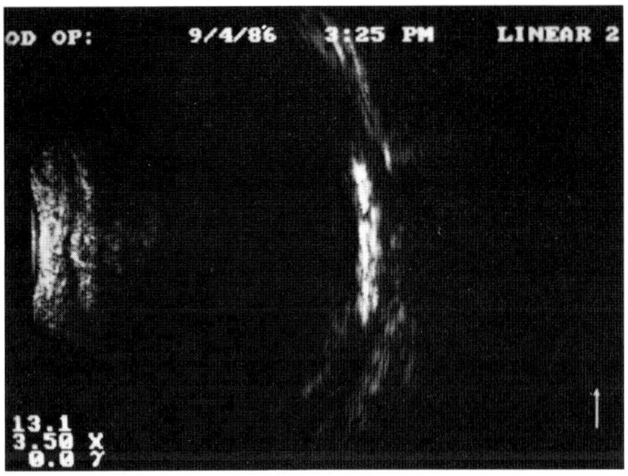


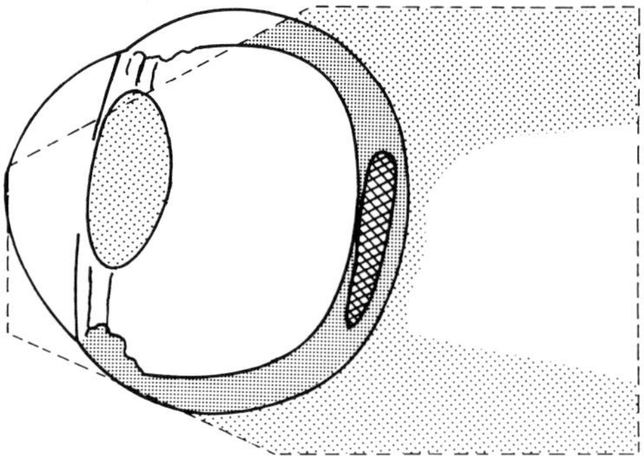
c

Fig. 4.**14a–c** Circumscribed calcification of the ocular coats in advanced phthisis bulbi. With progressing phthisis, there may be calcification or ossification on the choroid
**a** Echographically we find highly reflective changes in the ocular coats. These cast a shadow on the soft tissue behind them
**b** These strong echos can be presented selectively by reducing the amplification
**c** Schematic drawing

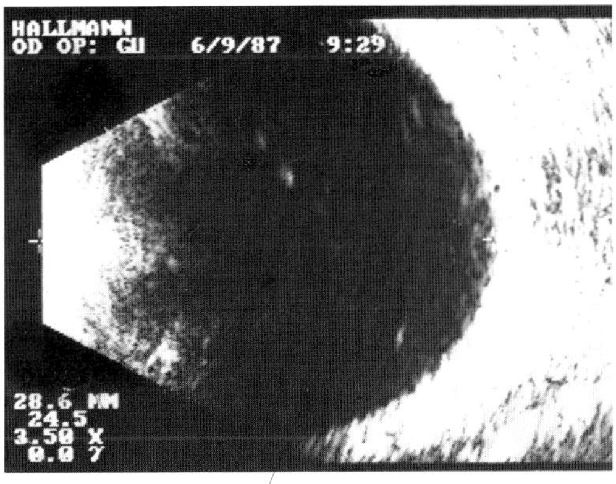


Fig. 4.**15** Vitreous opacities. In maximal amplification, small heterogenous spots can be seen echographically, even though the vitreous appears optically clear. They act as dot-like reflectors

of the total volume of the ocular coats (Fig. 4.**63**). It is reasonable to assume that the degree of thickening of the ocular coats in chronic hypotony could be an indication of an impending phthisis of the globe; however, no exact measurements are available.

### 4.2.2 Vitreous Opacities

Occasionally, we can image vitreous opacities as they normally occur as floaters, provided we use maximal amplification. They appear as dot-like reflectors and are more pronounced in a myopic or senile vitreous (Fig. 4.**15**).

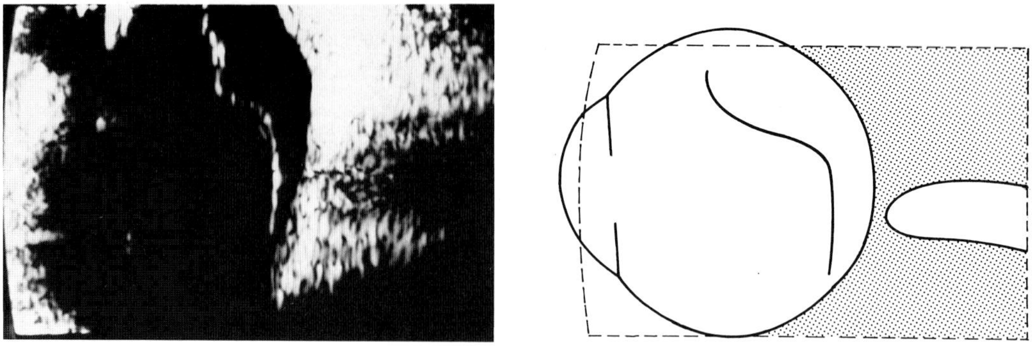

Fig. 4.**16a, b**

**a** Detached posterior hyaloid membrane. In a symptomatic posterior vitreous detachment, we can occasionally image a freshly detached and occasionally blood-tinged posterior hyaloid membrane as a floating structure of low reflectivity

**b** Schematic drawing

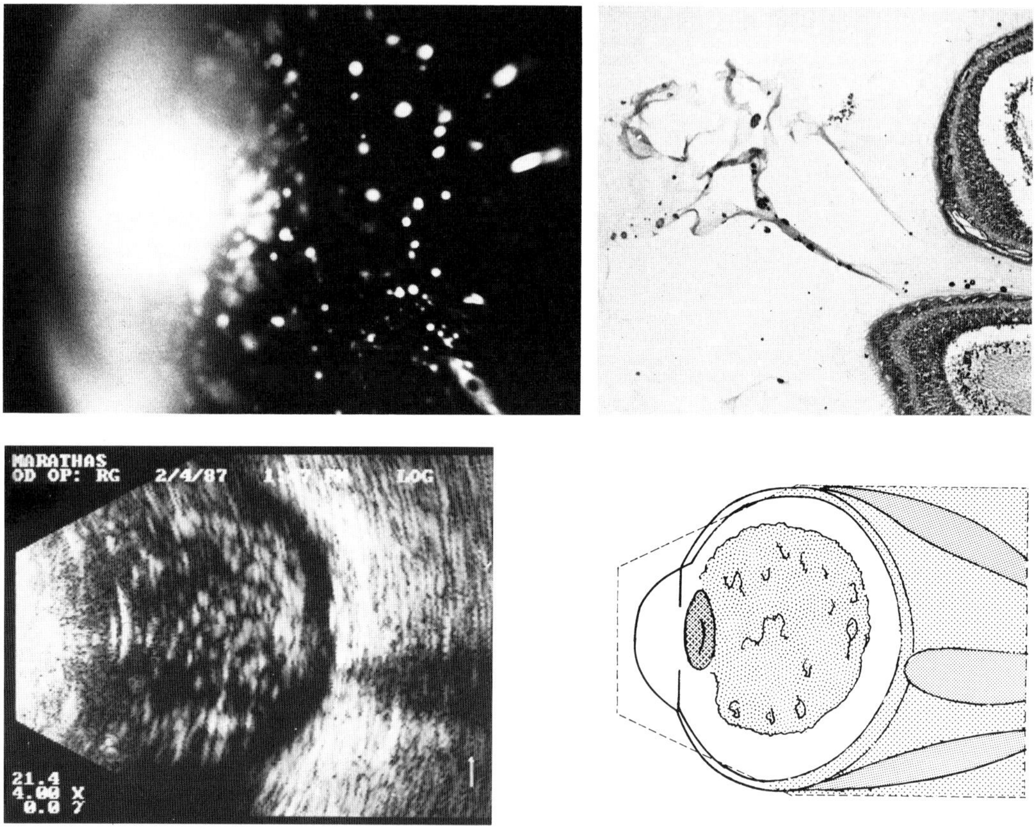


Fig. 4.**17a–d** Asteroid hyalosis. The calcium crystals adhere to the vitreous scaffold and represent good reflectors for the ultrasound

**a** Slit lamp microscopic photo of the anterior vitreous space

**b, c** There is a discrepancy between the conspicuous and impressive echographic picture and the slight optical difficulties experienced by the patient. Close to the ocular wall there is always an echo-free retrovitreal space. **d** Schematic drawing

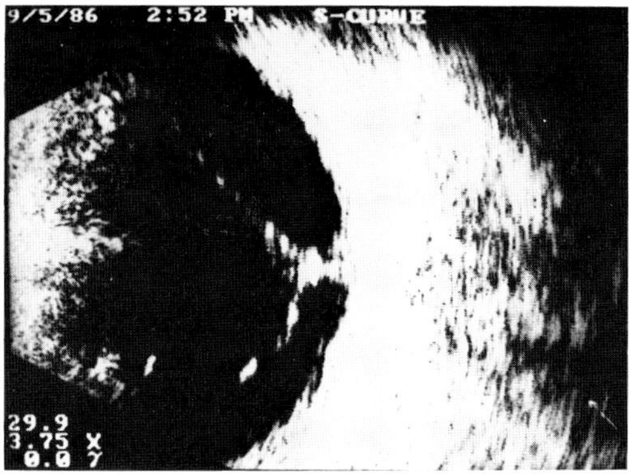


Fig. 4.**18** Fresh vitreous hemorrhage. In a cross sectional echogram the vitreous framework converges towards the ocular wall. Blood precipitates increase the acoustic reflectivity of the vitreous. Traction has to be assumed where the vitreous is in contact with the ocular wall

During a symptomatic posterior vitreous detachment, the B-mode echogram may demonstrate various stages of the condition and, possibly, remaining adhesions of the hyaloid membrane to the retinal surface (Gärtner et al. 1967, 1968, Oksala 1975) (Fig. 4.**16**).

### 4.2.3 Asteroid Hyalosis/Synchysis Scintillans

In asteroid hyalosis and in synchysis scintillans there is a conspicuous discrepancy between the mild optical difficulties of the patient and the conspicuous optical and echographic findings (McLeod et al. 1977).

The calcium-containing lipids (asteroid hyalosis) are suspended in the vitreous framework and constitute perfect reflectors (Fig. 4.**17**). They demonstrate the dynamics of vitreous movements especially well. Characteristically, there is a posterior vitreous detachment and therefore an acoustically empty retrovitreal space. In synchysis scintillans we are dealing with cholesterol crystals which are not suspended, but float freely in the vitreous space. When the globe moves, the clinical picture may resemble asteroid hyalosis, but after a few seconds the cholesterol crystals sink down toward the bottom of the liquified vitreous, thereby removing the numerous echos. In the A-mode echogram we see characteristic flickering spikes as they otherwise occur only in Coats' disease.

### 4.2.4 Vitreous Hemorrhages

An acute **vitreous hemorrhage** represents an especially important indication for echography.

If the hemorrhage occurs within the framework of a symptomatic posterior vitreous detachment, the erythrocytes frequently precipitate on a pre-existing vitreous strand. This strand may be responsible for the development of a retinal tear, and its traction can be demonstrated directly in an acoustic cross section (Fig. 4.**18**). A circumscribed thickening of the ocular coats in cross section may indicate the presence of a retinal operculum. This area should be carefully scrutinized with the ophthalmoscope (Fig. 4.**19**). If the retina cannot be evalu-

a

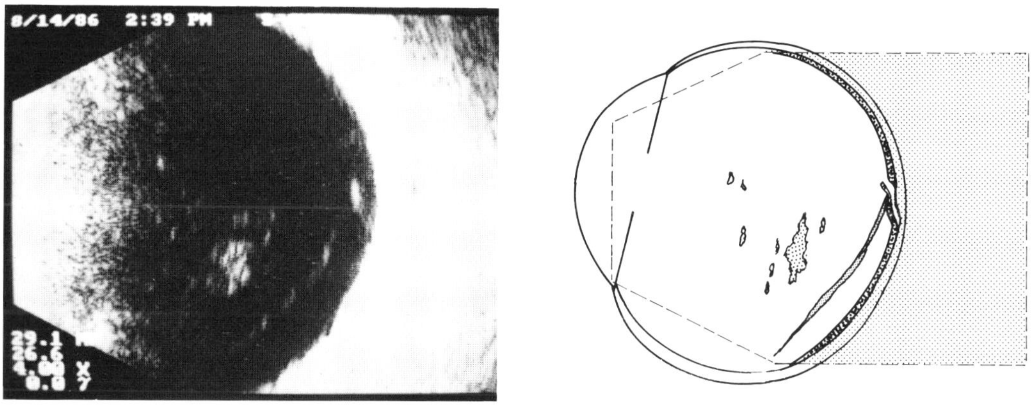


b

Fig. 4.**19a, b**
**a** Recent vitreous hemorrhage. On ocular motion the slightly reflecting membranes float freely. Where they contact the ocular wall a newly formed horseshoe tear may be present. **b** Schematic drawing

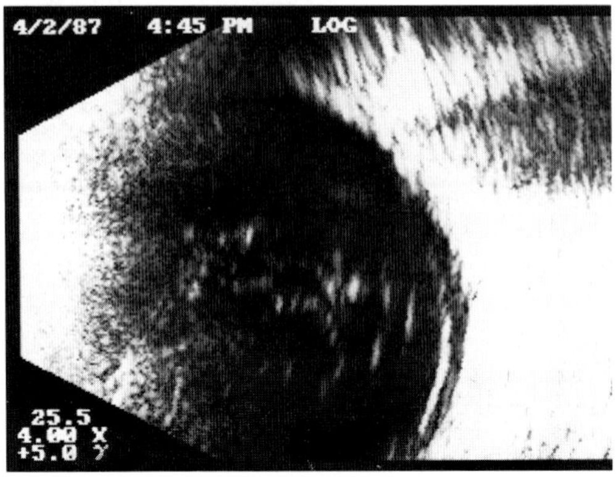


a

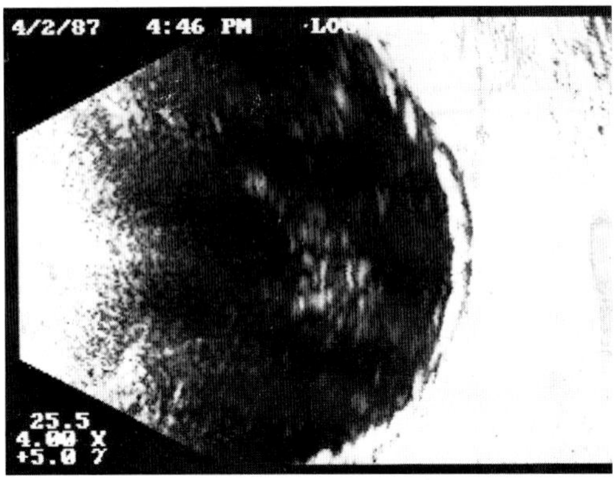


b

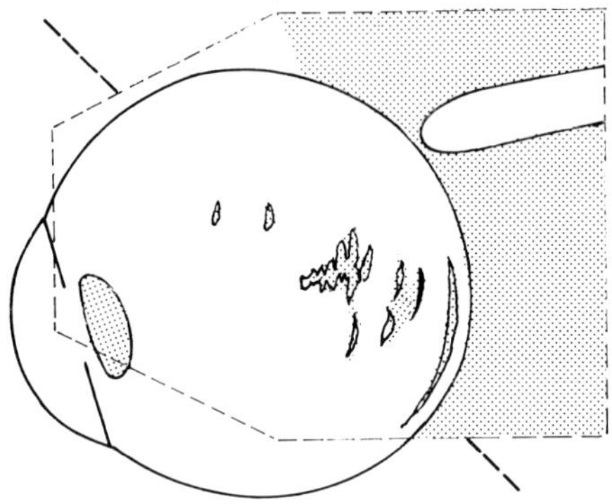

c

Fig. 4.**20** **a–c**
**a, b** Recent vitreous hemorrhage. Erythrocytes have precipitated onto the partly detached posterior hyaloid membrane, increasing its acoustic reflectivity
**c** Schematic drawing

ated ophthalmoscopically, the echographic examination should be repeated after a few days et al. so that a beginning retinal detachment can be diagnosed as early as possible (Coleman 1974, Tso 1976, Kolozsvary 1981). Smaller hemorrhages appear as erythrocytic precipitates on the posterior hyaloid membrane, which can then be well demonstrated echographically (Fig. 4.**20**).

Bleeding into a syneretic vitreous may give a static picture resembling a solid mass. However, when the globe moves, the clearly visible flowing motions indicate that we are dealing with disseminated opacities in a liquified vitreous. These opacities usually accumulate after a few hours in the lower circumference of the vitreous base (Fig. 4.**21**).

### Vitreous Hemorrhage and Diabetic Retinopathy

Hemorrhages from newly formed vessels of a proliferative **diabetic retinopathy** will always be accompanied by pathologic changes in the vitreous. The erythrocytes precipitate on interfaces which, up to then, produced only weak echos. The echogram emphasizes the danger of a shrinking vitreous. Vitreous membranes tent rectilinearly between adhesions to the retina. The typical aftermovements after changing the position of the globe are lacking here. We frequently find vitreous adhesions circling the posterior pole, whereby the detached vitreous membrane is as taut as a springboard. The first signs of a diabetic traction detachment appear at these circular adhesions (Fig. 4.**22**) between retina and vitreous.

### Terson Syndrome

After blunt trauma to the skull or to the brain, the retinal vessels at the posterior pole may bleed without direct injury to the globe. This is usually accompanied by a subarachnoidal hemorrhage. If the posterior hyaloid membrane is still attached, the preretinal bleeding will slowly diffuse into the formed vitreous and with it, the underlying retina

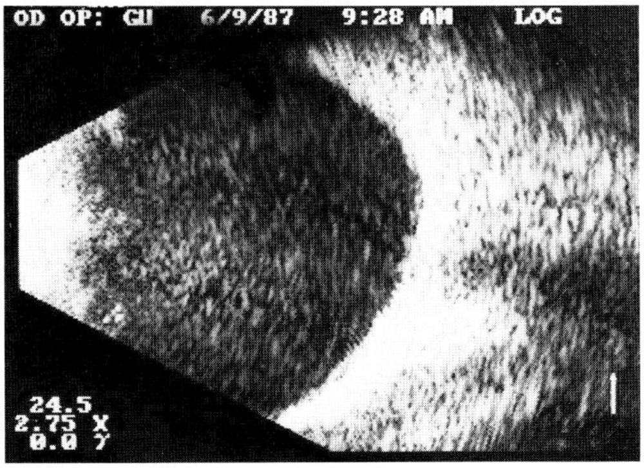


a

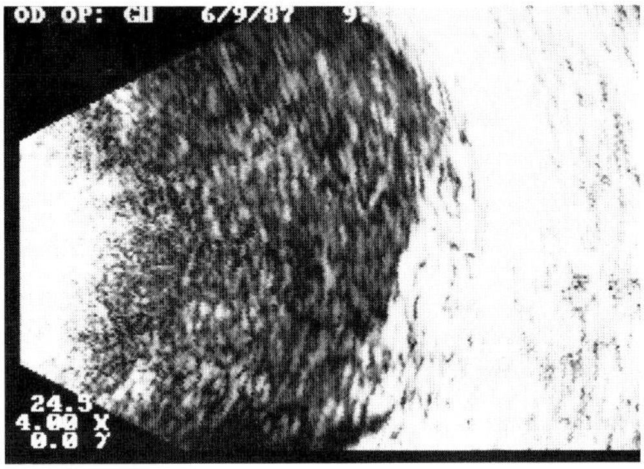


b

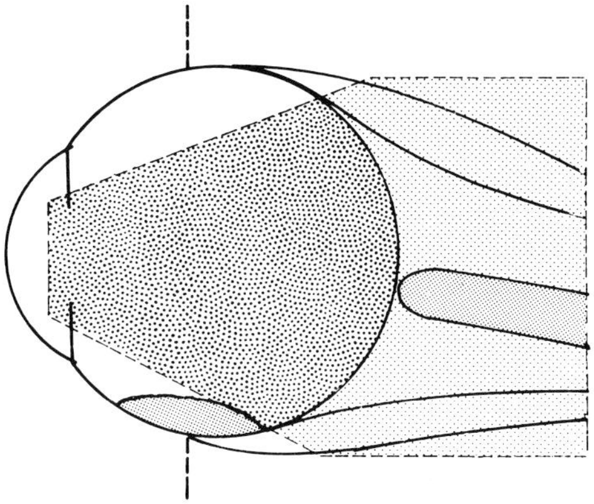

c

Fig. 4.**21 a–c**
**a, b** Conspicuous bleeding into a syneretic vitreous. A static picture may give the impression of a solid lesion. After a few hours the opacities usually accumulate in the lower aspect of the vitreous cavity
**c** Schematic drawing

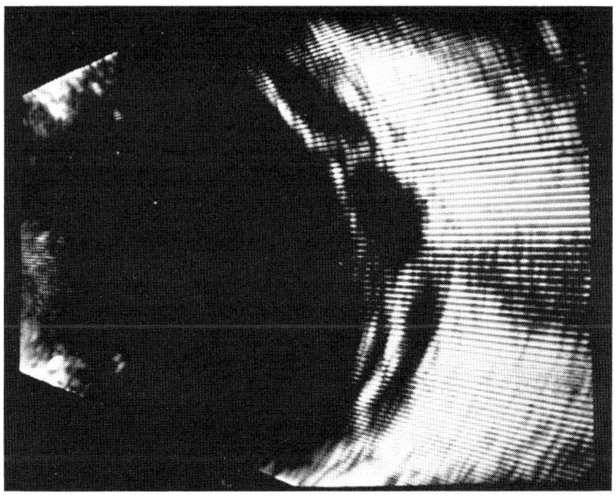

a

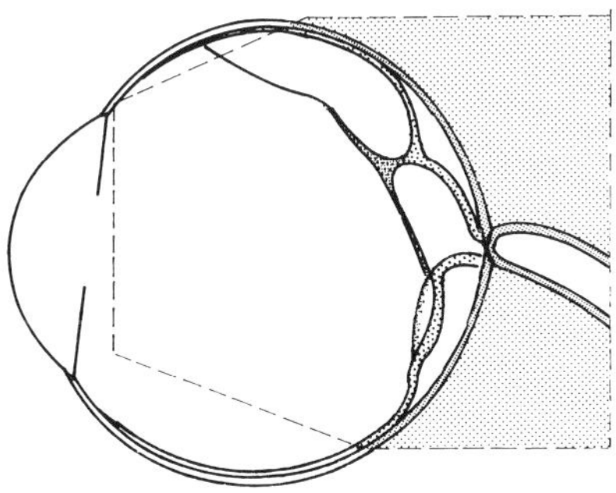

b

Fig. 4.**22 a, b**
**a** Beginning traction detachment at the posterior pole with vitreous contraction and proliferative diabetic retinopathy, which is hidden behind a diffuse vitreous hemorrhage. A springboard-like, taut, detached hyaloid membrane is still adherent to the retina at the posterior pole and has led to a traction detachment in several places
**b** Schematic drawing

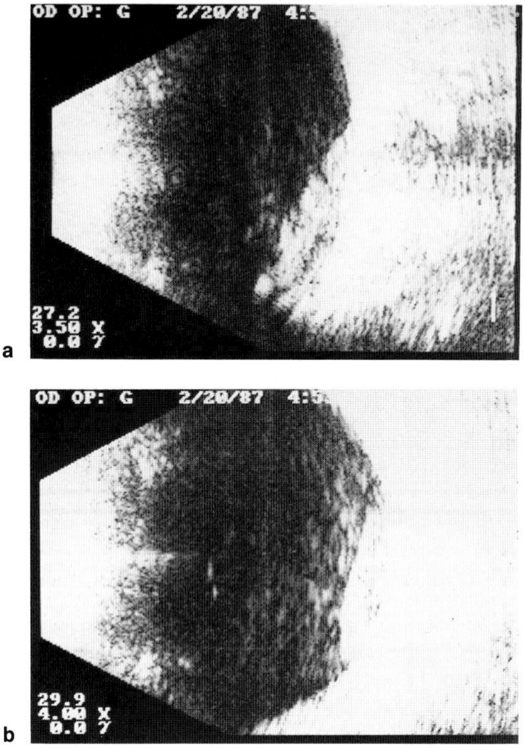


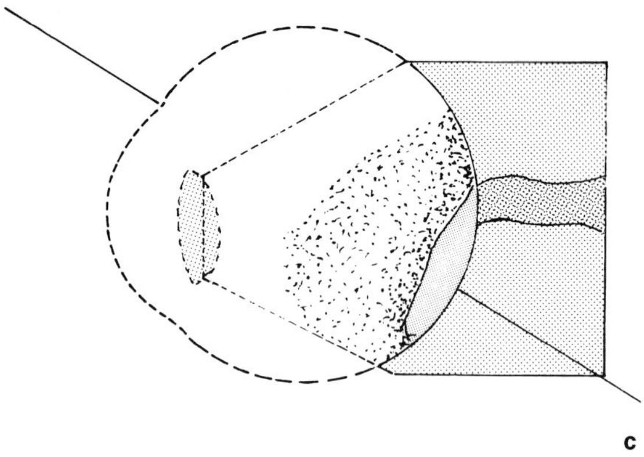


Fig. 4.**23** **a–c**
**a, b** Retrovitreal bleeding associated with a subarachnoidal hemorrhage (Terson syndrome). The bleeding originates from the area of the optic nerve head; if the posterior hyaloid membrane is still attached, blood will diffuse into the formed vitreous body
**c** Schematic drawing

may be damaged (Fig. 4.**23**). Many authors believe that this condition is an indication for an early vitrectomy (Schmidt et al. 1970, Kahn et al. 1975).

#### Vitreous Hemorrhage After Vitreous Detachment

If a detachment of the posterior hyaloid membrane precedes a vitreous hemorrhage, several compartments will be available for the dissemination of blood. In the early phase the erythrocytes collect in the retrovitreal space (Fig. 4.**24**). Slight bleeding leads only to a densification of the posterior hyaloid membrane, which then becomes echographically well visible. With severe hemorrhages a diffusion of blood into the formed vitreous occurs, thereby enhancing the normally present interfaces (Fig. 4.**25**). The retrovitreal space may completely clear after a few days or weeks, due to its high fluid exchange rate. Blood on the vitreous framework absorbs much more slowly (Till et al. 1975, Oksala 1979, Cennamo et al. 1981) (Fig. 4.**26**).

### 4.2.5 Endogenous Uveitis

Inflammatory and hemorrhagic vitreous changes cannot, in principle, be differentiated on the basis of echographic findings. Both conditions may cause densification of pre-existing vitreous structures with subsequent shrinkage of the vitreous and traction detachment of the retina (Fig. 4.**27**). This is especially the case if there are post inflammatory adhesions between the vitreous and the ocular coats. If there is an early, complete posterior vitreous detachment in a case of chronic uveitis, the formed vitreous shrinks to a frontal membrane which extends from the vitreous base (Fig. 4.**28**). If this membrane adheres to the ciliary body, it may detach the ciliary body, producing a subsequent ocular hypotony (Jaffe 1969).

### 4.2.6 Intraocular Infections

When a beginning intraocular infection is suspected, treatment should be initiated immediately, without waiting for a definite diagnosis. Echo-

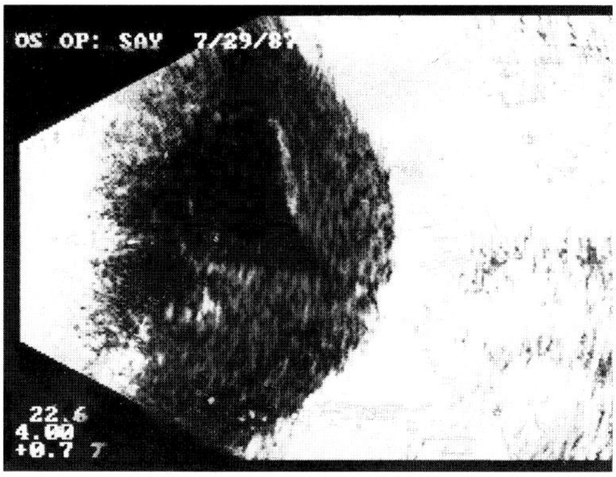


a

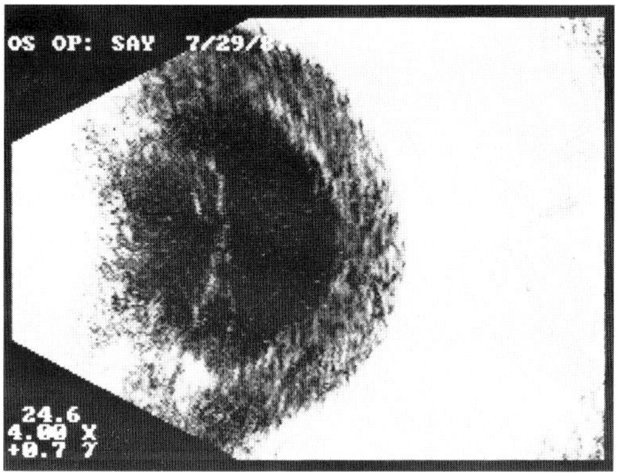


b

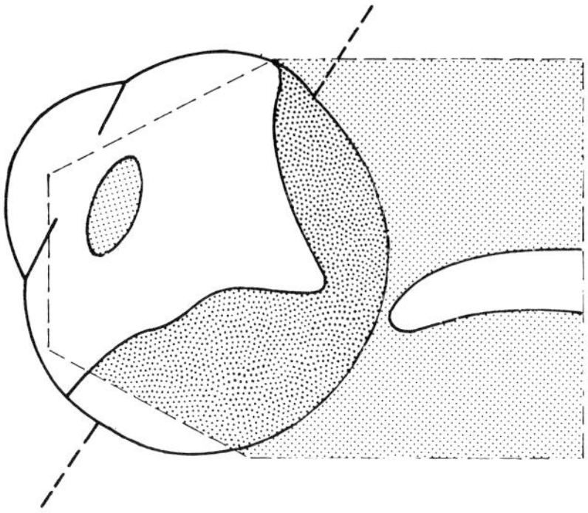

c

Fig. 4.**24a–c**
**a, b** Vitreous hemorrhage with posterior vitreous detachment emphasizing the retrovitreal space. In the early stage after the hemorrhage, erythrocytes accumulate in the retrovitreal space. They may ensheath the part of the vitreous which is free of blood and has a normal structure
**c** Schematic drawing

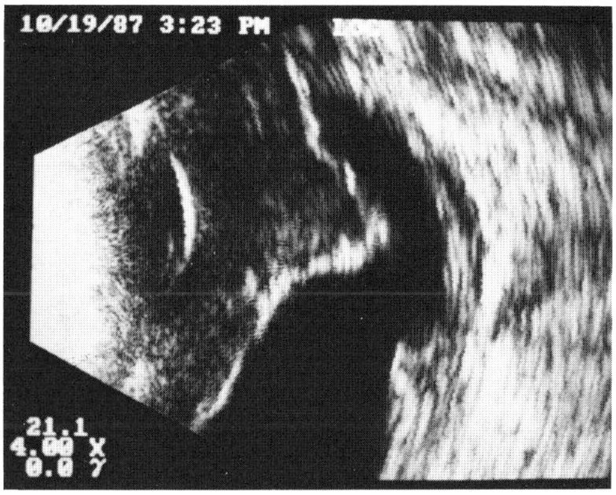


a

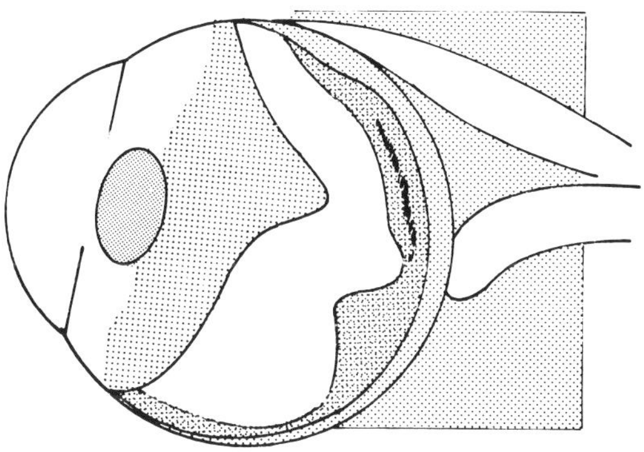

Fig. 4.**25a, b**
**a** Extensive bleeding from a disciform macular degeneration the presence of which was known. The bleeding disseminates onto the ocular coats and the formed vitreous. The retrovitreal space is already clear because of its high fluid exchange
**b** Schematic drawing

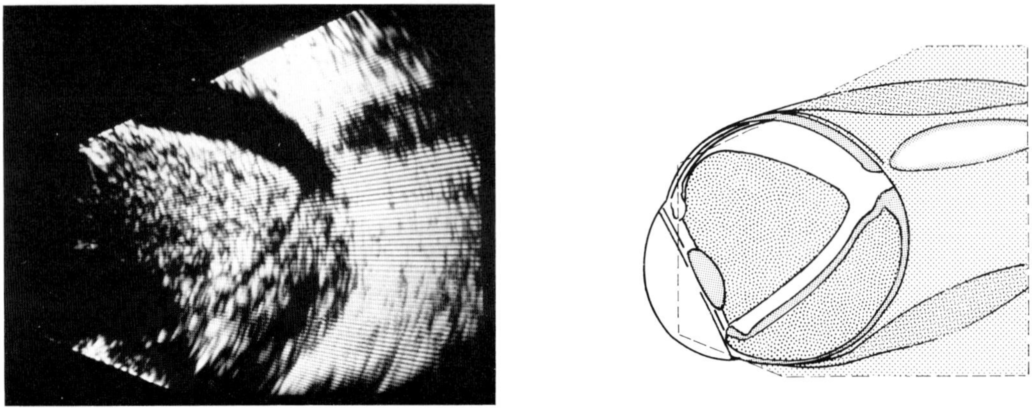

Fig. 4.**26a, b**
**a** Extensive vitreous hemorrhage from a disciform macular degeneration. The blood dissipates into the preretinal or intrachoroidal space, into the area of the macular lesion and into the detached vitreous. The retrovitreal space is echo-free
**b** Schematic drawing

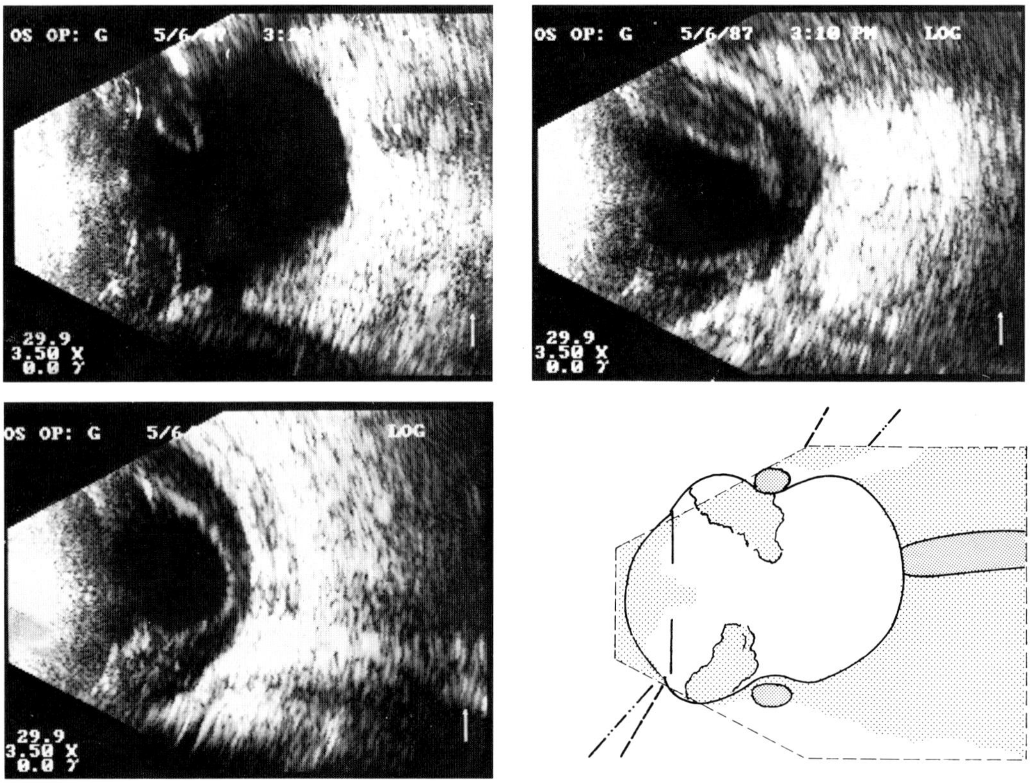


Fig. 4.**27a–d** Chronic uveitis with massive vitreous infiltration refractory to medical treatment. Subsequent pars plana vitrectomy and scleral buckle
**a** Remnants of the infiltrated vitreous can be seen at the vitreous base anterior to the scleral buckle
**b, c** Cross sections approximately at right angle to (**a**) through the vitreous base
**d** Schematic drawing

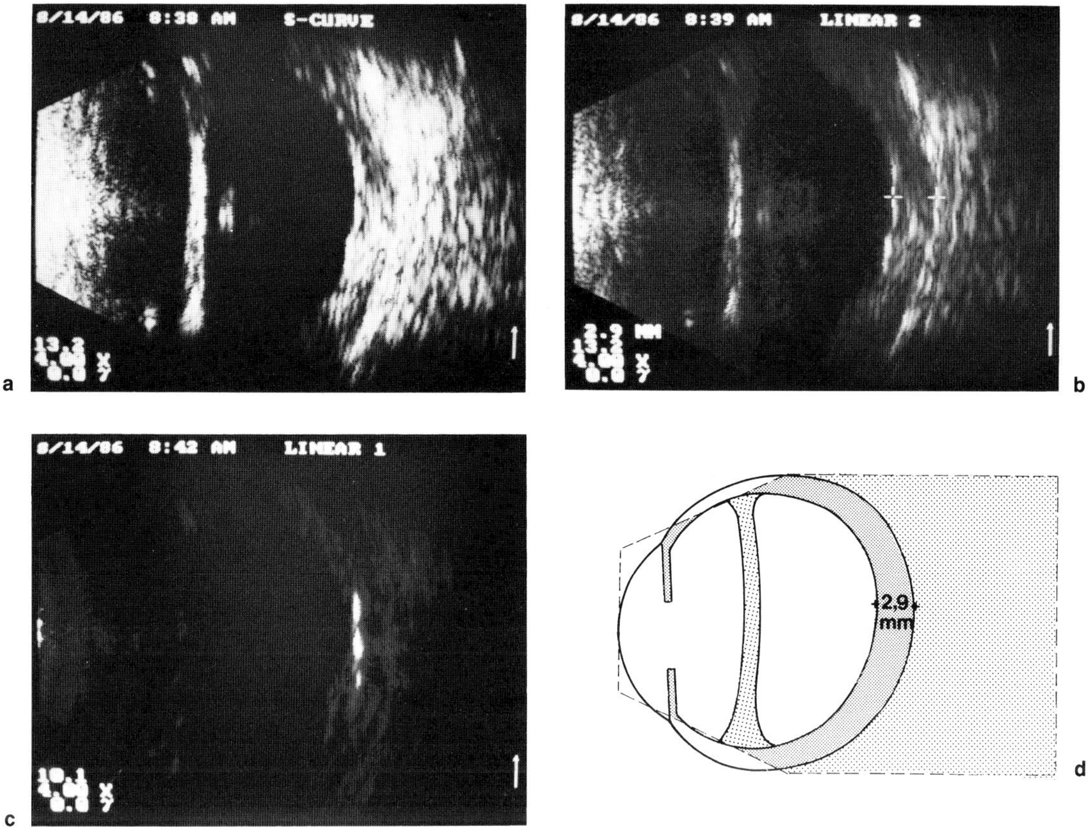


Fig. 4.**28a–d** Phthisis oculi in chronic panuveitis.
**a** The vitreous has shrunk to a frontal membrane of high acoustic reflectivity; the ocular wall is widened to 2.9 mm
**b** Using linear amplification, the various layers of the ocular coat become especially clearly outlined
**c** Isolated areas of the ocular coat with high acoustic reflectivity indicate calcification on the choroid or in the sclera
**d** Schematic drawing

graphically, we can follow the expansion of the inflammation, depending upon the site of the infection.

If the infection extends toward the anterior segment, echographically demonstrable structures will develop in the anterior vitreous space, together with the formation of a hypopyon. The changes in the anterior part may, after a few hours, involve the entire vitreous (Diamond et al. 1977, Hasenfratz 1987). Occasionally, we find thickening of the ocular coats once the inflammation has reached the ocular walls (Fig. 4.**29**).

If a panophthalmitis follows a perforating injury, we may occasionally echographically see a local reaction at the entrance port of the infection (Fig. 4.**30**). Once infection has been diagnosed, we can follow the course of the disease echographically and when the findings change, they may help us decide whether to perform a vitrectomy or not.

### 4.2.7 Intraocular Foreign Bodies

If we keep in mind that differences in acoustic impedance of various media are responsible for the intensity of the echo, we may anticipate that intraocular foreign bodies, regardless of the material, should be imaged conspicuously (Figs. 4.**31–33**). In practice, however, we find that other parameters, which cannot be easily defined in an individual case, participate in the image formation

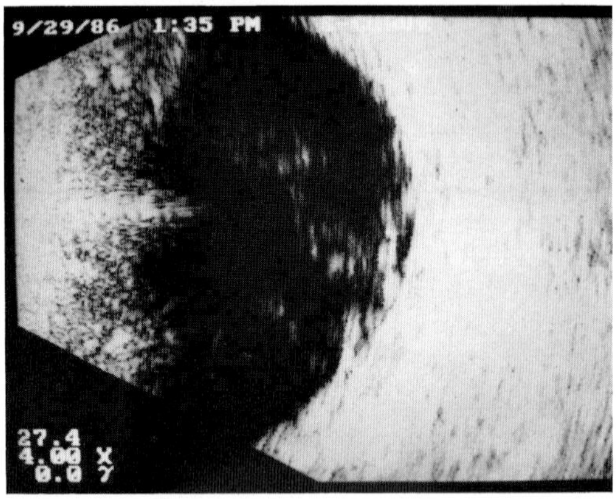


a

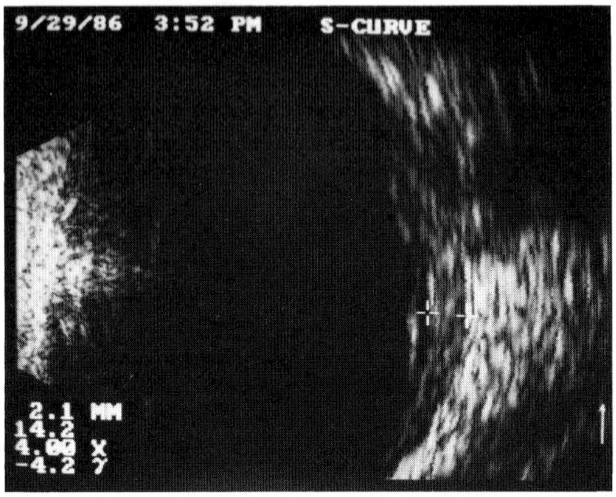


b

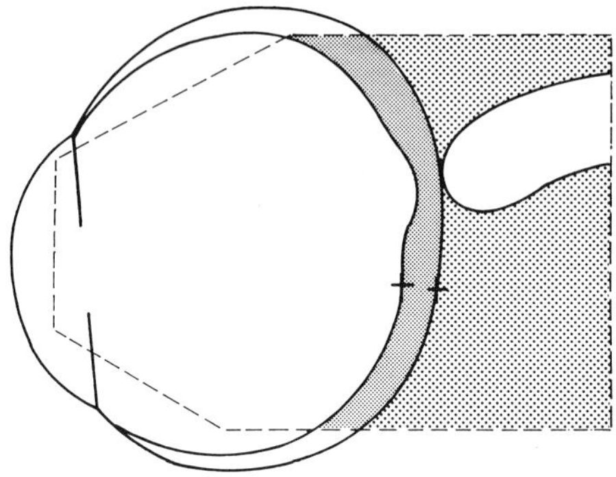

c

Fig. 4.**29a–c** Panophthalmitis after an intraocular operation
**a** Together with an hypopyon, echographically demonstrable structures appear in the vitreous
**b** Widening of the ocular coats to about 2.1 mm indicates inflammatory choroidal infiltrates
**c** Schematic drawing

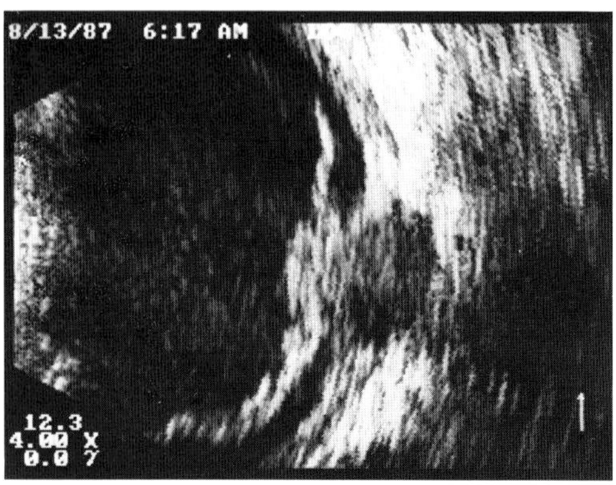


a

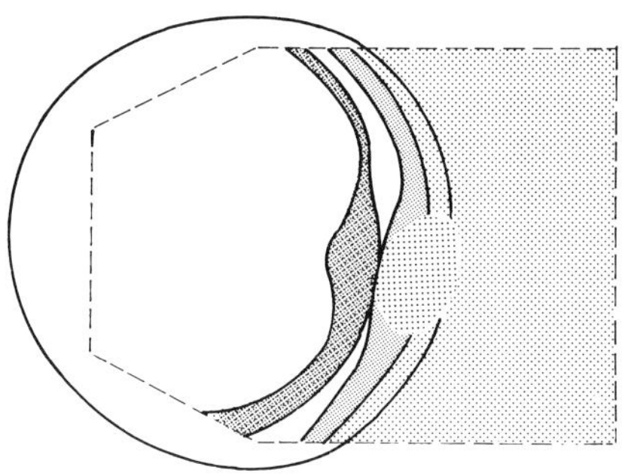

b

Fig. 4.**30a, b**
**a** Beginning panophthalmitis after perforating injury. The circumscribed thickening of the ocular wall corresponds to the posterior extensin of the perforating wound. The vitreous is filled with inflammatory cells and blood; the posterior hyaloid membrane is thickened
**b** Schematic drawing

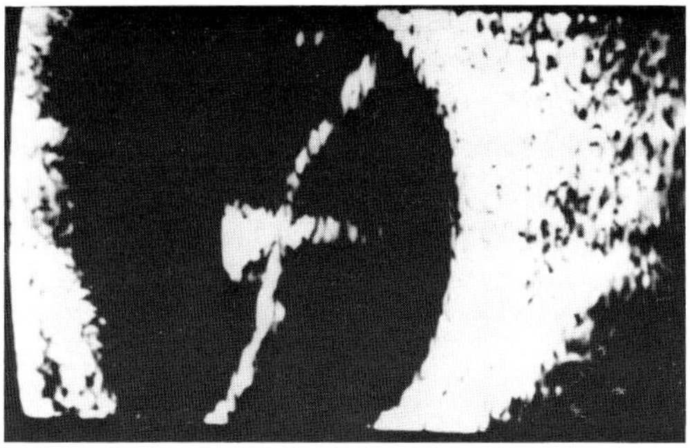
a

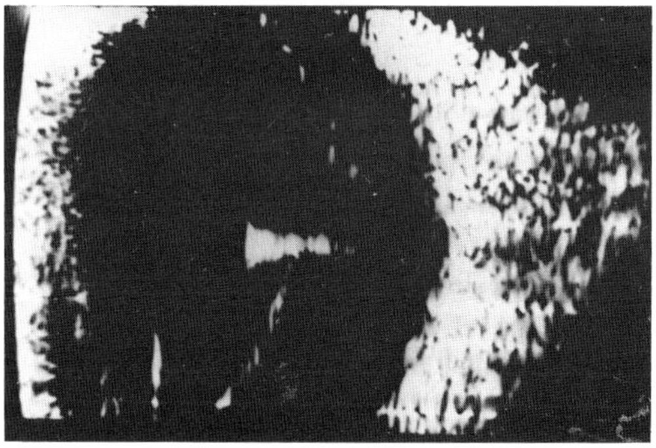
b

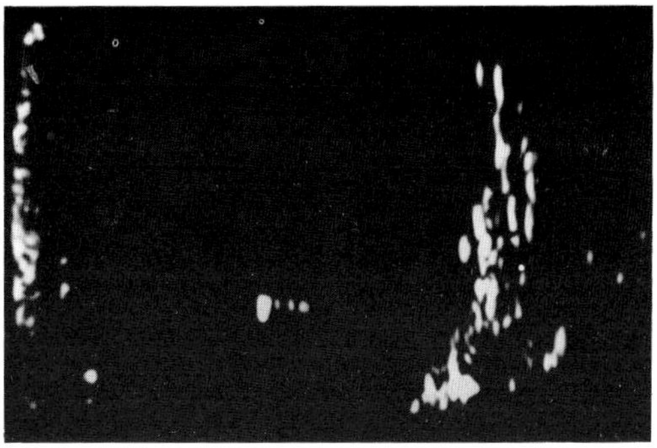
c

Fig. 4.**31a–c** Metallic foreign body in the vitreous with total retinal detachment. The foreign body spike is characterized by its high amplitude and repetitive echos. With reduced sensitivity the foreign body can be imaged as a nearly isolated echo

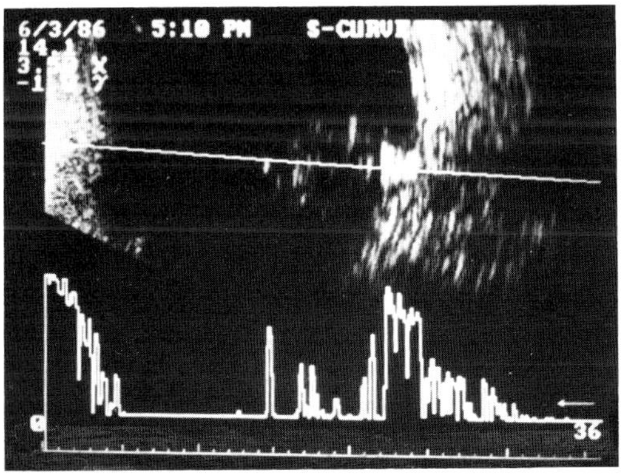

a

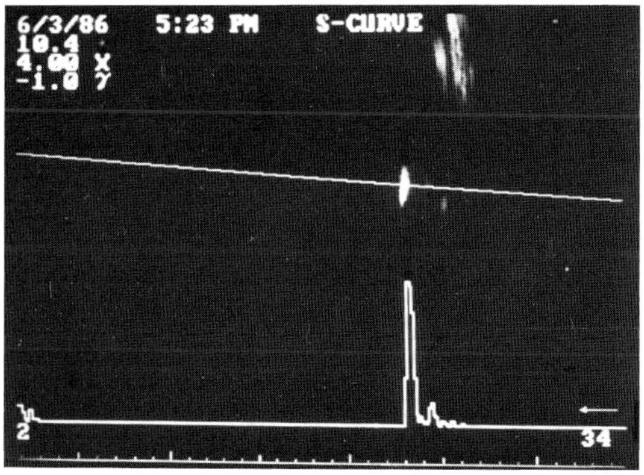

b

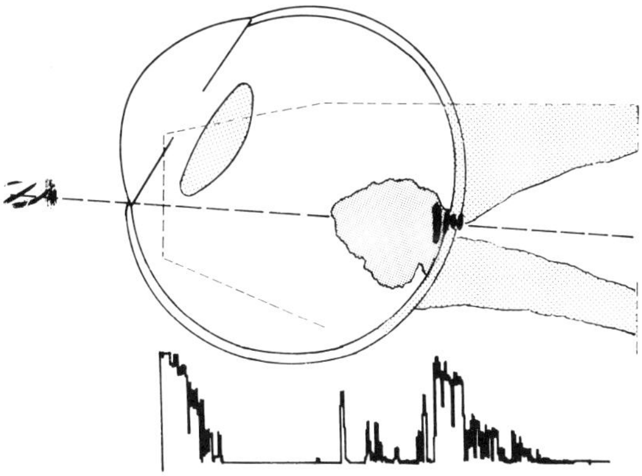
c

Fig. 4.**32a–c** Acute perforating injury with intraocular metallic foreign body. The X-ray localization after Comberg gives equivocal results concerning the location of the foreign body in regard to the ocular coats

**a** Echographically, there is a typical foreign body echo with repetitive spikes in the vitreous, about 2 mm in front of the ocular wall

**b** With decreasing amplification the foreign body echo remains as the only intraocular structure. During the operation a foreign body wedged into the sclera was found

**c** Schematic drawing

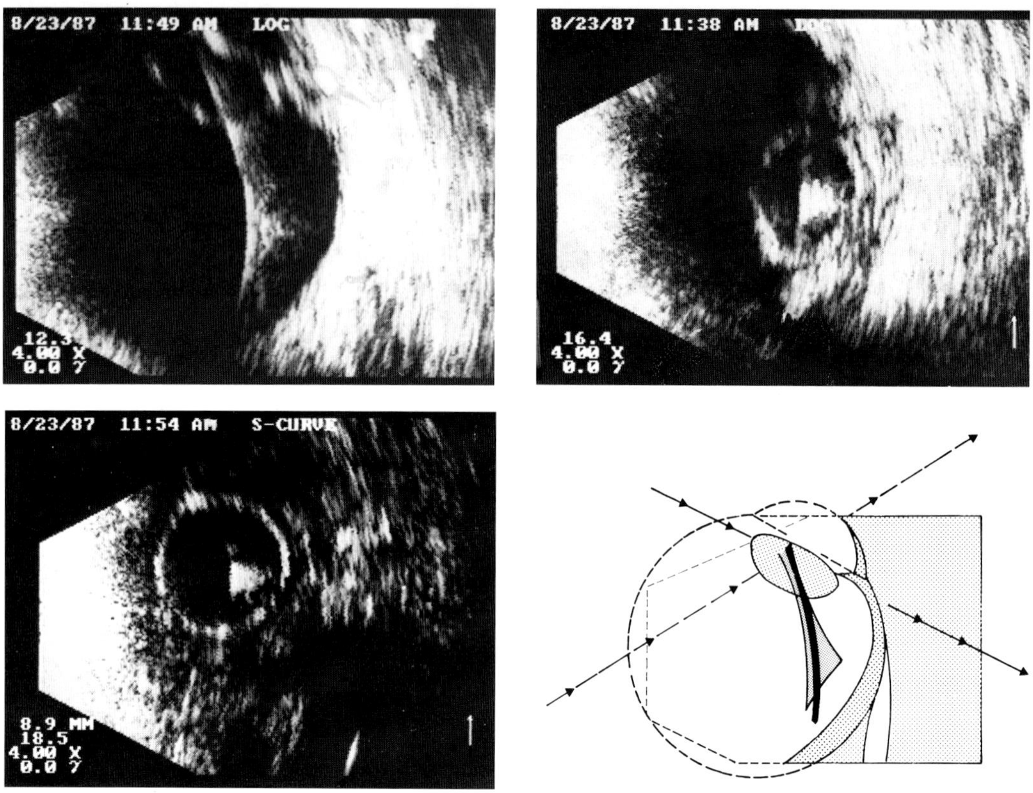


Fig. 4.**33a–d** Intraocular foreign body (wire piece). The anterior end of the wire remained visible in the lens
**a** Cross section from temporal with maximal adduction of the globe
**b** Cross section at right angle to **a**
**c** Frontal section through iris and lens
**d** Schematic drawing

Table 4.**2** **Factors influencing the echographic imaging of an intraocular foreign body**

1. Sound impedance within the foreign body
2. Size of the foreign body
3. Surface characteristics of the foreign body
4. Shape of the foreign body (direction of the foreign body in the sound field)

(Ossoinig et al. 1969, Rüssmann 1975, Tane et al. 1983).

Thin-layer computer tomography has proven valuable in doubtful cases. We have to keep in mind that large metallic foreign bodies may lead to artifacts which may make it difficult to obtain exact localization. An air bubble in front of the foreign body will produce an echo which cannot be differ-

Table 4.**3**

Suspected intraocular foreign body
↓
Plain X-ray survey
↙ ↘

| | |
|---|---|
| No foreign body found<br>↓<br>If the history points toward foreign body, think of non-metallic material:<br>↓<br>B-mode echography ± thin layer CT-scan | Foreign body found<br>1.: CT (minimal slice thickness)<br>2.: Comberg localization (consider a possible axial ametropia)<br>↓<br>If the foreign body lies close to the ocular wall and unequivocal localization is not possible:<br>B-mode echography ± thin layer CT-scan |

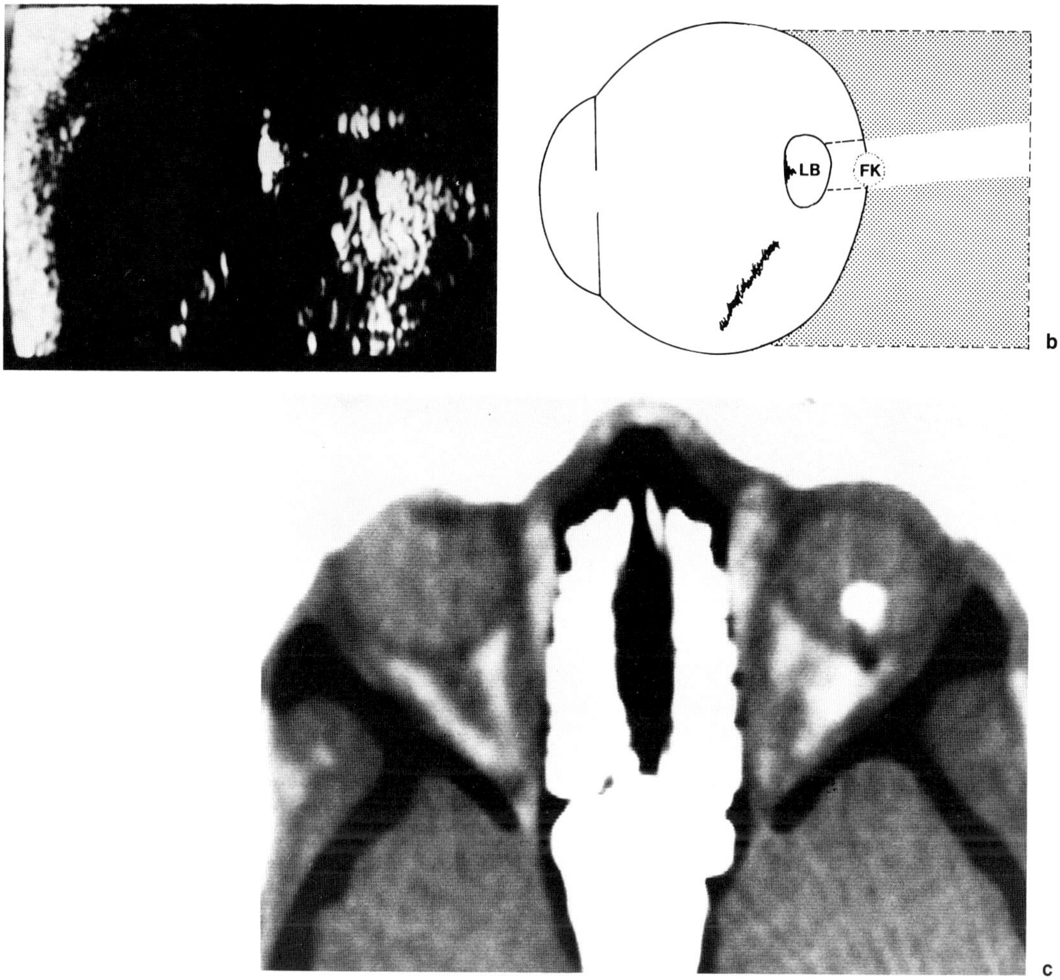


Fig. 4.**34a–c** A metallic foreign body wedged into the ocular wall with an air bubble in front of it
**a** On echographic localization a foreign body echo was found in the vitreous
**b** Schematic drawing
**c** After an unsuccessful attempt of a magnet extraction was made, the CT scan showed the foreign body in the area of the ocular wall
The erroneous echographic localization was caused by an air bubble in front of the foreign body. The great difference in acoustic impedance between the vitreous and air is capable of creating spikes similar to those of a metallic foreign body, so that the foreign body itself lies in the acoustic shadow and cannot be imaged

entiated from the foreign body itself; the latter may then remain undetected in the sound shadow (Fig. 4.**34**).

### 4.2.8 Persistent and Hyperplastic Primary Vitreous (PHPV)

In these cases the primary vitreous (tunica vasculosa lentis) regresses incompletely. In severe forms there will be microphthalmus, cataract and a connective tissue strand between the back surface of the lens and the area of the optic nerve head (Fig. 4.**35**). Clinically, the picture is that of a leukokoria, and, from a differential diagnostic point of view, retinoblastoma has to be considered (Foerster 1987). PHPV is echographically characterized by:

1. a strand extending between the posterior surface of the lens and the area of the optic nerve head (directly demonstrable);

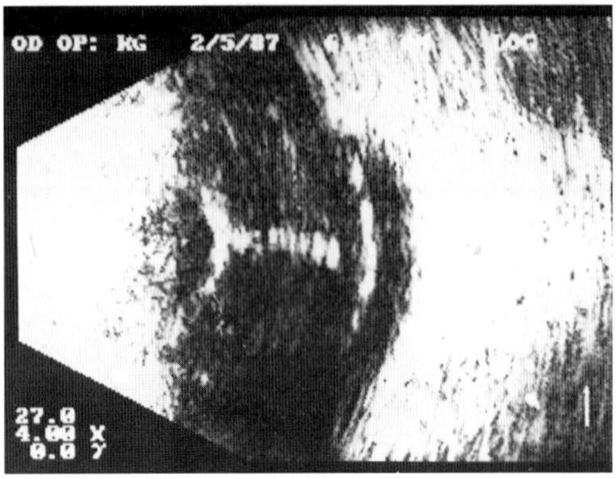
a

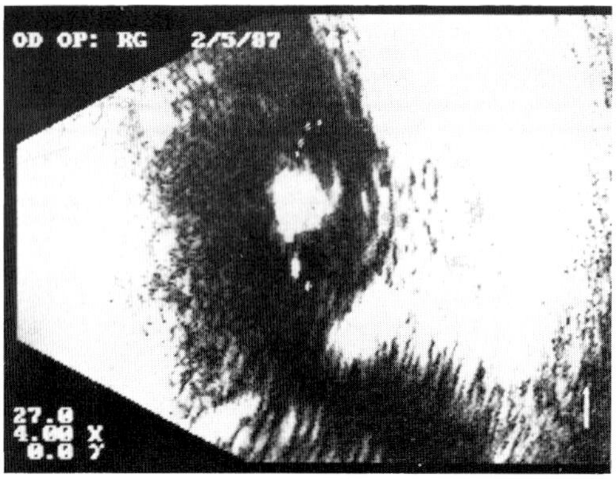
b

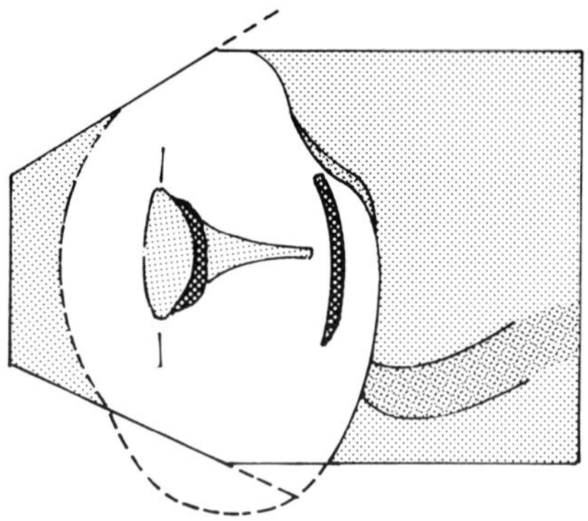
c

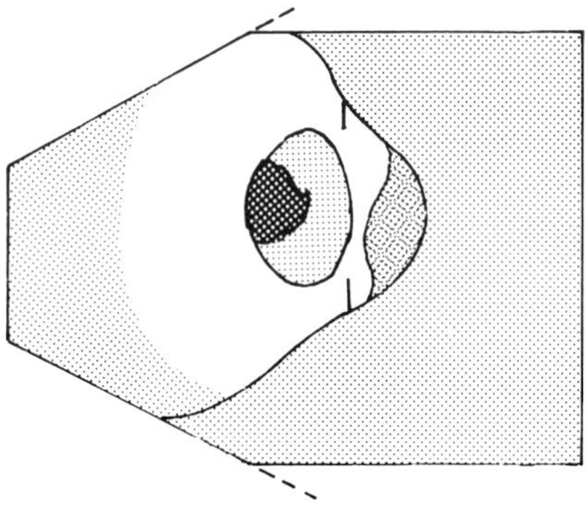
d

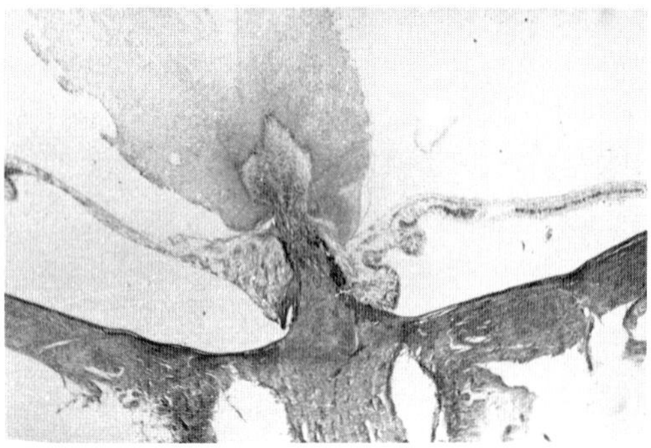
e

Fig. 4.**35 a–d** Posterior polar cataract in persistence and hyperplasia of the primary vitreous (PHPV). In infantile cataracts the retrolental space has to be scrutinized carefully. Occasionally, an echographically demonstrable strand attached to the posterior lens pole points toward a PHPV
**a** Sagittal plane
**b** Nearly frontal plane from temporal, with maximal adduction of the globe
**c, d** Schematic drawings. The dark, hatched parts correspond to the opaque area of the posterior cortex and posterior capsule in a child with severe PHPV
**e** Loupe magnification of a section demonstrating posterior PHPV

2. reduced axial length of the globe (can be proven by ultrasound biometry).

Schroeder stressed this connection already in 1976 with the help of A-mode echography. Nowadays, contact B-mode is the simplest method. If the anomaly is only mild, the lens may be clear at birth and will become cataractous after the posterior lens capsule has been ruptured. The cataract will then make the malformation obvious.

In formes frustes the PHPV may be limited to a paracentral thread at the posterior lens capsule or to a glial sheath around the optic nerve head (Bergmeister papilla). Both conditions can be demonstrated echographically, but they do not present any differential diagnostic problems; the eyes are usually of normal size and have normal vision.

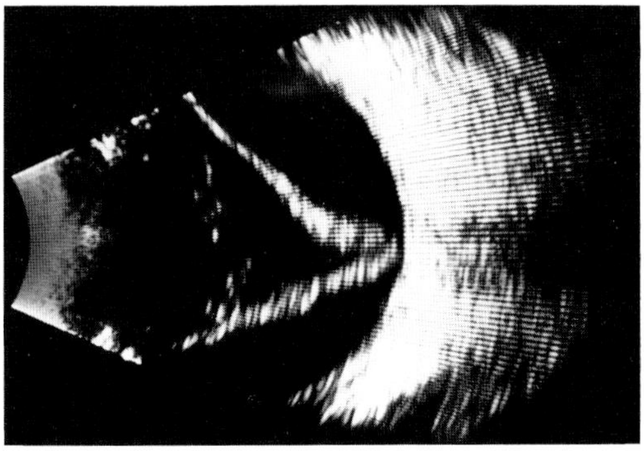

a

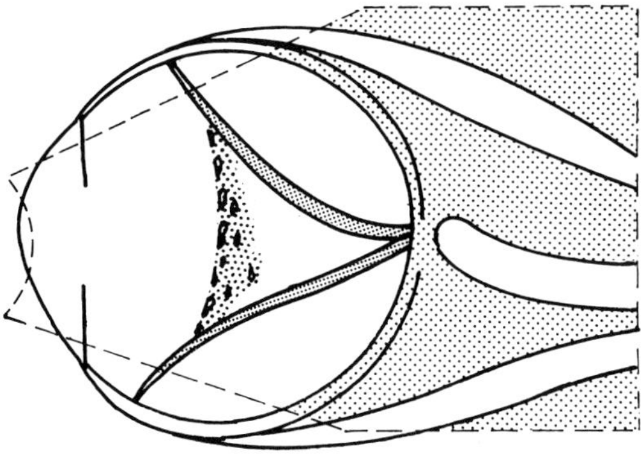

b

Fig. 4.**36a, b**
**a** Complete retinal detachment extending between the optic nerve head and the ora serrata. Heterogenous material in the anterior vitreous is a sign of vitreous reaction. **b** Schematic drawing

## 4.3 The Retina

Retinal diseases are often complicated by vitreous changes which make it difficult or impossible to visualize the fundus. The subretinal space is difficult to see, even if the media are clear, so that echography is especially important here.

Echography is a diagnostic aid in the following retinal diseases:

Retinal detachment
Retinoschisis
Coats' disease
Retinal malformations
Retinoblastoma.

### 4.3.1 Retinal Detachment

In a typical case of complete retinal detachment extending from the optic nerve head to the ora serrata, the diagnosis can be made within a few seconds by using contact B-mode echography (Fig. 4.**36**).

Identification of the retina may be difficult or impossible if there are different membranous structures in the vitreous, especially when they are complicated by strands and floating opacities (Fig. 4.**37**).

Depending on the clinical importance of this question, we can with a definite degree of uncertainty, make or suspect a diagnosis. The desired decisive diagnosis can often not be achieved, even when all techniques have been utilized. From a physical point of view, we are trying to evaluate the acoustic reflectivity and the mobility of these membranes. In spite of the difference in histologic structure, a vitreous membrane and a detached, taut retina may reflect ultrasound in an identical way.

#### Practical Procedures to Differentiate Various Membranes

It has been proven reasonable to ask the following questions when differentiating membranous structures:

1. What is the spatial extent of the membrane? At which point is there contact with the ocular wall?
2. What is the shape of a cross section of the membrane, especially in the optic nerve head area?
3. Which aftermovements occur?
4. How great is the difference of the spike from the membrane in question to the scleral standard or to the echo from a standard reflector?

These questions should be clarified in the following way:

**With regard to 1.** An acute rhegmatogenous retinal detachment characterized in cross section by a membranous structure of high reflectivity which converges in an acute angle toward the ocular wall. If the posterior pole is in the acoustic section, then the optic nerve head will present the border of the detached retina, and contact with the ocular wall will obviously be present there (Figs. 4.**39**, 4.**40**).

**With regard to 2.** In order to appreciate the extent of a retinal detachment, the performance of echographic examinations in various planes is indicated. This will facilitate orientation if the optic

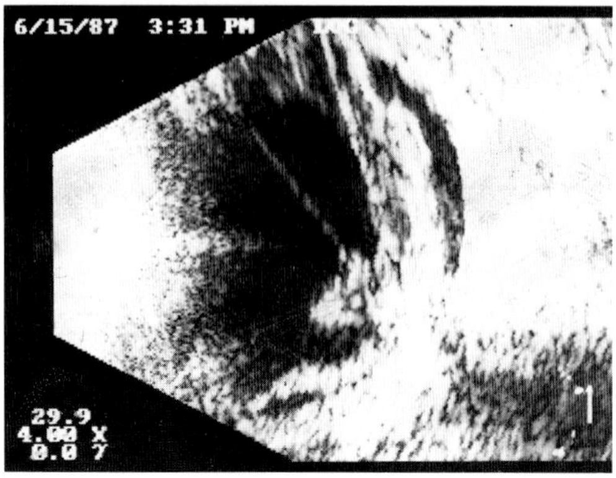


a

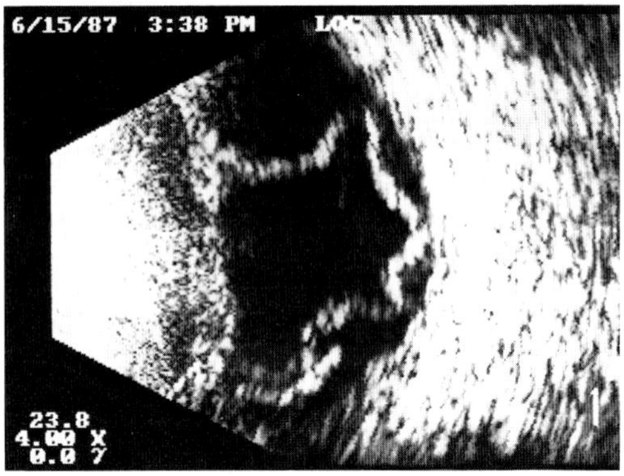


b

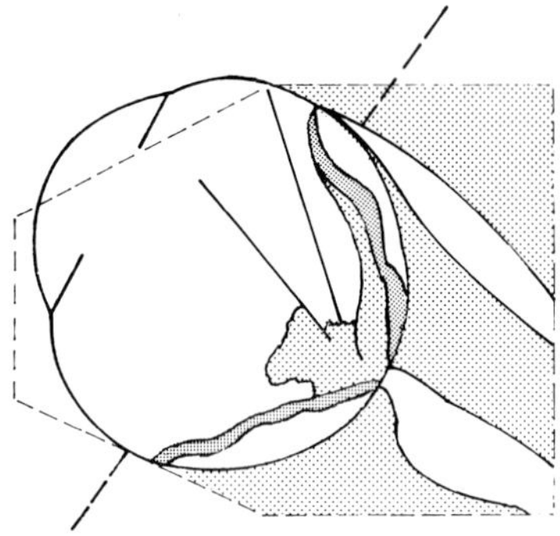

c

Fig. 4.**37** **a–c** Development of a traction detachment with massive vitreous retraction
**a** Flat subtotal retinal detachment with folds; rigid vitreous strands
**b** In a frontal section, multiple contacts of the retina to the ocular wall can be demonstrated
**c** Schematic drawing

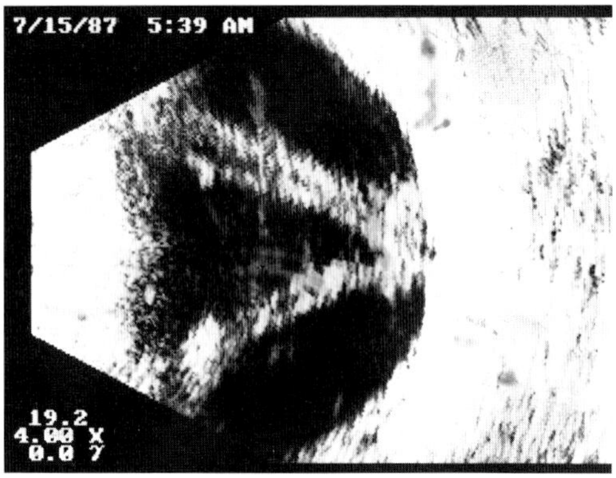


a

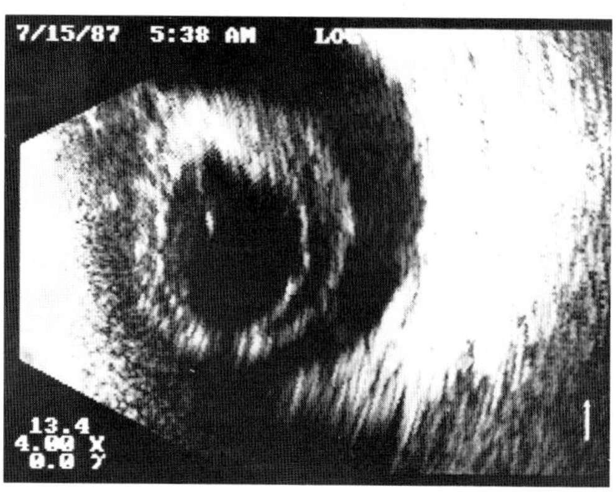


b

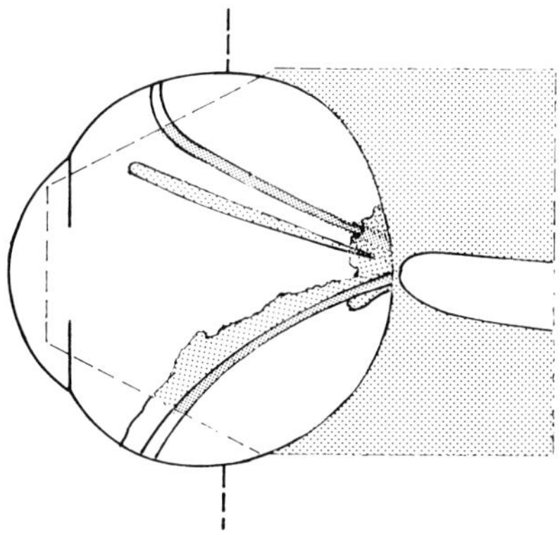

c

Fig. 4.**38** **a–c** Total traction detachment (same patient as in Fig. 4.**37**, four weeks later)
**a** Advanced shrinkage of the vitreous with total retinal detachment
**b** In a frontal section the concentric layers of vitreous and retina can be identified
**c** Schematic drawing

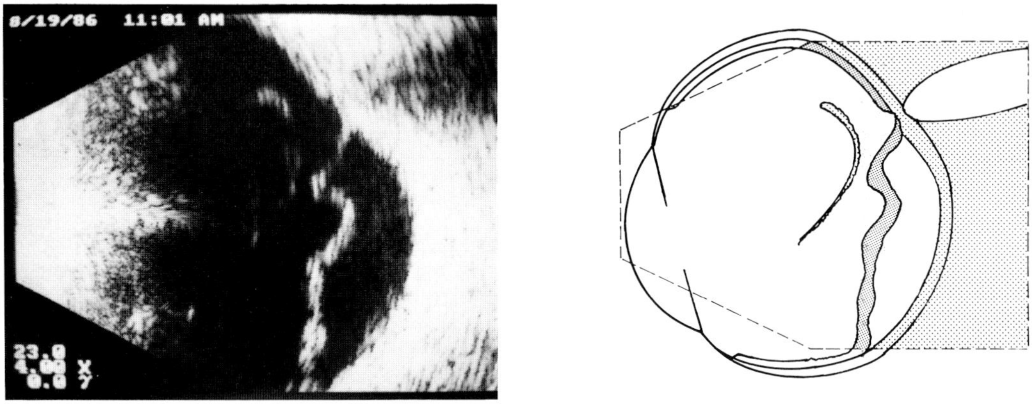


a b

Fig. 4.**39** **a, b**
**a** Sector retinal detachment. In acute retinal detachment short-lasting aftermovements appear when the globe moves. These aftermovements extend like a whiplash from the area of the contact to the ocular wall
**b** Schematic drawing

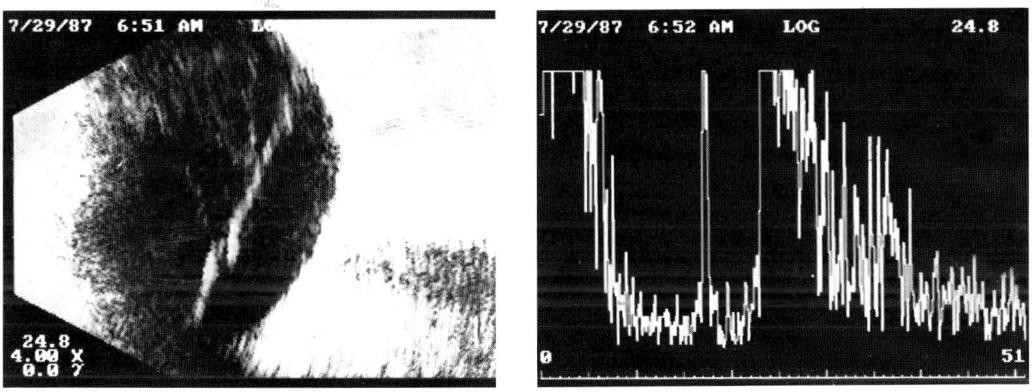


a b

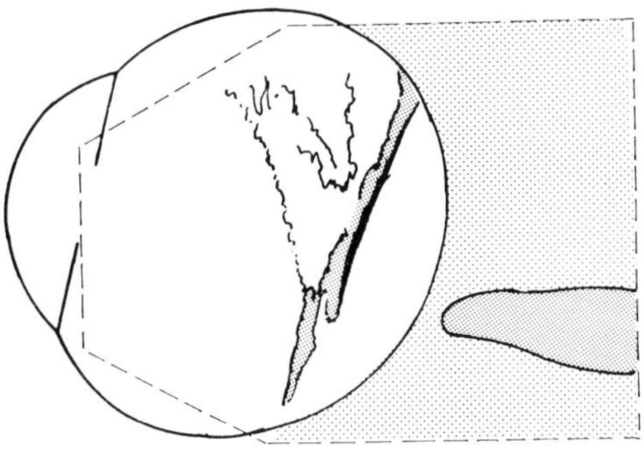

c

Fig. 4.**40** **a–c**
**a, b** Detached and dense posterior hyaloid membrane. Vitreous membranes may reach an acoustic reflectivity similar to that of the retina. If the membrane tents over the posterior pole without reaching the optic nerve head, we can, on the basis of these echographic findings, exclude a retinal detachment in that area
**c** Schematic drawing

nerve head area is initially included in the plane of the acoustic section.

In a sagittal section a total detachment looks like an isosceles triangle which is open toward the anterior segment, and the sides of which may be unevenly tented.

If the location of the disk in relation to the retinal detachment in question has been clarified, it is recommended that sectional planes be selected which are at right angles to the previously described ones. In these frontal examination planes (most easily obtained by placing the transducer in the temporal part of the lid fissure when the globe is maximally adducted), the conical shape of the detachment will appear in various sections from oval to nearly circular (see Figs. 4.**37**, 4.**38**). A complete serous choroidal detachment will, on the other hand, incorporate the ciliary body in the pathologic process (Fig. 4.**59**).

**With regard to 3.** An acute rhegmatogenous retinal detachment shows aftermovements of short duration which extend like a whiplash from the area where the retina is still attached (usually the optic nerve head) to the ocular wall (see Fig. 4.**39**). The amplitudes of these aftermovements are smaller and less extensive than those seen in the sinusoidal

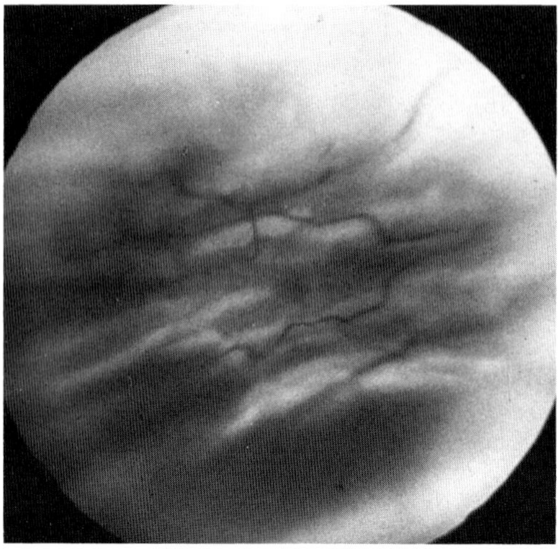

a

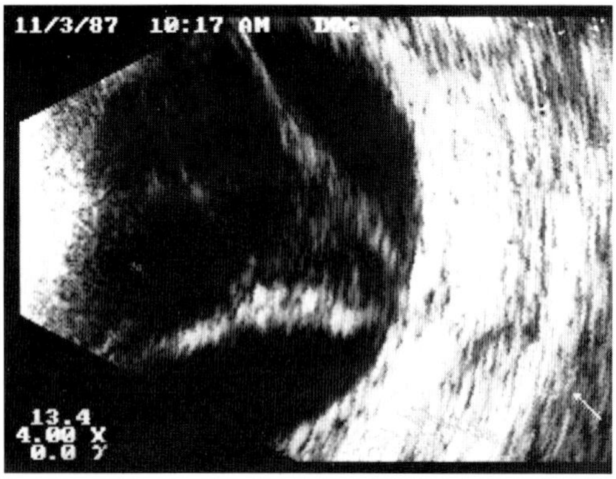


b

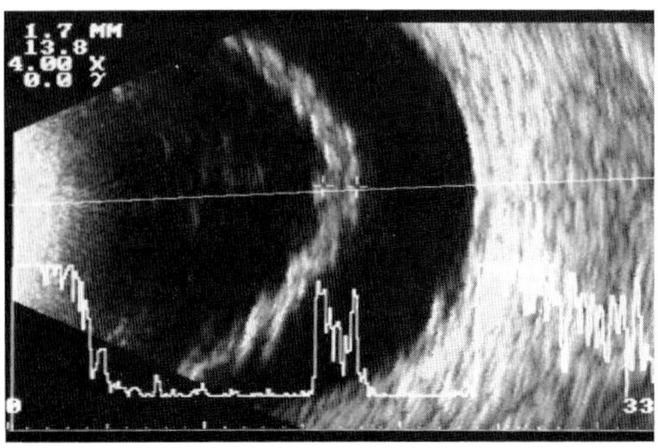


c

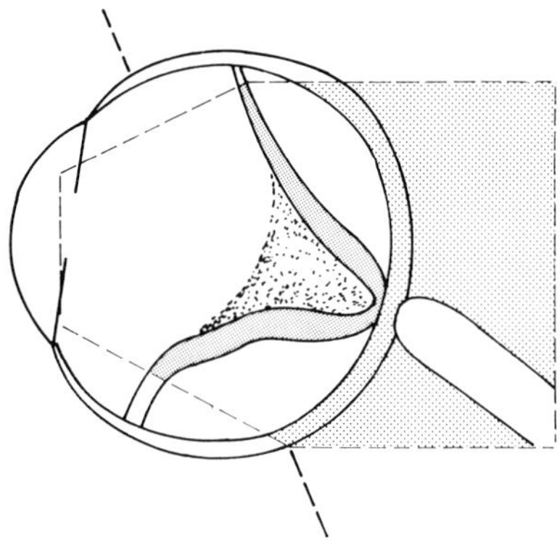

d

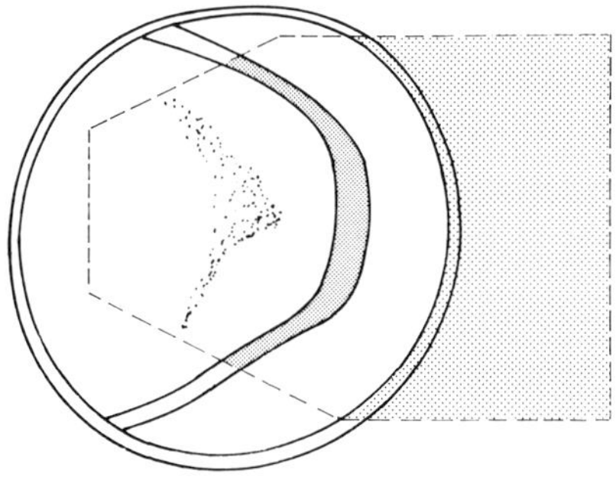

e

Fig. 4.**41 a–e** Recurrent retinal detachment with massive vitreous retraction
**a** Clinical picture
**b** Axial cross sectional echogram. The amplitudes of the aftermovements decrease; high-frequency flicker of the taut membrane appears after the eye changes position
**c** Frontal section toward 6 o'clock. Pucker of the retinal surface appears echographically as an apparent widening of the retina
**d, e** Schematic drawing

movements of a vitreous hemorrhage or in asteroid hyalosis (McLeod 1981, Restori et al. 1981). In a typical case, the subretinal space does not produce any echos. If there are subretinal echoes present, a tumor has to be excluded.

**With regard to 4.** With quantitative echography we find, according to Ossoinig (1983), a difference in the echo of the retina and that of the sclera extending from 8 to 15 decibels; between retina and the HEMA standard reflector, according to Buschmann (1981), from 25 to 30 dB (see Fig. 2.**14**). Unfortunately, these measurements provide only guidelines in doubtful cases. Well-developed connective tissue membranes may show reflection properties quite similar to those of a detached retina. In complicated cases it may be difficult to correlate an isolated A-spike to the multiple membrane structures as they appear on B-mode.

### Influences of Duration of Detachment on Echographic Findings

Depending on the duration of the detachment these changes affect:

- the thickness and mobility of the retina;
- the shape and mechanical properties of the vitreous base;
- the contents of the subretinal space.

These changes help us to plan treatment and estimate the prognosis of the disease process.

### Changes in Thickness and Mobility of the Retina

A proliferation of Müller cells and astrocytes will lead to changes in the mechanical properties of the detached retina already after a few weeks. When a massive periretinal proliferation (MPP) develops, the amplitudes of the aftermovements decrease and the large excursions are replaced by a high-frequency flicker. Occasionally the retina appears thickened (Fig. 4.**41**). Commercially available instruments do not allow us to differentiate a true retinal thickening from a retinal pucker in a cellophane maculopathy (Takeuchi 1981). Macroscopically visible retinal folds may appear early and indicate a poor prognosis (Fig. 4.**42**).

After a long-standing retinal detachment, we occasionally see enclosed, cyst-like cavities within the detached retina (Fig. 4.**43**). These are typically not affected when pathologic changes, e.g., hemorrhages or cholesterol deposits, occur in the vitreous. They may remain as the only intraocular

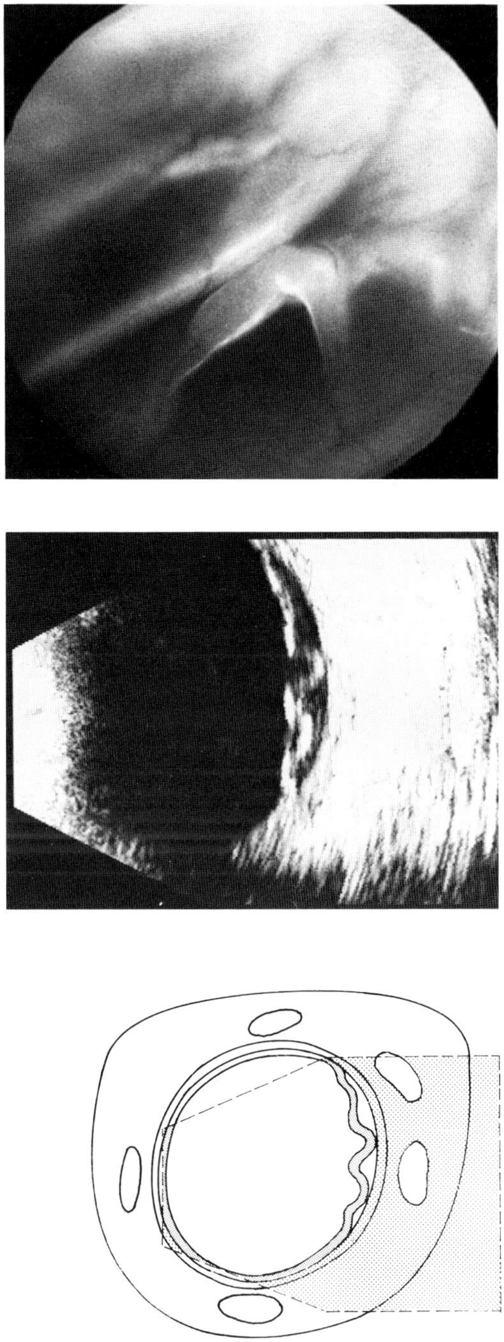

a

b

c

Fig. 4.**42a–c** Massive periretinal proliferation with large retinal folds
**a** Ophthalmoscopic picture with large horseshoe tear
**b** Rigid, fixed retinal folds echographically demonstrable
**c** Schematic drawing

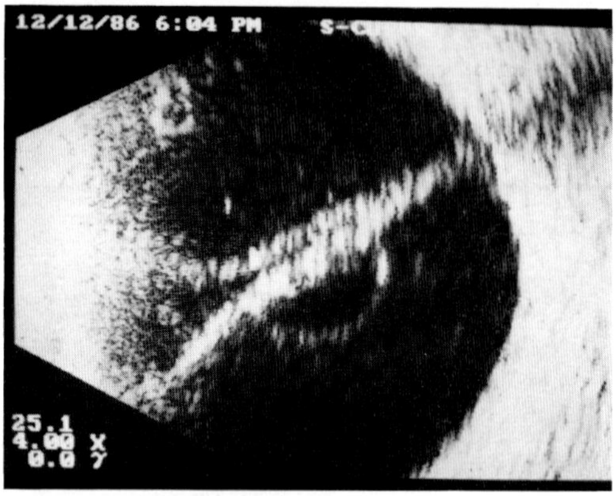


a

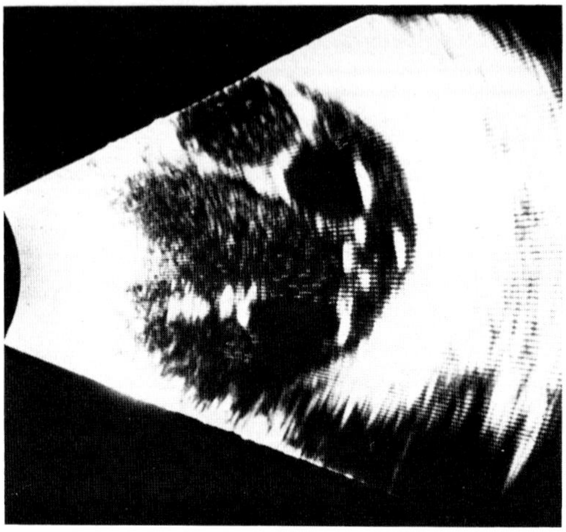

b

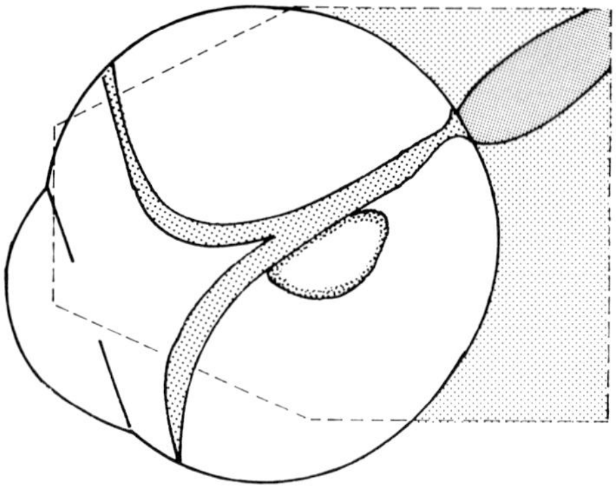

c

Fig. 4.**43a–c** Long-standing total retinal detachment
**a** Intraretinal cyst in the axial area (coalescing microcystoid degeneration)
**b** These cavities will not be involved in secondary vitreous changes, e.g., hemorrhages or cholesterol deposits
**c** Schematic drawing

structures free of any acoustic interfaces. Histologically, we are dealing here with coalescing microcystoid degenerations (Zimmerman et al. 1969).

#### Changes in the Form and Mobility of the Vitreous

An epiretinal connective tissue proliferation may, during the late stages of a retinal detachment, involve the vitreous and lead to shrinkage of its framework (Fig. 4.**37**). This process creates new acoustic interfaces which increase the echo spikes from the vitreous space, which is surrounded by the detached retina (Fig. 4.**44**). The increasing vitreous shrinkage can be followed by a narrowing of the retinal funnel. This funnel will gradually fill with membranous structures. The process begins in front of the optic nerve head and will finally obliterate the remaining vitreous space. Frontal "cyclitic membranes" can often be seen early, extending from the vitreous base (Fig. 4.**36**). In the further course the peripheral retina is pulled closer to this membrane so that finally, in cross section, the morning glory retinal detachment does not show any recognizable cavity of the original funnel (Fig. 4.**45**). In frontal sections the shrunk retina appears as a strand, only a few mm in diameter (Fig. 4.**46**). Occasionally, few retinal folds can be observed (Fig. 4.**47**).

If there is still traction once this stage has been reached, the ciliary body may be detached, leading to persistent hypotony and subsequent phthisis bulbi (Zimmerman 1961, Rentsch 1977).

#### Changes in the Subretinal Space in Long-Standing Retinal Detachment

In long-standing retinal detachment the protein content of the subretinal fluid will increase and

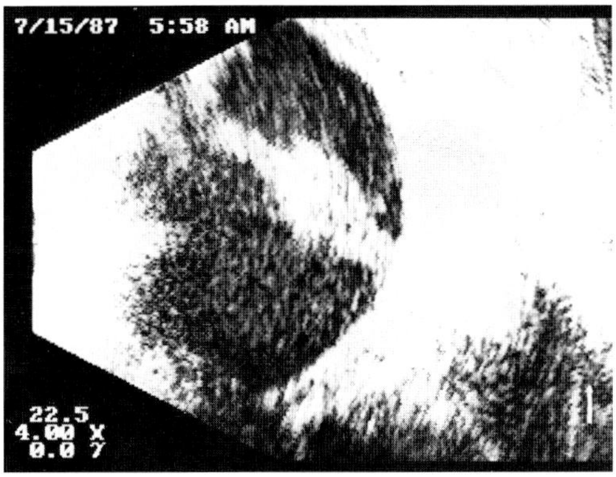

a

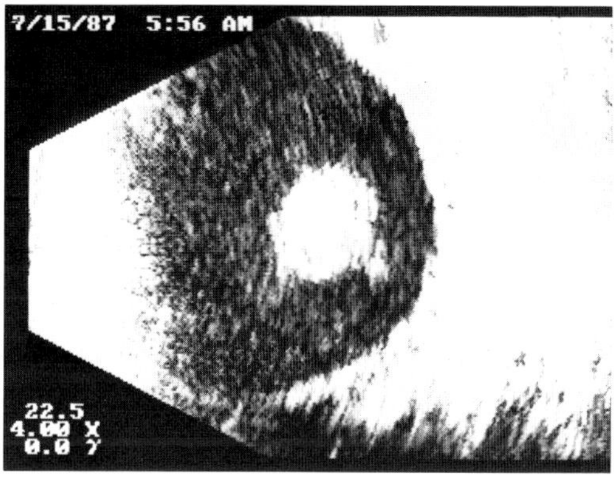

b

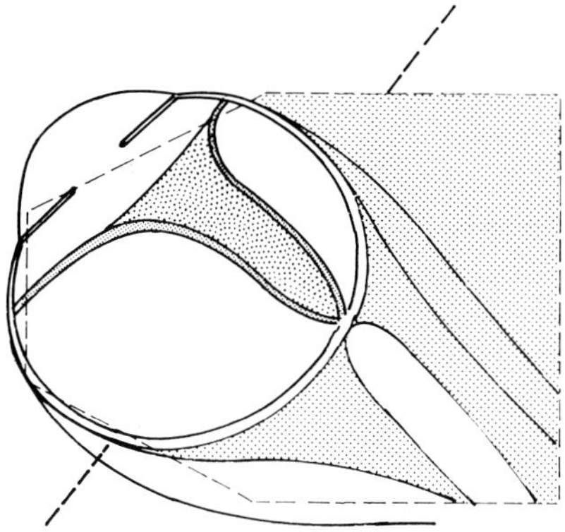
c

Fig. 4.**44a–c**
**a, b** Long-standing retinal detachment with increased connective tissue in the vitreous funnel. Free-floating opacities accumulate in the subretinal space (hemorrhages? cholesterol crystals?)
**c** Schematic drawing

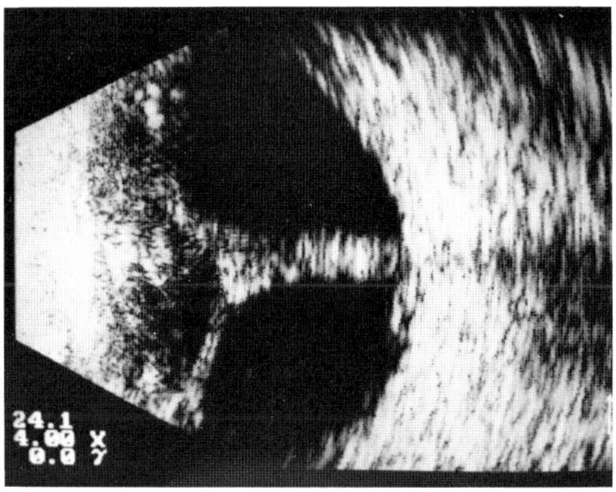

a

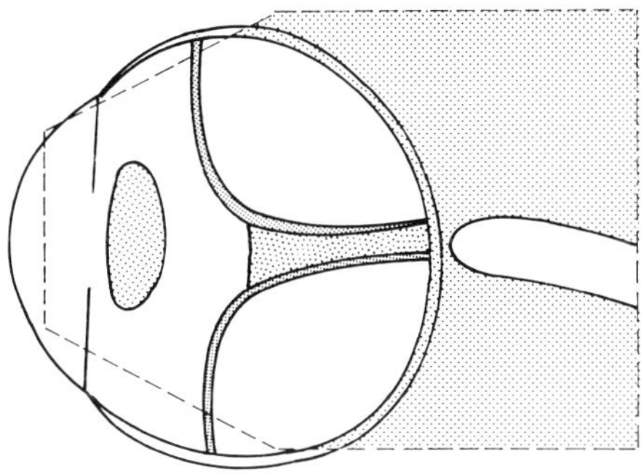
b

Fig. 4.**45a, b**
**a** Morning glory total retinal detachment. With persisting connective tissue proliferations in the vitreous body, a morning glory retinal detachment will develop; the retinal leaves attach to each other, forming an axial strand
**b** Schematic drawing

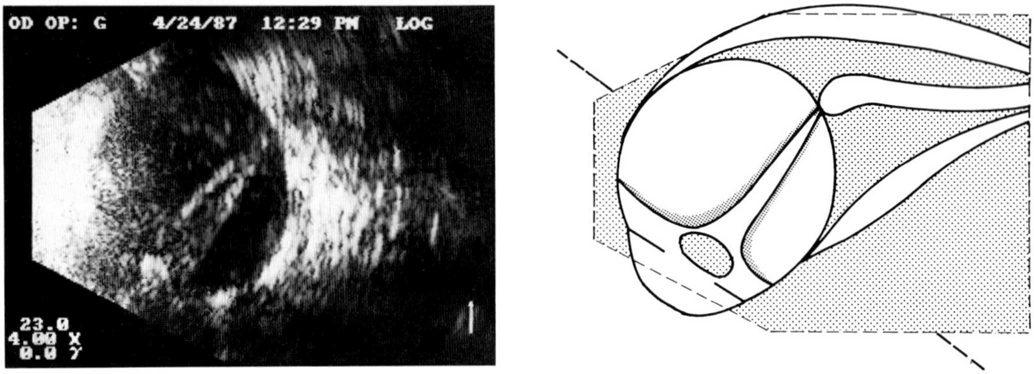


a

b

Fig. 4.**46** **a, b**
**a** Long-standing total retinal detachment. Occasionally, we see a tube-like remnant of the vitreous within the shrunk retinal funnel
**b** Schematic drawing

may precipitate (Gärtner et al. 1967). This will lead to free-floating opacities (Fig. 4.**48**). On the other hand, if these opacities remain in one location and do not show any aftermovements when the eyeball changes position, an intraocular tumor has to be excluded (Fig. 4.**49**). Under these circumstances, echography acquires a special differential diagnostic importance.

> **Key Statement:** Subretinal echos which remain in one location have to be regarded as a sign of a malignant tumor until proven otherwise.

### 4.3.2 Retinoschisis

It is not possible to differentiate retinoschisis from a retinal detachment echographically; nor does quantitative echography indicate unequivocal differences of reflectivity between the split and the detached retina. In a cross section echogram certain shapes of the membranes in question will point toward retinoschisis:

- A beginning peripheral retinoschisis appears as a well-visible membranous structure in the far periphery, with a convex border toward the vitreous (Fig. 4.**50**).
- Aftermotions are less conspicuous than in a retinal detachment of similar extent. This is because the retina is attached and there are no vitreous adhesions.

### 4.3.3 Coats' Disease

Coats' disease (external exudative retinopathy) mainly affects boys at the end of the first decade of life. A clinical diagnosis can be made if aneurysmatic malformations of retinal vessels and white subretinal plaques are associated with an exudative detachment. Echography can differentiate this condition from retinoblastoma by evaluating the subretinal space. The exudative detached retina often gives especially strong echos caused by the cholesterol deposits (Fig. 4.**51**). The crystals floating in the subretinal space produce the picture of floating opacities as they occur in synchysis scintillans. These appear in an A-mode echogram as flickering spikes (Till et al. 1975). On photographs these high-frequency motions of the spike produce a blurred pattern in the subretinal space.

### 4.3.4 Retinoblastoma

Retinoblastoma is, with leukemia and neuroblastoma, the most frequent malignant tumor of childhood. About 1% of all tumor deaths before the age of 15 are caused by retinoblastoma. Following choroidal melanoma and metastatic carcinoma, it is the third most frequent intraocular neoplasm. About 1 out of 20–40000 live births is affected with this disease.

In a typical case the echogram will provide a nearly pathognomonic picture (Till et al. 1975). The

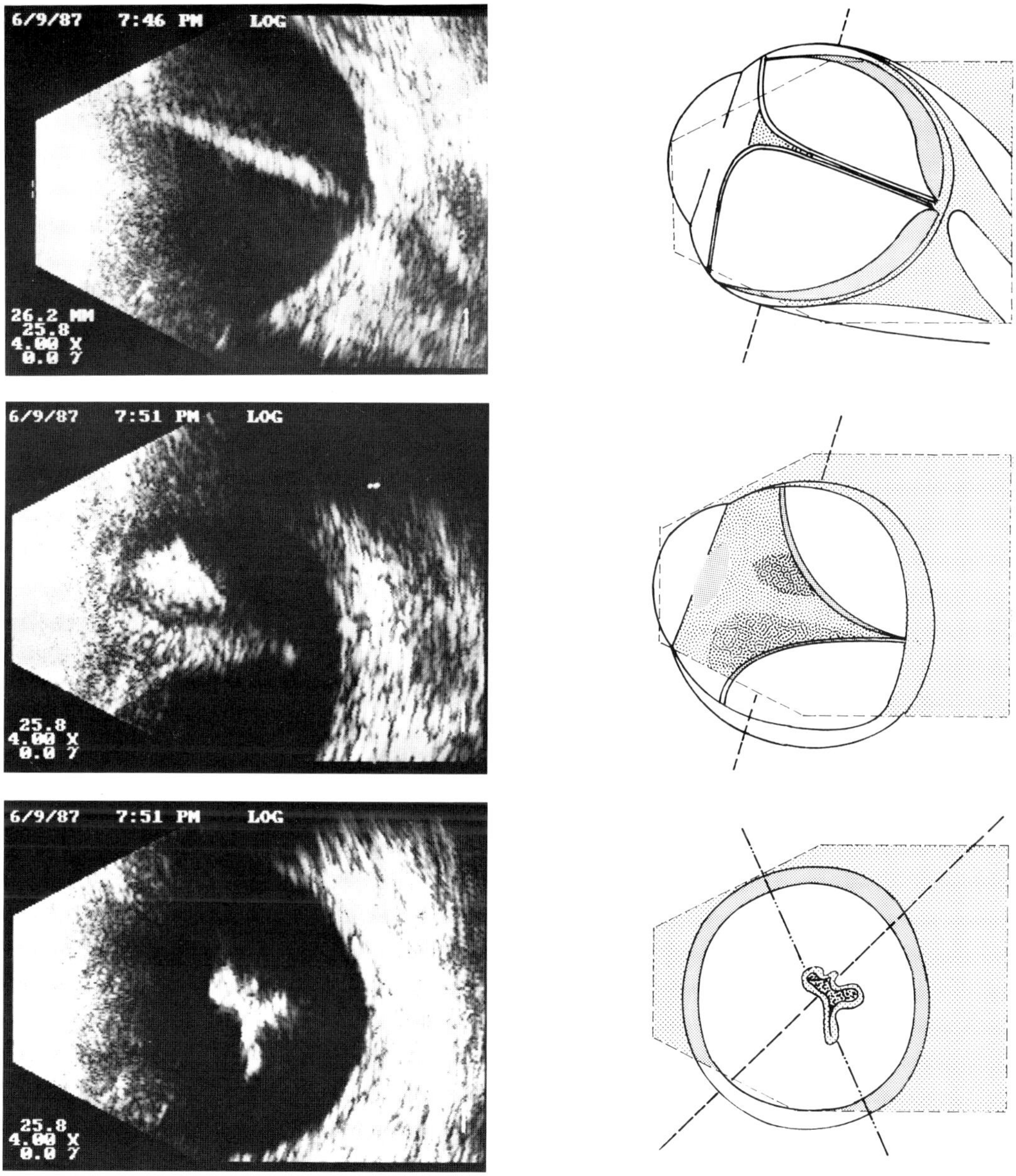


a b c d e f

Fig. 4.**47a–f** Long-standing retinal detachment with completely obliterated vitreous space
**a, b** In sagittal sections the extensive adhesions of the retinal leaves produce various acoustic sections
**c** A frontal section demonstrates the shrunk retinal funnel. **d–f** Schematic drawings

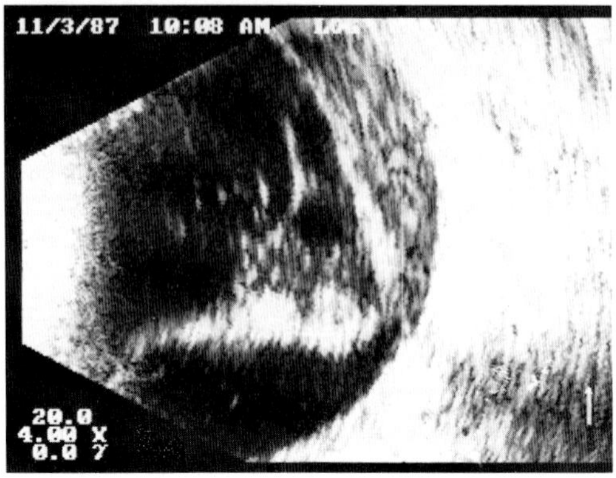


a

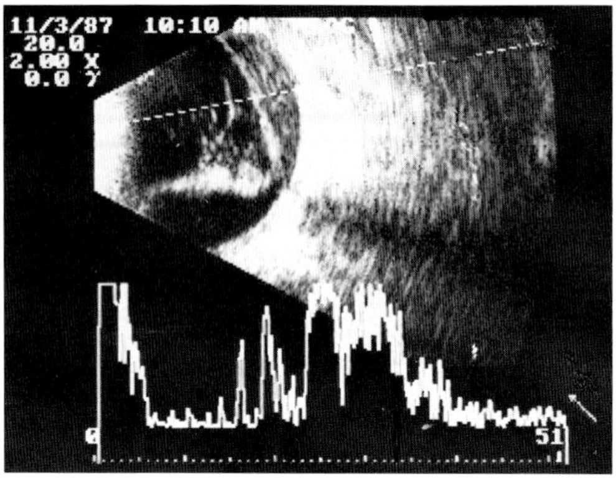


b

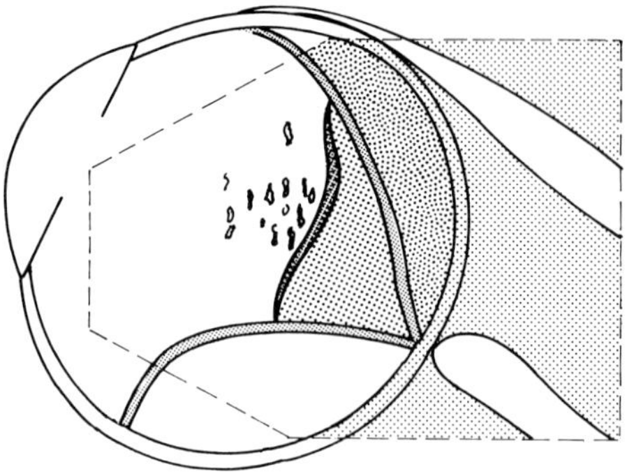

c

Fig. 4.**48a–c**
**a, b** Long-standing retinal detachment with floating opacities in the subretinal space. The densifications in the vitreous space indicate a tendency for shrinkage
**c** Schematic drawing

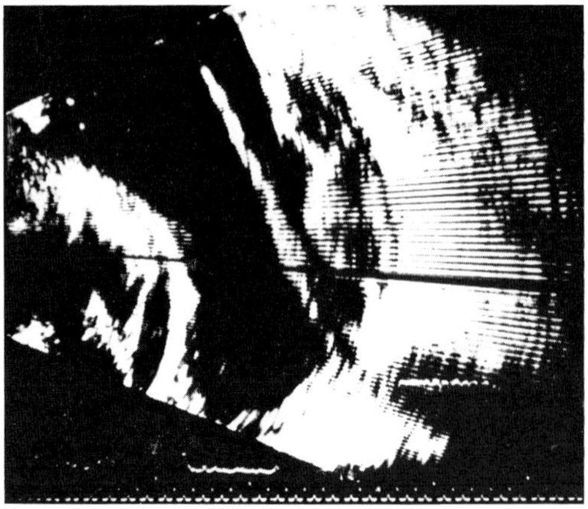

a

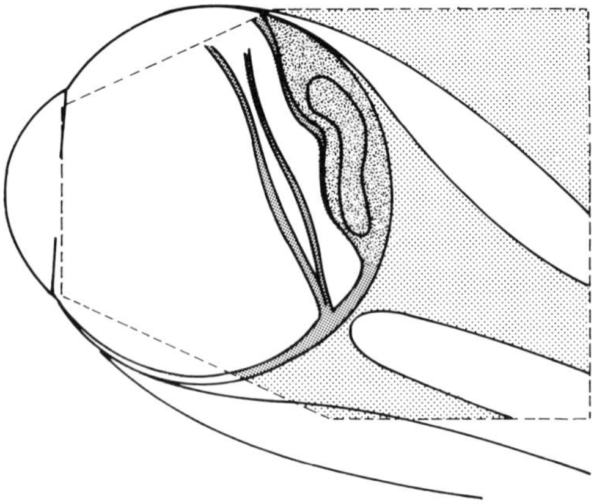

b

Fig. 4.**49a, b**
**a** Total retinal detachment in an eye with extensive disciform macular degeneration. Beneath the completely collapsed retinal leaves, heterogenous, partly strongly reflecting thickened ocular coats can be observed
**b** Schematic drawing

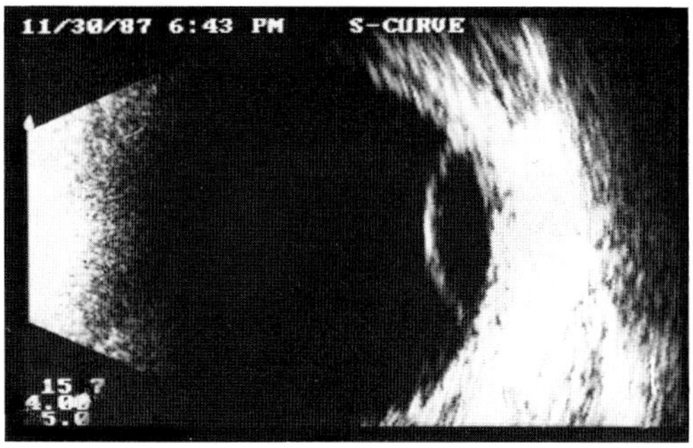

a

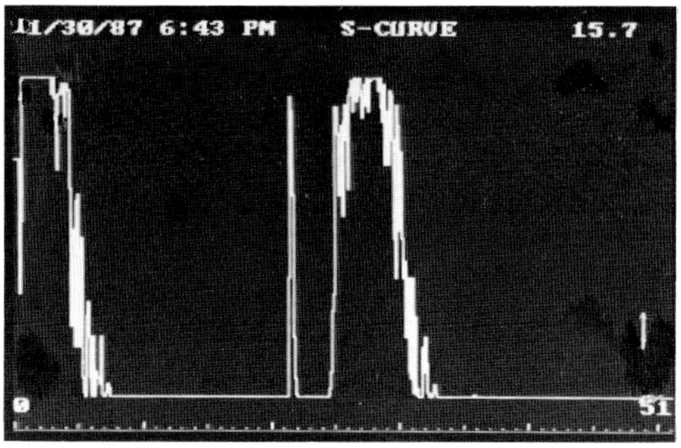

b

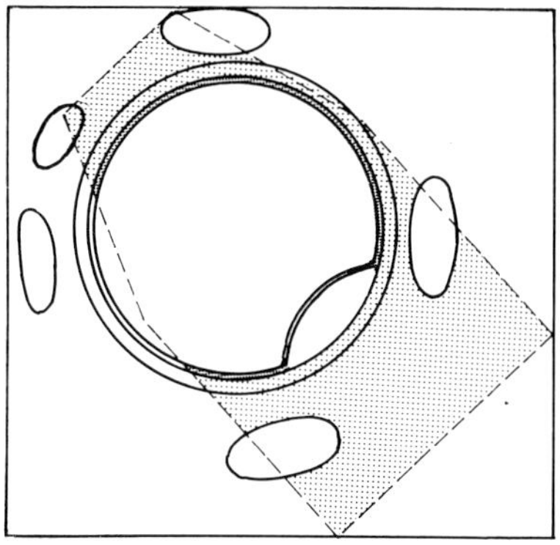
c

Fig. 4.**50 a–c**
**a, b** Senile retinoschisis in the temporal lower quadrant. Its acoustic reflectivity corresponds to that of a detached retina. The typical biconvex sectional image in association with slight aftermovements supports a tentative diagnosis
**c** Schematic drawing

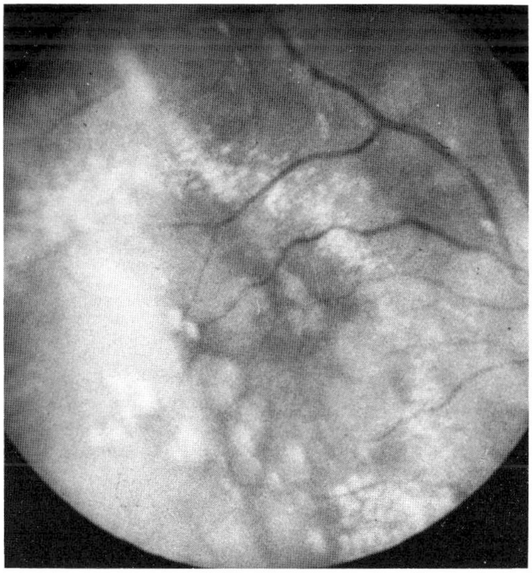
a

Fig. 4.**51 a–c** Circumscribed, strongly reflecting retinal detachment in Coats' disease
**a** Clinical photo
**b, c** The strongly reflecting membrane in association with floating opacities in the subretinal space corroborates the diagnosis

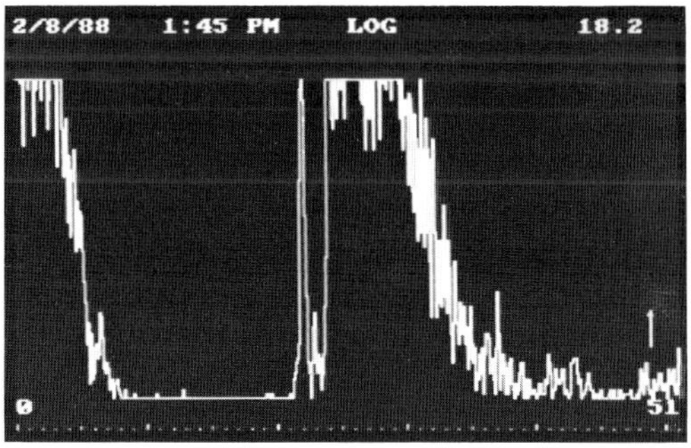

b

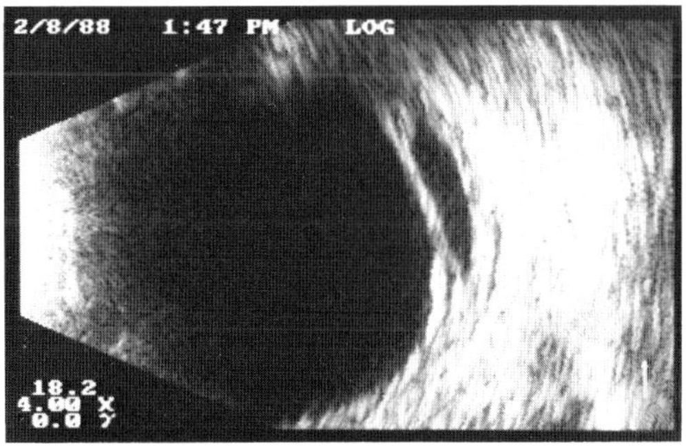

c

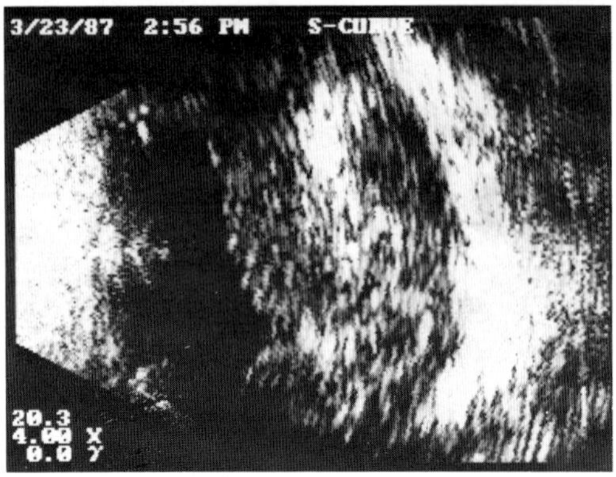


a

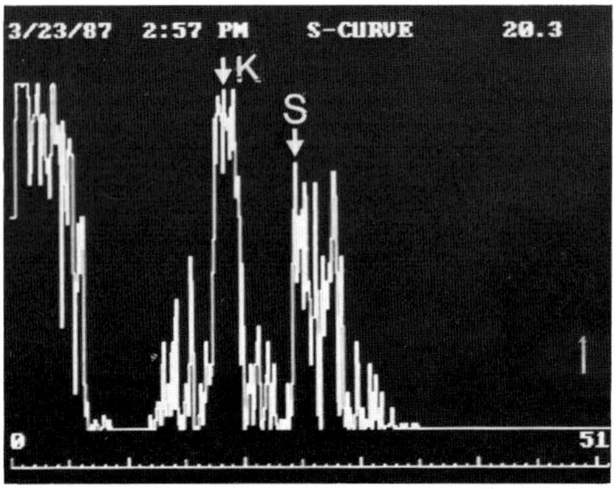


b

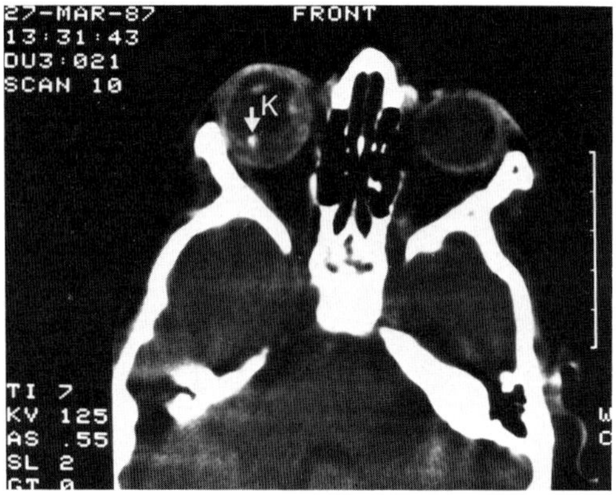


c

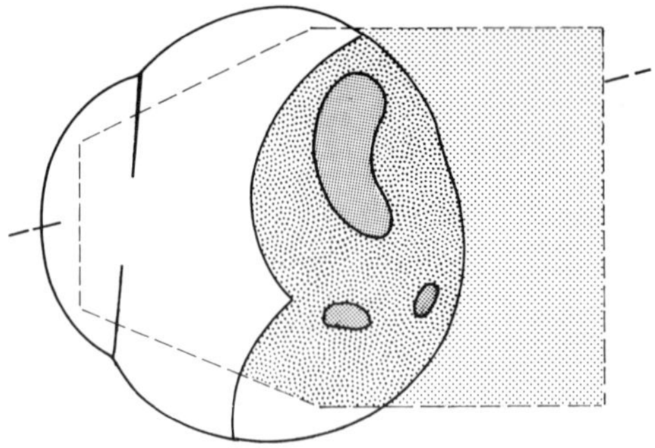

d

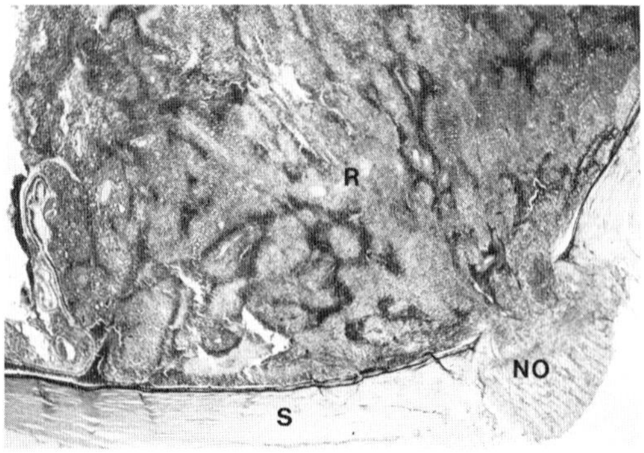


e

Fig. 4.**52a–e** Extensive retinoblastoma
**a** In cross sectional echographic images the tumor is characterized by areas of high acoustic reflectivity alternating with areas of low reflectivity
**b** The differences in reflection can be quantified on A-mode echography: calcified parts of the tumor (K) have markedly higher amplitudes than the sclera (S)
**c** In a CT scan the calcified parts of the tumor can be identifed with greater certainty than in a plain X-ray picture
**d** Schematic drawing
**e** Already under loupe magnification the heterogenous structure of the tumor with calcium deposits can be recognized. These structures explain the nearly pathognomonic echogram. Tumor invasion of the anterior optic nerve can be echographically demonstrated only exceptionally by a widening of the dural diameter (NO = optic nerve, R = retinoblastoma)

echographic cross section is characterized by a few areas of extremely high reflectivity (Fig. 4.**52**). It is assumed that calcifications within the tumor produce these signals. This characteristic echographic pattern may be produced by small areas of calcification which cannot be seen in a plain X-ray picture (François et al. 1971, Koch et al. 1983, Lopez et al. 1983, Till et al. 1969) (Fig. 4.**53**).

These calcifications can also be demonstrated in a computed tomography (CT) scan. If the clinical and echographic findings are unequivocal, we have to decide whether it is really necessary to obtain a CT scan under general anesthesia. By quantitative echography the reflectivity of the tumor calcification is markedly higher than that of the sclera or the retina. This high sound reflection produces a

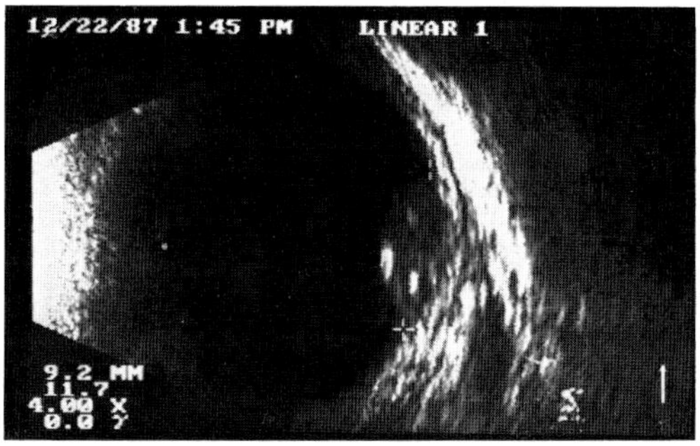


a

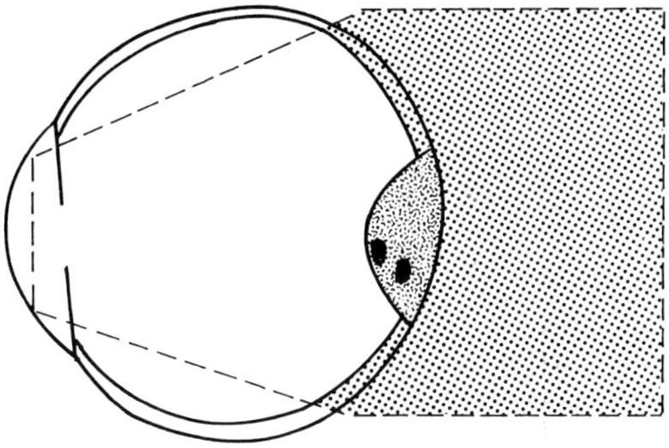

b

Fig. 4.**53** **a, b**
**a** Small retinoblastoma (elevation 3 mm) with circumscribed calcium deposits. Even small tumors may show calcium deposits due to rapid tumor growth. These deposits are especially well demonstrable in linear amplification
**b** Schematic drawing

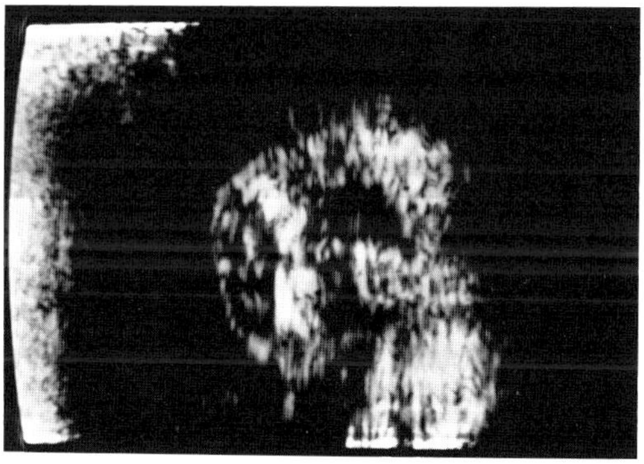

a

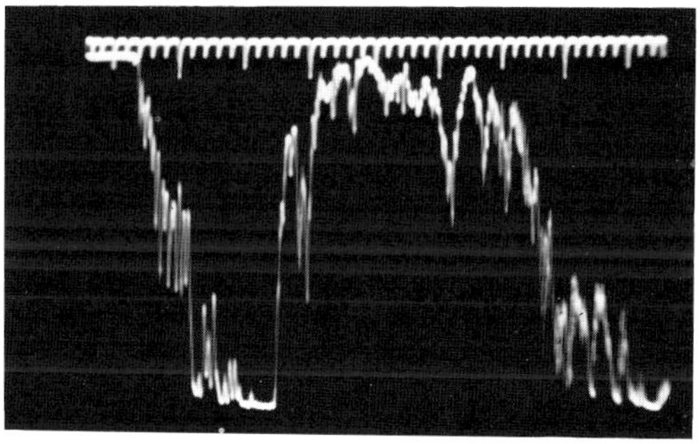

b

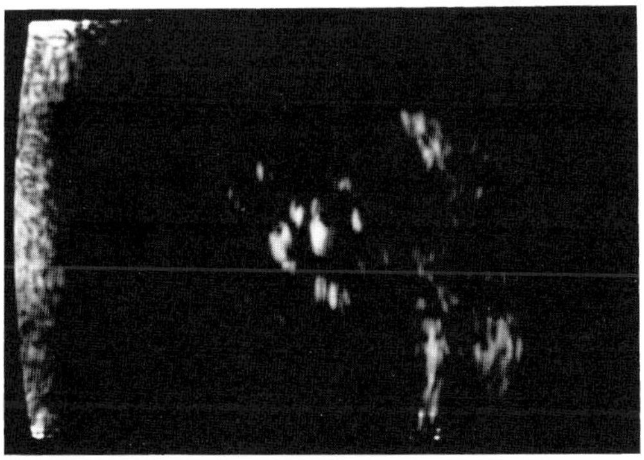

c

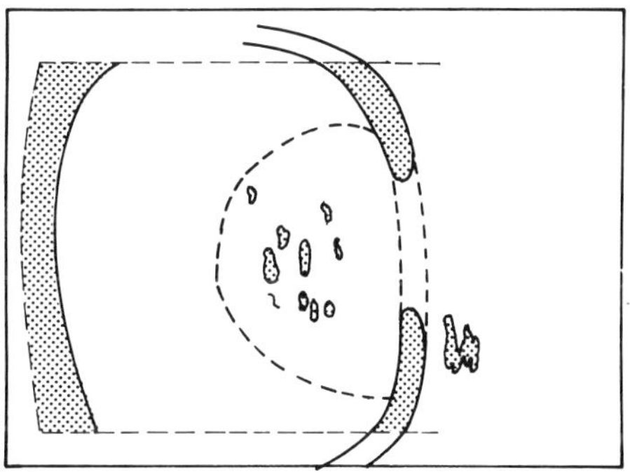

d

Fig. 4.**54** **a–d** Large retinoblastoma with calcifications and acoustic shadow cast on the adjacent sclera and orbit
**a, b** The calcifications light up in cross sectional echograms. In A-mode echograms they can be quantified as the strongest reflecting structures in the examined area
**c** With reduced amplification, the calcified areas are the only visible signals
**d** Schematic drawing

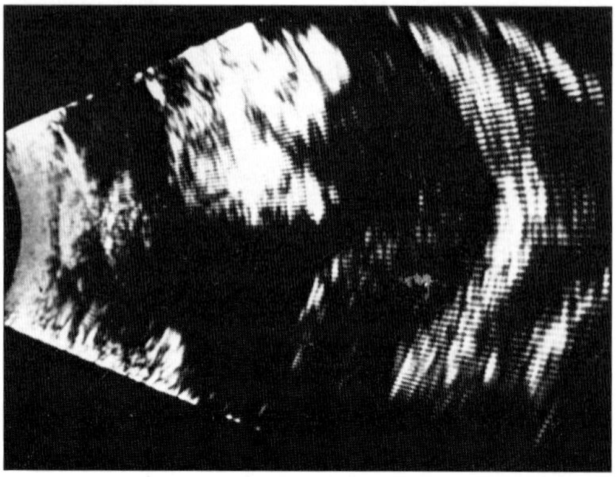

a

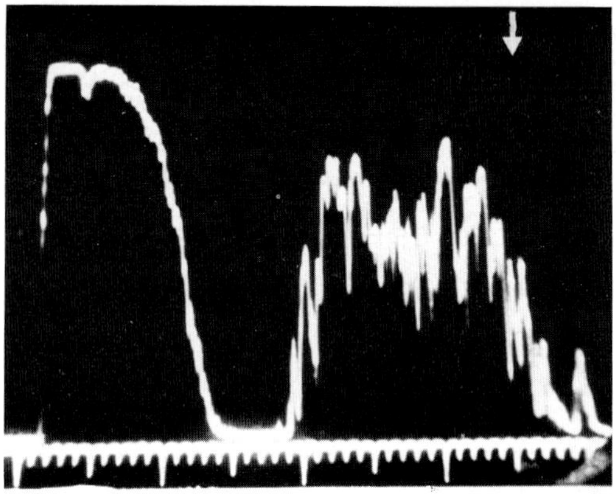

b

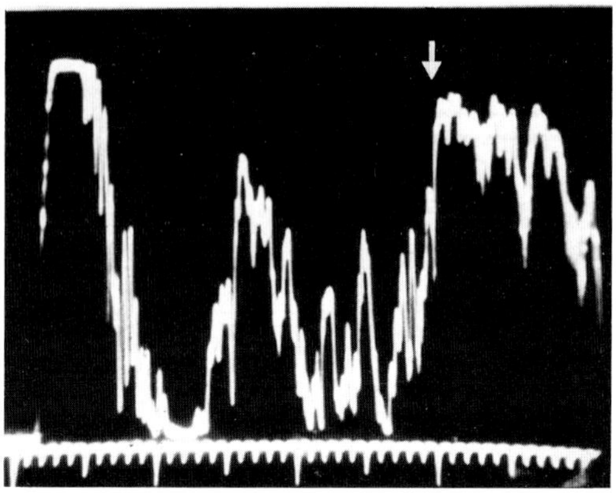

c

Fig. 4.**55** **a–c** Extensive retinoblastoma with varying histologic appearance
**a** The upper tumor parts as demonstrated in the cross sectional echogram show high acoustic reflectivity due to massive calcifications. The lower part of the tumor has less acoustic reflectivity than the adjacent sclera (the scleral spikes in **b** and **c** are marked by arrows)

shadow (Fig. 4.**54**) on more distant structures, e.g., sclera and orbit. With decreasing amplification we finally achieve a selective demonstration of the calcium deposits in the cross-section echogram until they are the only remaining tissue structure visible on the screen (Fig. 4.**54**). In some retinoblastomas the calcium appears only in few tumor areas. Even then this sign should be important for the diagnosis (Fig. 4.**55**).

The absence of echographically demonstrable calcifications does not exclude the presence of a retinoblastoma. It has been repeatedly pointed out (Koch et al. 1983, Förster 1987) that in doubtful cases, if there is enough clinical evidence, an enucleation should be performed (for the differential diagnosis of leukokoria, Sect. 4.6).

Extraocular tumor extension is of great prognostic and therapeutic importance. A perforation of the sclera with orbital invasion can be shown echographically; however, a beginning infiltration of the optic nerve cannot be established or excluded by any diagnostic examination method involving the soft tissues. A piece of optic nerve, as long as possible, should be excised during every enucleation for this type of neoplasm.

### 4.3.5 Retinal Malformations

Retinal malformations in incontinentia pigmenti (Bloch-Sulzberger), retinal dysplasia and Norrie's disease have to be considered in the differential diagnosis of retinoblastoma. The clinical manifestations of these disease entities vary a great deal and therefore make it difficult to present a systematic description of echographic findings. In addition to varying degrees of retinal detachment, there may be retinal cysts, intraocular cartilage and late calcifications, all of which produce a variety of echographic images.

In our experience, the calcification in a phthisical eye or with retinal malformations does not show the distribution pattern of a retinoblastoma characterized by diffusely disseminated calcium deposits. In these nonneoplastic cases, we usually find dense calcium plaques in the ocular coats.

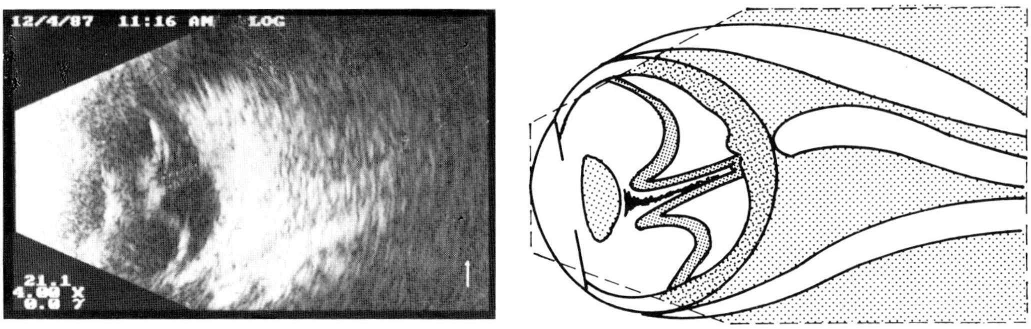


a

b

Fig. 4.**56** a, b
**a** Stage V of retinopathy of prematurity. In cross sectional images we see a complete retinal detachment with a widening of the avascular peripheral retina toward the subretinal space.
**b** Schematic drawing

### 4.3.6 Retinopathy of Prematurity

Because of the improved survival rate of prematurely born children, we will see this condition more frequently than previously. Mild cases show axial myopia with scars in the temporal fundus periphery; in stages IV and V we find, in addition, traction detachments of the retina. If the fundus can be visualized, we gather all information for diagnosis and for a planned treatment with the opthalmoscope. If in stages IV and V the fibrovascular masses become extensive, echography is valuable in order to plan treatment and to evaluate the prognosis of a surgical intervention. Machemer (1981) has emphasized the indispensable information obtained by cross-section echography in these stages. Of essential importance is the diameter of the nearly strand-like shrunk retinal funnel in the retrolental space (see Fig. 4.**56**).

### 4.3.7 Coloboma of the Ocular Fundus

Such colobomas have been mentioned in the differential diagnosis of retinoblastoma (Shapiro et al. 1985). These lesions can be seen clearly by echography even if the fundus cannot be visualized optically (Fig. 4.**57**). In our experience, even large glaucomatous excavations of the optic nerve head cannot be reliably diagnosed by echography. This is in contrast to the reports by other authors.

### 4.3.8 Assessment of Optic Nerve Cupping

The lateral resolution of B-scan equipment has only recently reached a standard capable of displaying the optic cup reproducibly (Darnley-Fisch et al. 1990). This method has also proven to the author its clinical relevance in detecting glaucomatous cups in patient with opaque media.

For optimal results the probe should be placed temporal to the limbus, so that it scans the optic disc vertically as first described by Darnley-Fisch and coworkers.

Fig. 4.57 c–d gives an example of a physiological cup with a C/D ratio of 0.5.

## 4.4 The Choroid

### 4.4.1 Changes in the Ocular Coats due to Hypotony

In order to preserve normal choroidal structure, sufficient blood supply and a physiologic relation between intra- and extravascular pressure are necessary. If in acute hypotony the pressure within the choroidal vessels predominates, an exudation into the suprachoroidal space will follow and lead to a choroidal detachment.

This situation is echographically characterized on a cross section by a detachment of the ocular coats with a convex border. This detachment begins in the ciliary body (Fig. 4.**58**). Occasionally, we get the impression that the detached pars plana of the ciliary body is touching the lens equator (Fig. 4.**59**). At the posterior pole the detached choroid meets the outer ocular coat at a blunt angle, but never extends to the optic nerve head. In severe cases, the two parts of the choroidal detachment meet in the optical axis ("kissing choroidals"). In typical cases the subchoroidal space is free of echos; only rarely

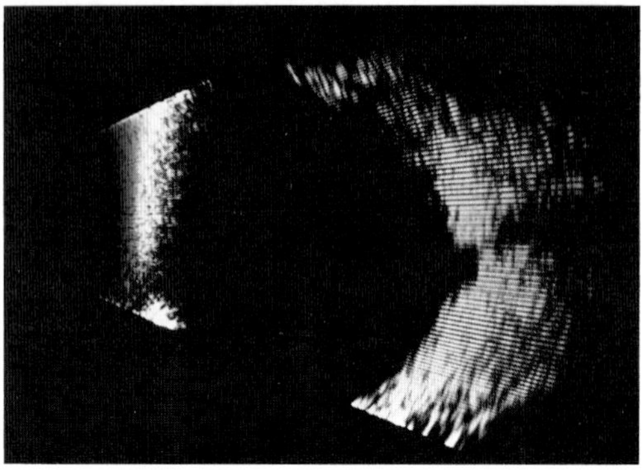

a

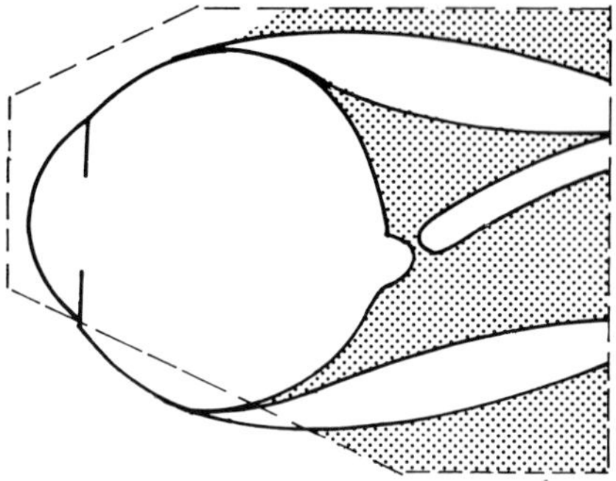

b

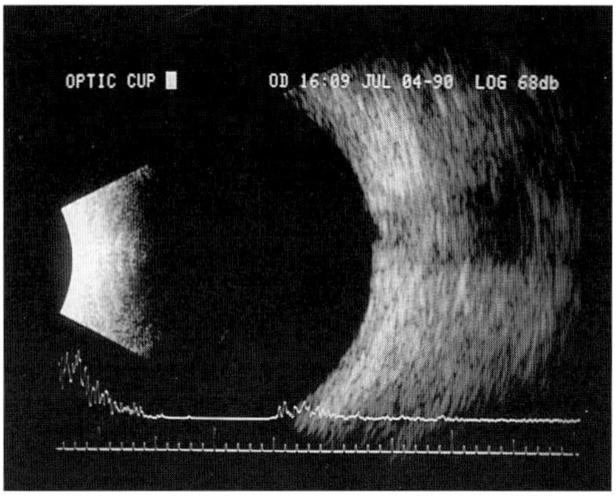


c

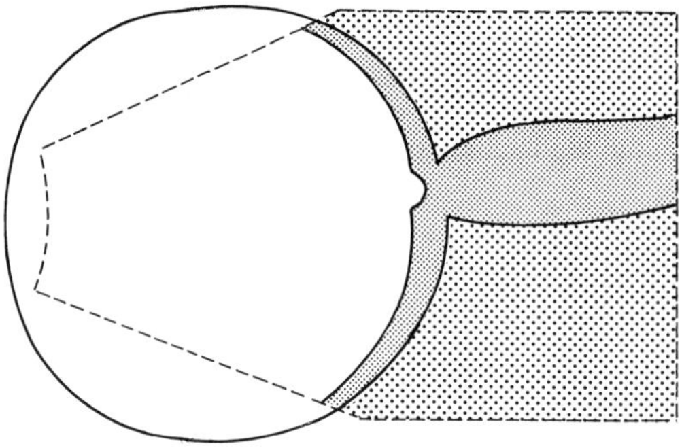

e

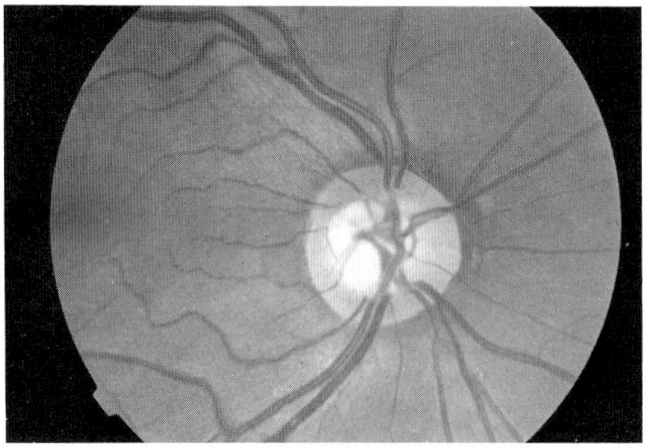

d

Fig. 4.**57 a–e**
**a** Small coloboma of the optic nerve with a diameter of about 2.5 mm. Recently, the identification of glaucomatous excavations by B-mode ultrasound was described (Darnley-Fisch et al. 1990)
**b** Schematic drawing
**c** B-scan section through physiological cupping of an optic nerve head (author's nerve head)
To obtain this vertical section a probe is placed temporal to the limbus, thereby avoiding any artifacts, caused by the lens
**d** Schematic drawing
**e** Fundus photograph showing the excavation displayed in 4.57 c

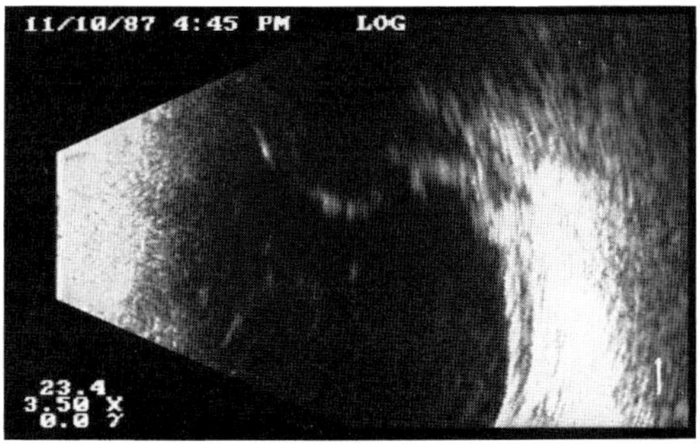


a

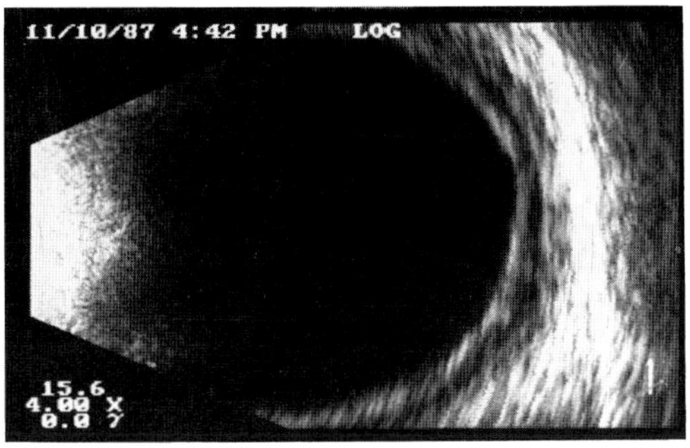


b

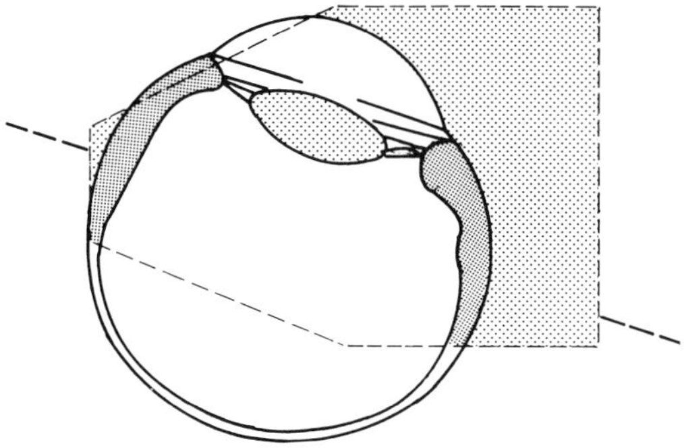

c

Fig. 4.**58** **a–c**
**a, b** Detachment of the ciliary body and the peripheral choroid due to hypotony. The thickening of the ocular coats begins in the area of the ciliary body and extends to the equator
**c** Schematic drawing

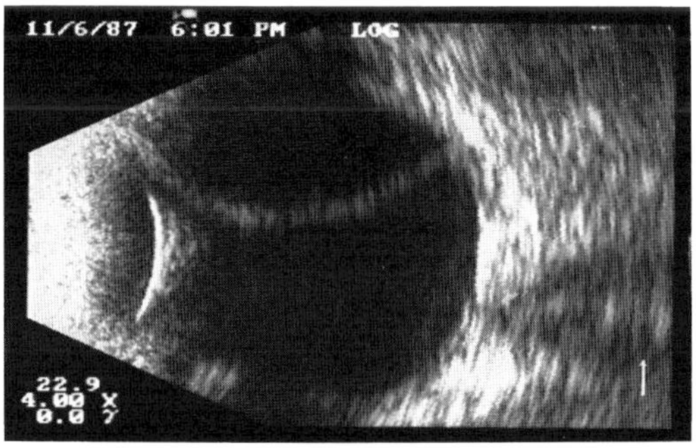


a

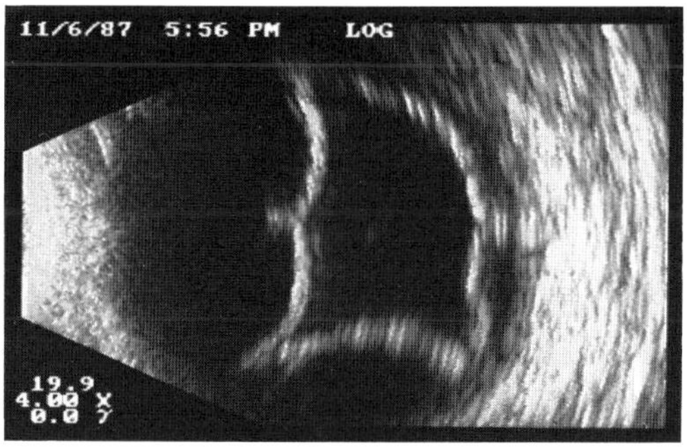


b

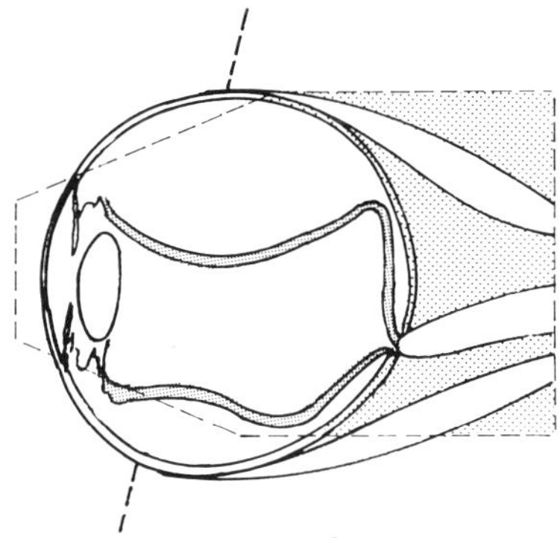

c

Fig. 4.**59** **a–c** Subtotal exudative choroidal detachment
**a** In contrast to a retinal detachment, the choroidal detachment extends beyond the ora serrata; the detachment extends from the iris diaphragm to the posterior pole without reaching the optic nerve head
**b** In frontal sections we see indentations which are caused by large vessels
**c** Schematic drawing

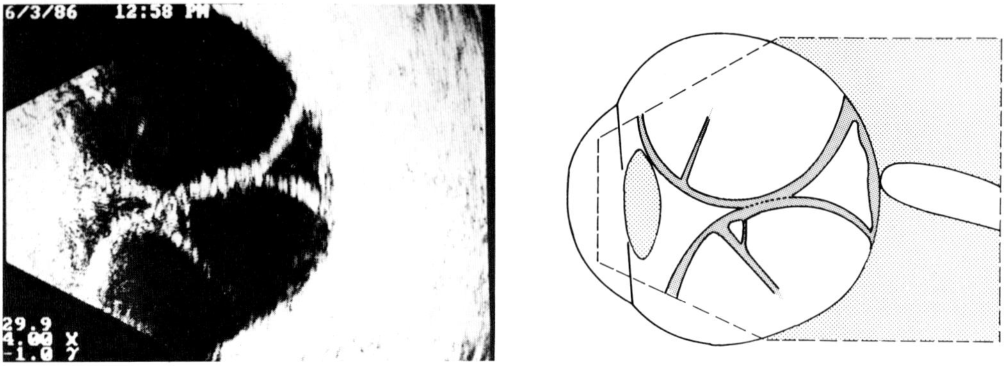


Fig. 4.**60** a, b
**a** Total exudative choroidal detachment in persisting hypotony after a fistulating operation. The choroidal leaves touch each other axially in the vitreous ("kissing choroidals"). Strand-like structures (taut vorticose veins?) course through the intrachoroidal space
**b** Schematic drawing

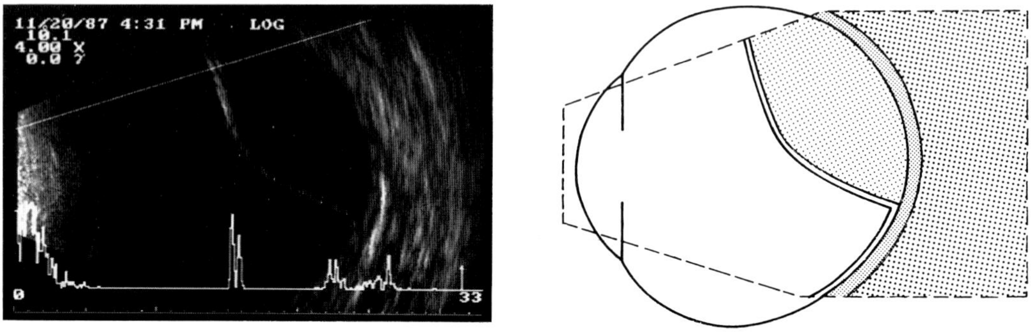


Fig. 4.**61** a, b
**a** Double contour of the detached choroid. Occasionally, the double contour or a double spike may be helpful in differentiating a choroidal from a retinal detachment
**b** Schematic drawing

do we see strands in this area (Fig. 4.**60**). It is possible that these are taut, large choroidal vessels.

As there are no connections between the subchoroidal space and the vitreous, here we do not see the aftermovements so typical of a retinal detachment. On A-mode we occasionally observe double spikes representing the thickness of the ocular coat (Fig. 4.**61**). In an expulsive hemorrhage the intrachoroidal space is filled with strongly reflecting blood clots (Fig. 4.**62**).

In a chronic and persistent hypotony of the globe, we only rarely find a bullous choroidal detachment. Most often the entire ocular coat appears concentrically widened (Fig. 4.**63**). In advanced stages of atrophy, the vitreous space may be reduced to a fraction of its original volume and the ocular coat may be thicker by many factors. It is not possible to differentiate the various parts of the ocular coat (Shapiro 1985). In such severely atrophic eyes, calcification and ossification may develop after many years, due to metaplasia of the pigment epithelium. These changes totally reflect the ultrasound and produce characteristic images. Such changes give all the signs of a foreign body of similar density (Howard et al. 1965, Naumann et al. 1976).

### 4.4.2 Disciform Macular Degeneration

Disciform macular degeneration (Kuhnt-Junius, macular pseudotumor) is regarded as the end stage of the proliferation form of an age-dependent

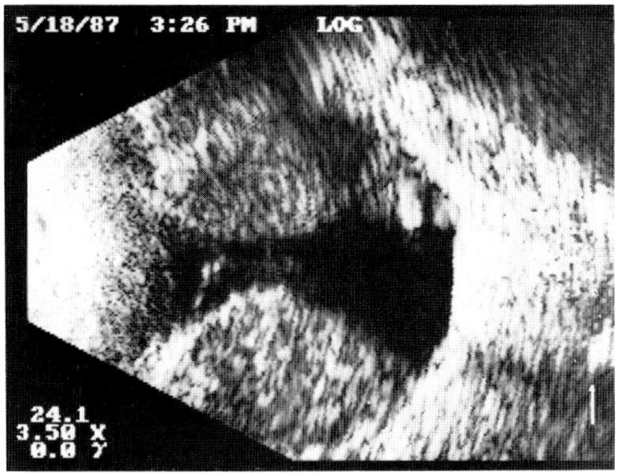


a

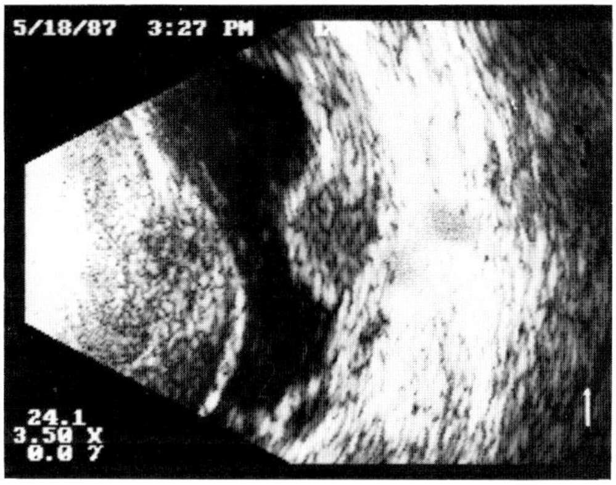


b

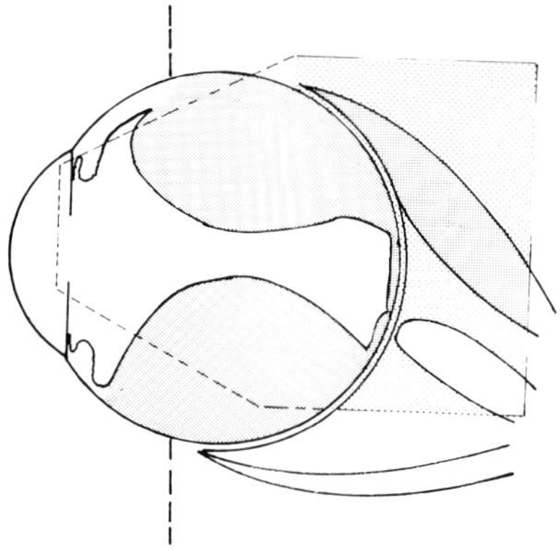

c

Fig. 4.**62 a–c**
**a, b** Extensive choroidal detachment in an eye with expulsive hemorrhage. The intrachoroidal space has acquired acoustic reflectivity due to the accumulation of blood. There may be anatomical healing after the absorption of the blood, but we cannot expect visual function to improve
**c** Schematic drawing

maculopathy (wet type of macular degeneration, according to Sautter). The histologic substrate is a protruding, vascularized connective tissue mound which extends from the choriocapillaris through defects of Bruch's membrane under the pigment epithelium or into the subretinal space (Fig. 4.**64**). These constituents produce an echographically heterogenous internal structure in which some parts without acoustic interfaces, e.g., recent exudates, alternate with good reflectors, e.g., connective tissue septa.

It is an individual decision whether and when a patient with a suspected disciform macular degeneration should undergo an echographic examination. In general, we assume that elevations of more than 3 mm are quite unusual for this disease entity. A high content of pigment, which is attributed to hemosiderin deposits, may make a differential diagnosis with a choroidal melanoma difficult. The

Table 4.4 **Differential diagnosis of choroidal detachment from retinal detachment**

| | Retinal Detachment | Choroidal Detachment |
|---|---|---|
| Shape | Varies | Convex toward the vitreous, posterior pole not involved |
| Borders | Optic nerve head/ ora serrata | Does not reach to the optic nerve head/iris lens diaphragm may be reached |
| Angle of insertion at the posterior pole | Acute | Blunt |
| Aftermovements | Present | Absent |
| A-mode signs | One spike | Double spikes |
| Intraocular pressure | Varies | Low |

a b c d

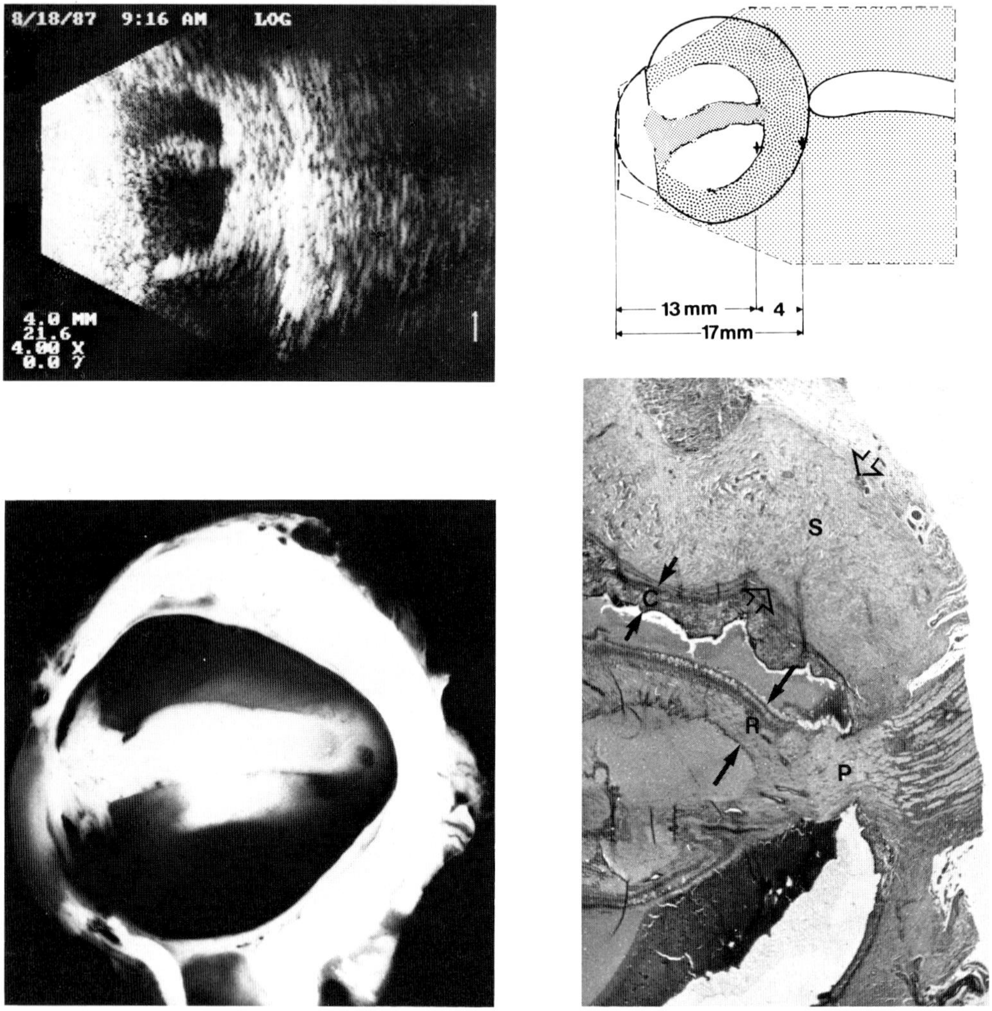


Fig. 4.**63 a–d** Advanced phthisis bulbi

**a** The ocular coats are widened to 4 mm; individual layers cannot be differentiated; the vitreous has shrunk to 13 mm. There is total retinal detachment

**b** Loupe magnification after enucleation: marked widening of all layers of the ocular coats; strand-like total retinal detachment

**c** Schematic drawing

**d** Histologic section through the optic nerve head of the same globe (S = markedly thickened sclera, C = choroid, R = retina, P = optic nerve head)

markedly different histological structure of these two lesions will give ultrasonograms which usually can be quite well differentiated because of their signal intensity (Freyler 1975, Ossoinig et al. 1969). A disciform macular degeneration is characterized by alternating areas of high and low acoustic reflectivity. The retinal echo is frequently separated from the connective tissue mound by a thin layer of fluid. The retina shows a wavy surface and is markedly thinned; it is therefore difficult to demonstrate as a maximal image.

If it can be echographically proven that the size of the lesion is decreasing, a malignant neoplasm can be excluded with a great degree of probability. An increase in size does not necessarily exclude the diagnosis of a disciform lesion. For the final evaluation of such an entity it is absolutely necessary to use all available information.

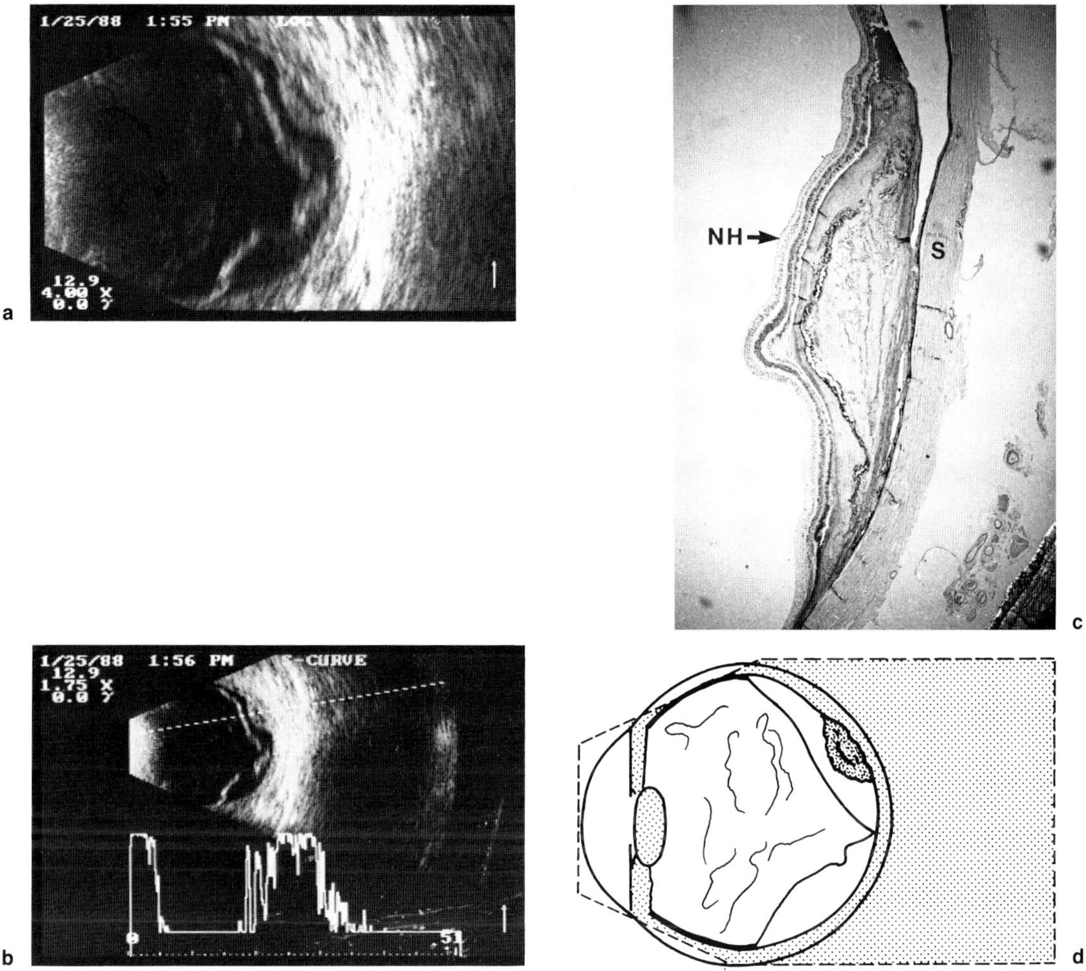


Fig. 4.**64 a–d** Disciform macular degeneration with exudative retinal detachment

**a** In cross sectional echogram the widened ocular coats in the macular area appear as a strongly reflecting, layered structure

**b** The acoustic interfaces of the macular degeneration produce high signals

**c** Histologic section of a disciform macular degeneration under loupe magnification: vascularized connective tissue scars with exudations without acoustic interfaces produce the substrate for the heterogenous nature of the echogram (NH = retina, S = sclera)

**d** Schematic drawing

### 4.4.3 Choroidal Melanoma

When evaluating a clinical situation in which a choroidal melanoma has to be considered, we have to use all available diagnostic procedures, especially for doubtful cases. In this way, the frequency of an erroneous diagnosis leading to an enucleation could be decreased from 20 to 5%.

Echography is especially important here. It provides information on certain physical properties of the tissue in question and thereby complements the routine optical methods (Nover et al. 1965, Ossoinig et al. 1969, Oksala 1974, Freyler 1975, Gonvers et al. 1979, Guthoff et al. 1981).

When using the customary ophthalmic amplifier transducer combinations (see Sect. 1.3), the tumor will reflect ultrasound in a typical manner. The signals produced within the tumor are more complicated than those we encounter when evaluating

a

b

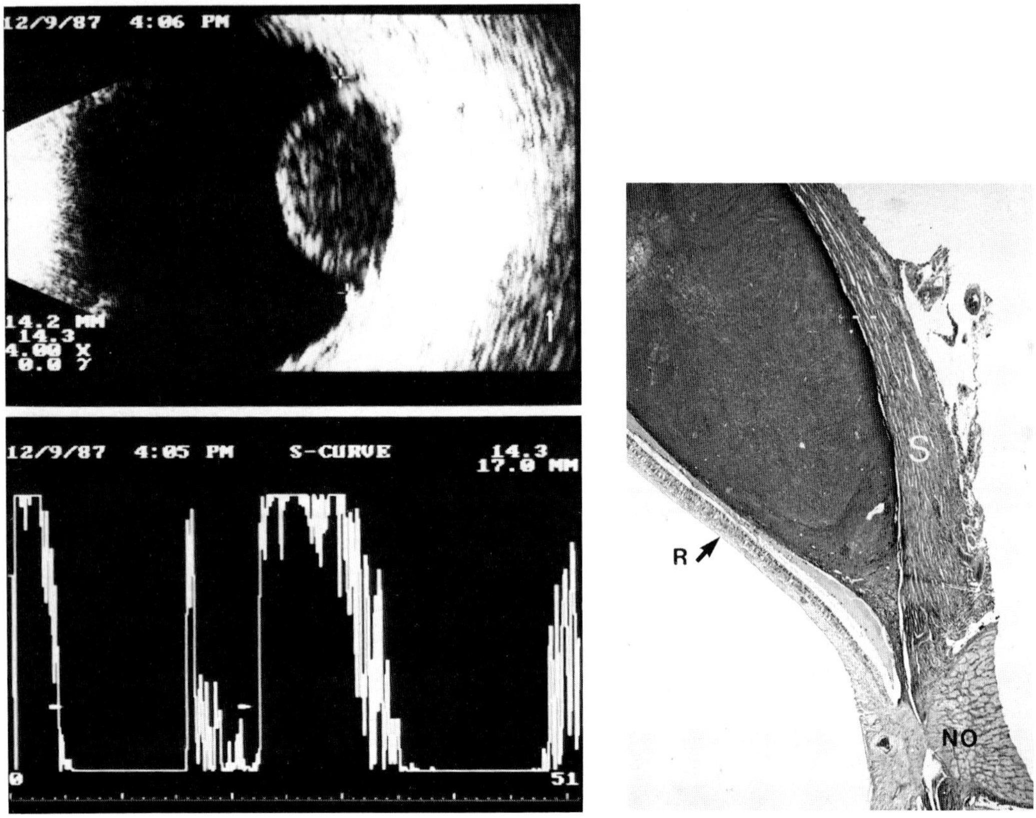


c

Fig. 4.**65a–c** Typical findings of a choroidal melanoma.
**a** In cross section the tumor is biconvex. The diameter of the base is 14 × 14 mm; elevation, 8.5 mm; calculated tumor volume, 750 cmm
**b** The spike amplitude within the tumor amounts, with standardized A-mode, to about 20% of the scleral spike
**c** Loupe magnification of a peripapillary choroidal melanoma. The reason for the low homogenous acoustic reflectivity of a choroidal melanoma is the densely packed tumor cells, the margins of which are separated by a distance much smaller than the wavelength of ultrasound (R = retina, S = sclera, NO = optic nerve)

membrane echoes in the vitreous body; overlapping and dampening processes play a decisive role in the echographic summation of signals, due to the densely packed tumor cells the cytoplasmic membranes of which are separated by a distance which is considerably smaller than the ultrasound wavelength. Connective tissue septa and vessels vary in their prominence and interfere with the signals from the tumor tissue.

The interpretation of echograms, either A- or B-mode, are based on experiences which were gathered during the pioneer time of ophthalmologic ultrasound diagnosis. Decisive reports on this topic were published by Oksala (1959), Baum (1964), Ossoinig (1967), Buschmann (1971), Till (1979, 1985), Poujol (1975) and Trier (1977).

We shall now attempt to discuss the role of an echographic diagnosis of choroidal melanomas in the clinical decision process.

### The Principles of Image Production in Choroidal Melanoma

After the ultrasound wave courses through the vitreous, it meets the first acoustic interface, the retina overlying the tumor. The intensity of the echo produced by this interface is physically characterized by the impedance difference between vitreous and

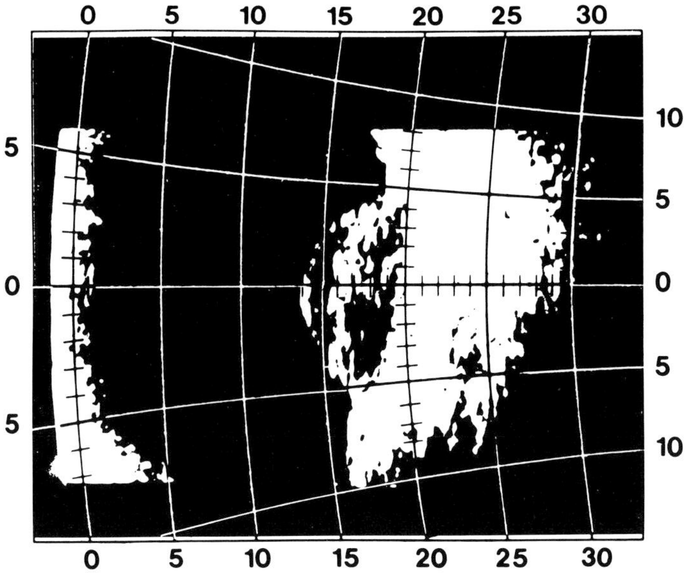


Fig. 4.**66** Choroidal melanoma with associated retinal detachment over the peak of the tumor. Tumor size: base, 9 × 9 mm; elevation, 3.5 mm. The detached retina lies about 2 mm in front of the tumor. The calculated tumor volume is about 150 cmm. If the retinal detachment were erroneously included, the volume would be about 230 cmm

retina; it is therefore not important for identifying the tumor itself (Fig. 4.**65**).

If the retina is attached to the tumor surface, no separate presentation of the two interfaces is possible. On the other hand, if the accompanying retinal detachment is also present over the peak of the tumor, then the retina will be imaged as a separate membranous structure lying in front of the lesion (Fig. 4.**66**). An exact localization of the peak of the tumor is especially important for measuring the elevation of the lesion when planning a treatment, or for follow-up examination after radiation therapy (Guthoff et al. 1975). The signals following that of the tumor surface or that of the retinal echo are produced by the interaction of the ultrasound with tumor tissue. The scleral echo is, as the posterior border, also in the tumor area the strongest signal for the specific direction of examination. When the tumor breaks through the scleral barrier, the continuity of this strong signal is interrupted at the site of perforation (Fig. 4.**67**).

### The Characteristics of a Choroidal Melanoma on B-Mode Echography

In B-mode echograms a melanoma appears as a biconvex area. The internal structure is relatively homogenous and produces markedly fewer signals than the tumor surface or the sclera. If the tumor has broken through Bruch's membrane, then the mushroom-shaped lesion (collar button) can be demonstrated in a cross section as a pathognomonic sign (Fig. 4.**68**). This perforation does not necessarily occur at the peak of the tumor. It should be carefully searched for because it is of great importance for the differential diagnosis (Fig. 4.**69**) (Hallermann et al. 1983).

Occasionally, the mushroom of a tumor may, in some section planes, simulate a tumor mass lying free in the vitreous (Fig. 4.**68b**). A tumor lying immediately beneath the sensory retina occasionally reflects ultrasound more than tumor parts beneath Bruch's membrane. Ossoinig uses sound attenuation, i.e., the continuous decay of spike altitudes, in the A-mode to characterize choroidal tumors. He calls this the angle kappa. This is probably not only an attenuation phenomenon (Guthoff et al. 1979), but can be explained additionally on the basis of echographic-histopathologic comparisons (Figs. 4.**70**, 4.**75**). The part of the tumor growing in front of Bruch's membrane will be drained less well because of the collar button effect, leading to a dilatation of the vessels in this part of the tumor (Naumann et al. 1980, Ossoinig et al. 1979, Shields et al. 1980). This creates new acoustic interfaces which are responsible for a high signal intensity (brighter dots in B-mode, higher spikes in A-mode).

In the area of the tumor base, we frequently see a "choroidal excavation" (Figs. 4.**71**, 4.**72**). This step

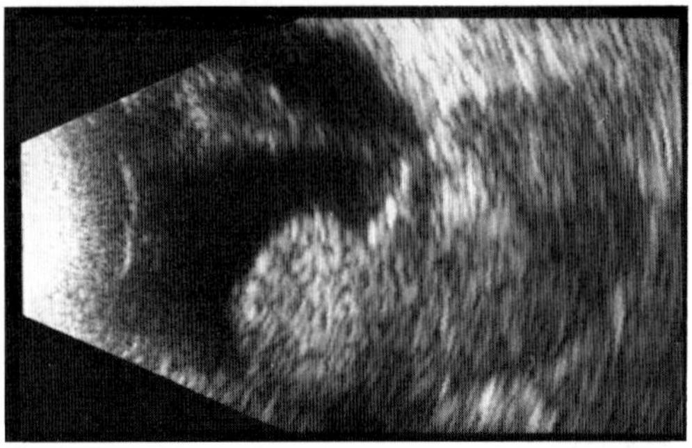

a

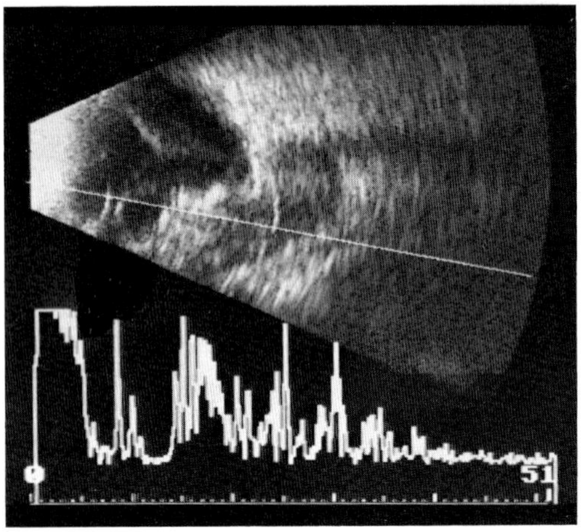


b

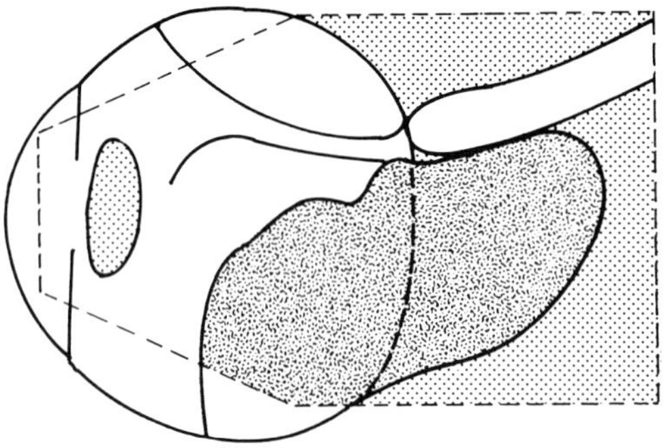

c

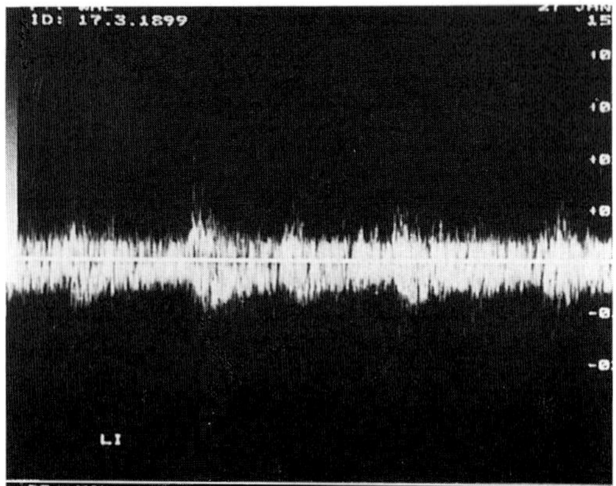


d

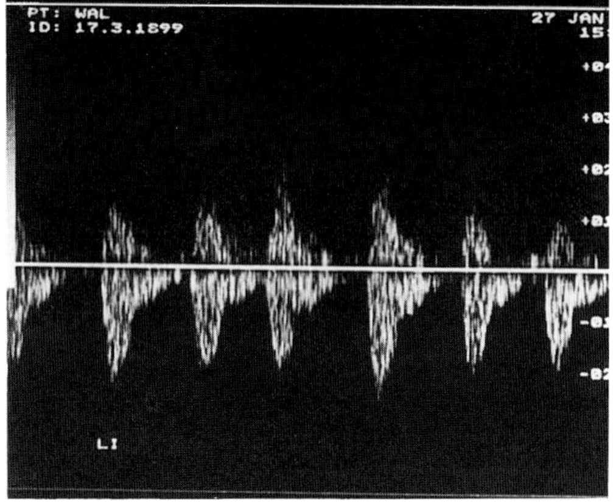


e

Fig. 4.**67 a–e**
**a, b** Choroidal melanoma with scleral perforation in a 65-year-old woman. Referral diagnosis: orbital cellulitis. Echographic findings: large intraocular tumor with wide invasion of the orbital tissues. Remnants of the sclera can be demonstrated within the tumor (both in A- and B-mode echograms) because of their strong acoustic reflectivity. Additional finding: total retinal detachment
**c** Schematic drawing
**d** Frequency shift from the intraocular tumor, maximum velocity: 10 cm/s;
**e** Frequency shift from the extraocular tumor, maximum velocity: 2 cm/s
With Doppler technique we see that the intraocular part of the tumor shows reduced blood flow compared to the extraocular part. The secondary glaucoma apparently compresses the intraocular tumor

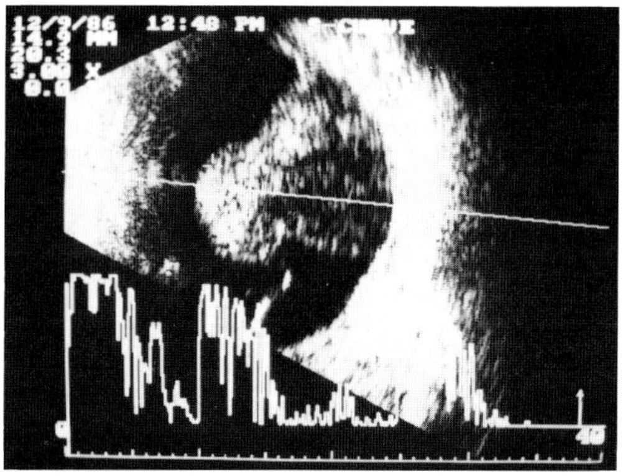

a

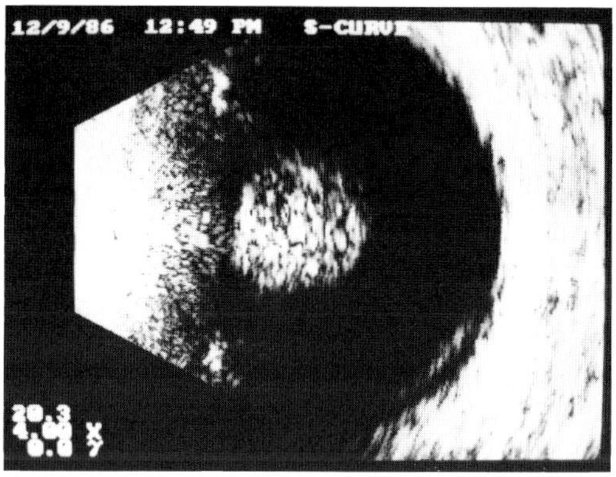


b

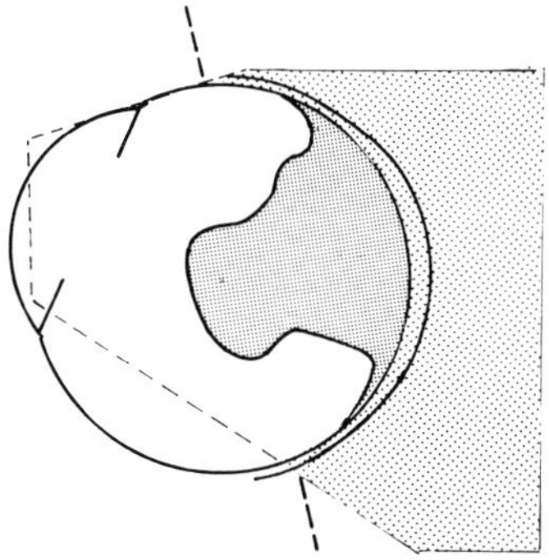

c

Fig. 4.**68 a–c** Large choroidal melanoma, mushroom-shaped after perforating Bruch's membrane
**a** Sagittal section
**b** Frontal section: in the frontal plane one part of the tumor does not seem to have contact with the ocular coats. In principle we have to request an examination in various sectional planes
**c** Schematic drawing

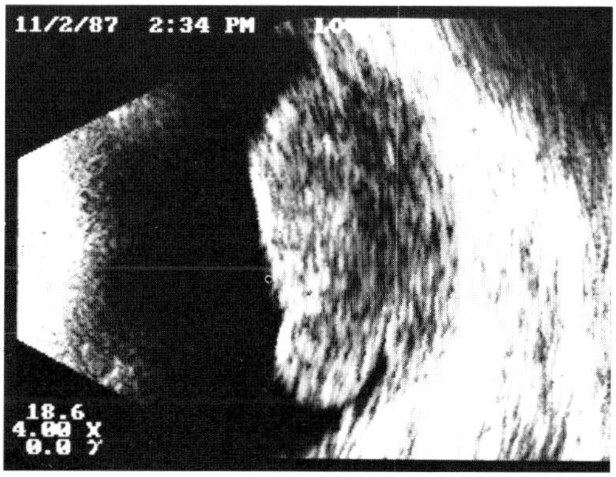


a

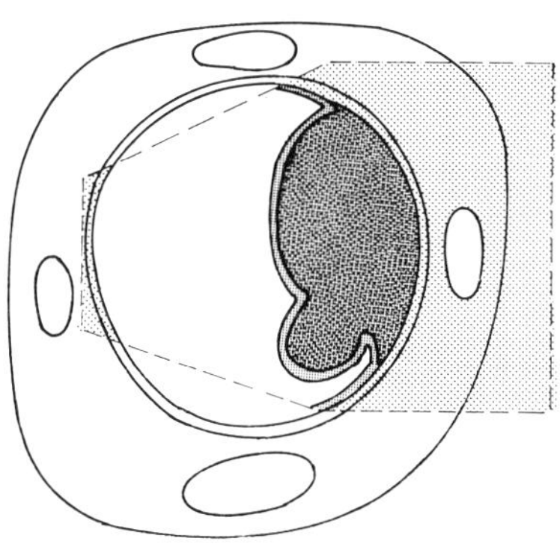

b

Fig. 4.**69 a,b**
**a** Choroidal melanoma with eccentric perforation of Bruch's membrane. We should search for a mushroom-like shape of the lesion, which is nearly pathognomonic for a melanoma and therefore of great differential diagnostic value
**b** Schematic drawing

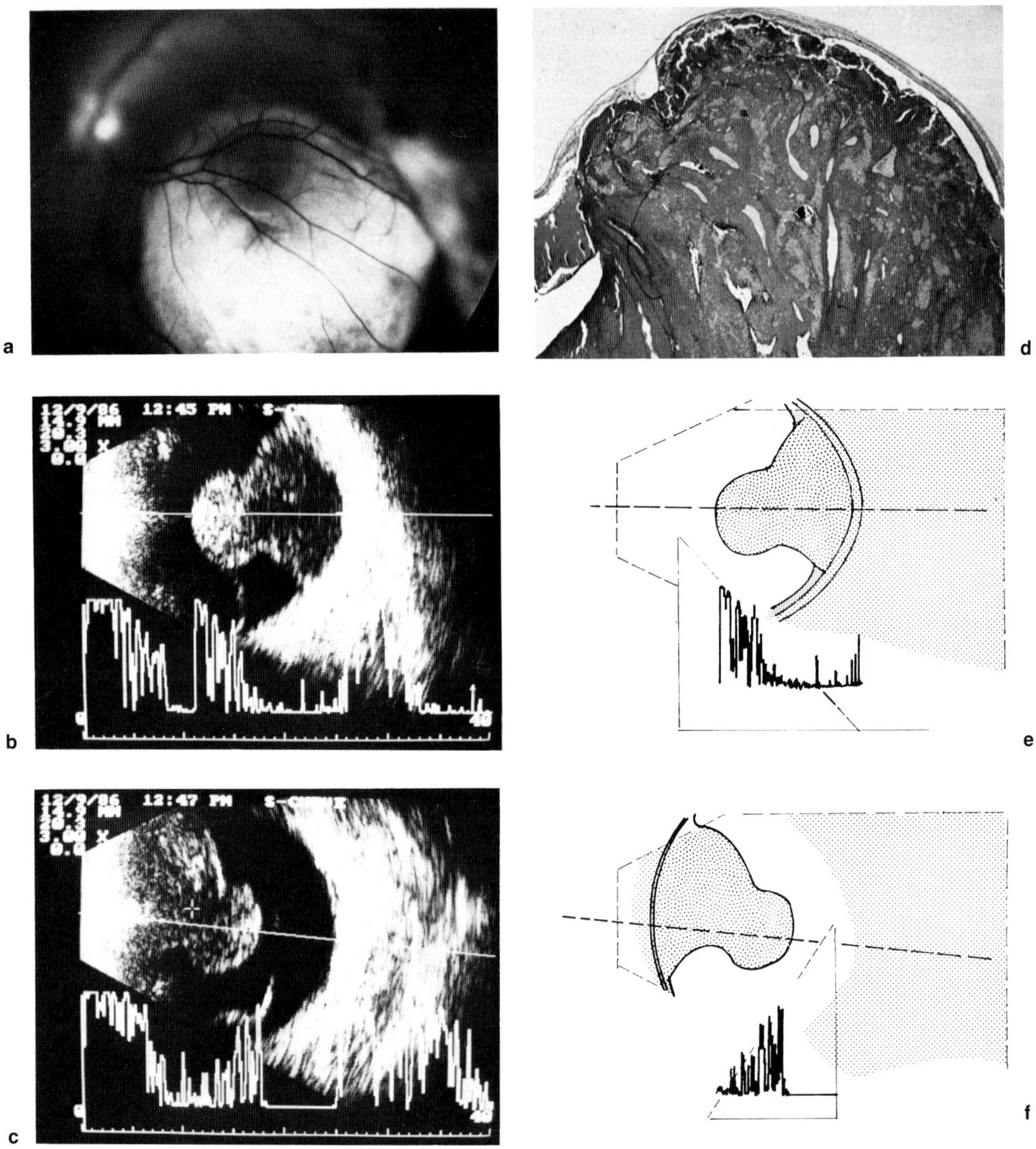


Fig. 4.**70a–i** Large mushroom-shaped choroidal melanoma with especially strong reflectivity in the area of the collar button
**a** Clinical picture
**b** Sagittal echogram: in cross sectional and A-mode echograms, there is markedly increased reflection in the area of the tumor peak
**c** Echogram from the tumor base (obtained with maximal adduction of the globe, and made possible because of the far temporal location of the tumor base). Also in this direction of examination, the part of the tumor anterior to Bruch's membrane shows a high reflectivity
**d** The part of the tumor in front of Bruch's membrane often shows dilated vessels which act as interfaces, increasing the acoustic reflectivity
**e, f** Schematic drawings
**g–i** See color plates

a

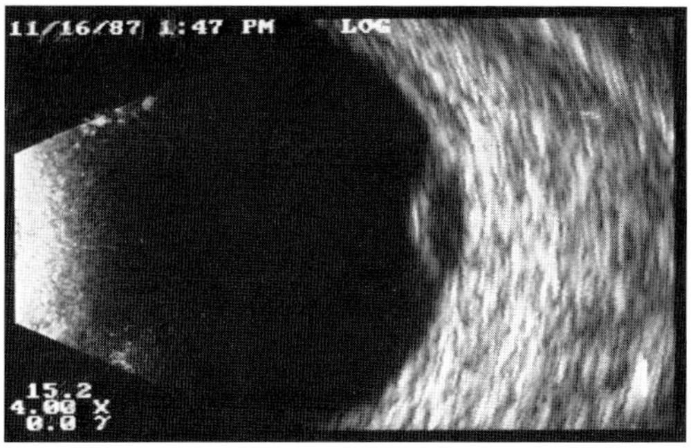


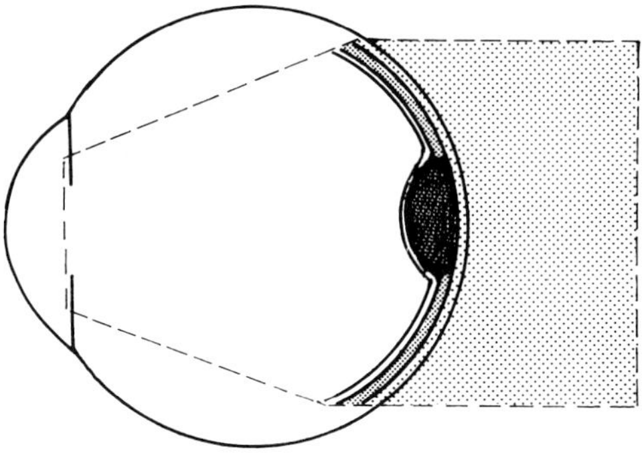

b

Fig. 4.**71 a, b**
**a** Small choroidal melanoma. Elevation 2.5 mm; base, 8 × 8 mm; calculated tumor volume, 66 cmm. The choroid at the tumor base has been replaced by tumor which has less acoustic reflectivity and provokes a choroidal excavation echographically
**b** Schematic drawing

a

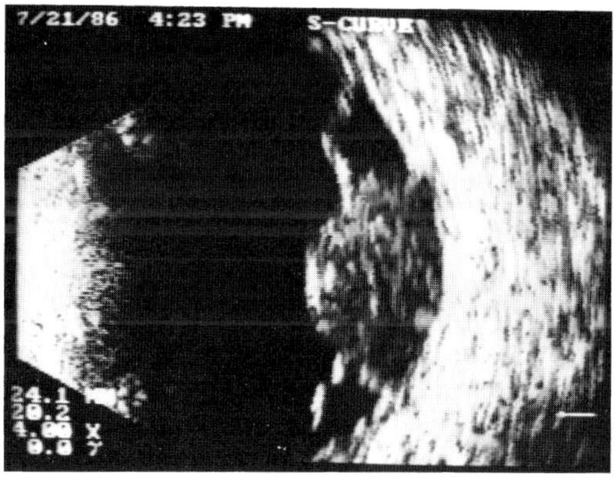


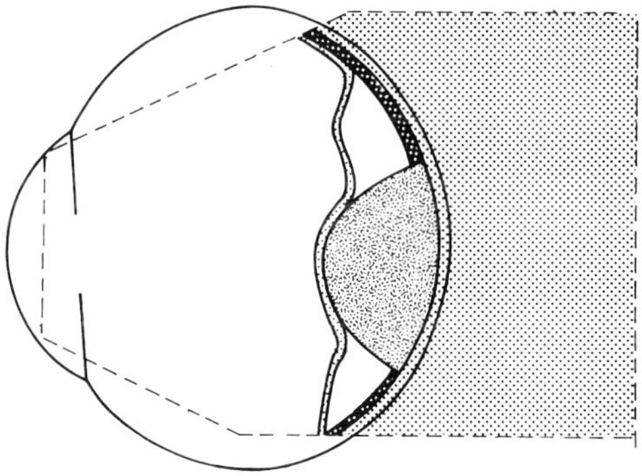

c

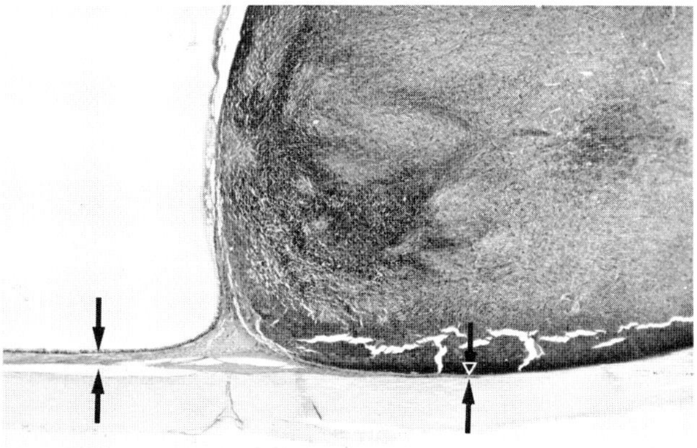

b

Fig. 4.**72 a–c** Choroidal melanoma of average size. Elevaton, 6 mm; diameter at the base, 11 × 12 mm; calculated tumor volume, 330 cmm
**a** The highly reflecting choroid has been replaced by the poorly reflecting melanoma, producing a choroidal excavation in the cross section
**b** Histologic section through the margin of a choroidal melanoma. At the base, normal choroid is replaced by tumor
**c** Schematic drawing

in the acoustic section develops at the edge of the tumor where melanoma tissue borders on adjacent strongly-reflecting intact choroid (Baum et al. 1967, Wolter et al. 1973).

### The Characteristics of Choroidal Melanoma on A-Mode Echography

The echographic internal structure of a tumor is quantitatively best described in the A-mode echogram.

When using an unfocused A-mode transducer, we obtain a summation signal from a large tissue area (see Sect. 1.2.2). For evaluation, a calibrated instrument is necessary. The type of instrument plays a minor role, but mode of amplification and accuracy of decibel adjustment have to be known. An amplification corresponding to tissue sensitivity according to Ossoinig (about 58 dB above the standard reflector echo W 38 of Buschmann) typically produces a complex of spikes in the tumor, the median altitude of which lies between 10 and 60% of the scleral spike amplitude. Within a biconvex tumor which has not extensively broken through Bruch's membrane, we find spikes of relatively uniform amplitudes (Fig. 4.**65**). This corresponds to the uniform histologic structure of a melanoma (Fig. 4.**65c**). Exceptions are secondary changes of large tumors, e.g., hemorrhages or necrosis (Coleman et al. 1974, Bujara et al. 1980). In the majority of cases we can establish the diagnosis with a great deal of certainty by considering all ophthalmologic findings. A preoperative correlation between the echographic pattern and the histopathologic findings is currently only speculative and lacks any clinical verification (Manschot 1981).

Table 4.5 **B-mode echographic characteristics of a choroidal Melanoma**

| |
|---|
| Highly specific signs:<br>1. Mushroom or hourglass shape<br>2. Choroidal excavation at the margin<br>3. Doppler shift inside the tumor? |
| With extraocular extension:<br>4. Widening of Tenon's space<br>5. Reduced scleral reflectivity at the tumor base |
| Less specific signs:<br>1. Biconvex tumor<br>2. Homogenous internal structure (uniform average steps of gray) |

The melanona consists of solid tissue and therefore *no aftermovements* can be expected as they might occur with a large subretinal or choroidal hemorrhage. *Flickering spike complexes* may be seen on the A-mode echogram within the tumor itself. Various authors interpret them differently. It is assumed that they are due to blood circulating in large tumor vessels. It has recently been possible to obtain Doppler signals from the interior of the tumor by using B-mode Doppler devices with a high resolution power and a frequency between 7 and 20 MHz. This method is apparently more sensitive than the purely visual evaluation of a time amplitude echogram (Guthoff et al. 1989) (Fig. 4.**73**).

Since 1988 we have examined 27 choroidal melanoma patients in our clinic, using not only the routine A- and B-mode techniques, but also the Duplex Scanner in order to receive Doppler signals from the interior of the tumor. Most of the examinations were made with the instrument ATL Ultramark 8. A few patients were also examined with the angiodynograph made by Philips, and with the instrument Acuson, which is equipped with a colorcoding device. The B-mode echograms were always obtained with a frequency of 7.5 MHz. The emitted frequency of the Doppler signal was 5 MHz.

In some patients it was possible to determine the angle of blood flow within the tumor using color coding technology; this is necessary to calculate flow velocity accurately. (Fig. 4.**70 g–i**).

The flow parameters in the central retinal artery and vein (Berger and Guthoff 1989) in an eye with a choroidal melanoma do not differ significantly from those in a normal eye.

We have meanwhile examined 42 eyes with melanoma. Doppler shifts could be detected in all patients excepting one. Tumor size varied between 80–1500 $mm^2$. The average blood flow velocity was 18.8 cm/s (SEM 7.6 cm/s).

In one patient the tumor perforated the sclera and invaded the muscle cone (see Fig. 4.**67**). A secondary glaucoma with an intraocular pressure of 45 mm Hg compressed the intraocular tumor; this influenced the maximal flow velocities, which could be measured by Doppler sonography (Fig. 4.**67d**).

At the present time the state of the art does not allow us to exactly measure specific maximal flow

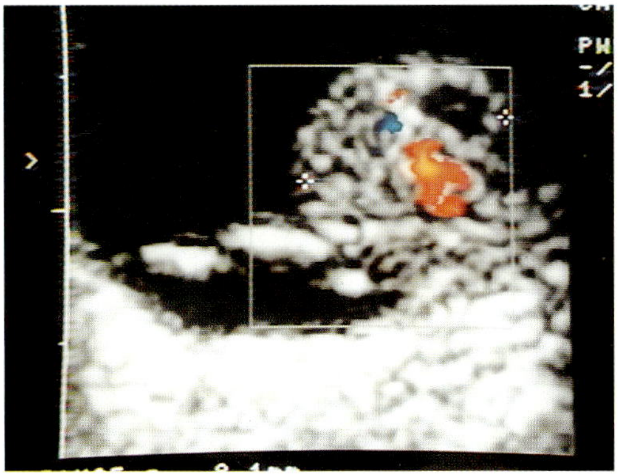

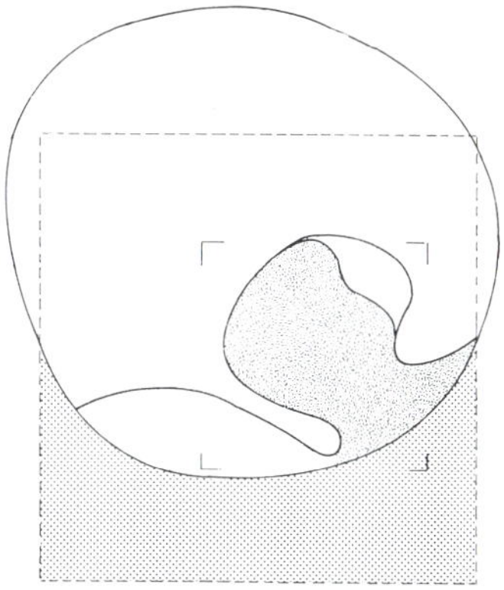

Fig. 2.**9c** Choroidal melanoma after breaking through Bruch's membrane, accompanying retinal detachment. The color Doppler sonography with the instrument Acuson (5 MHz examination frequency) reveals increased blood flow in the part of the tumor which is strangulated by Bruch's membrane. The red color coding corresponds to a blood flow toward the transducer; the blue color coding corresponds to a flow away from it

Fig. 2.**9d** Schematic drawing

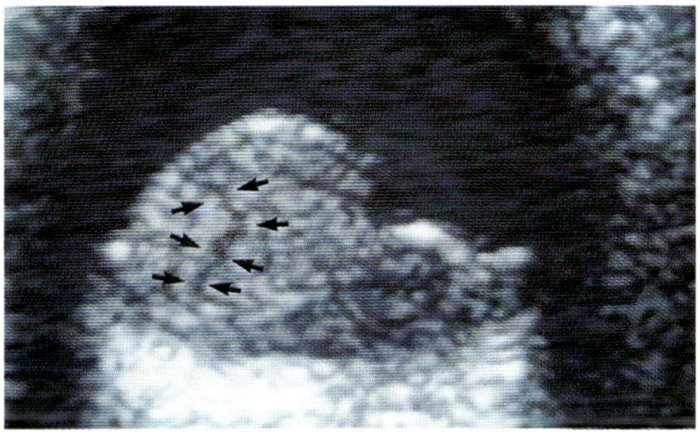

Fig. 4.**70g** Cross-sectional echogram through a choroidal melanoma with an elevation of 8 mm and several peaks. Close to the center is a band-shaped area of low reflectivity (black arrows)

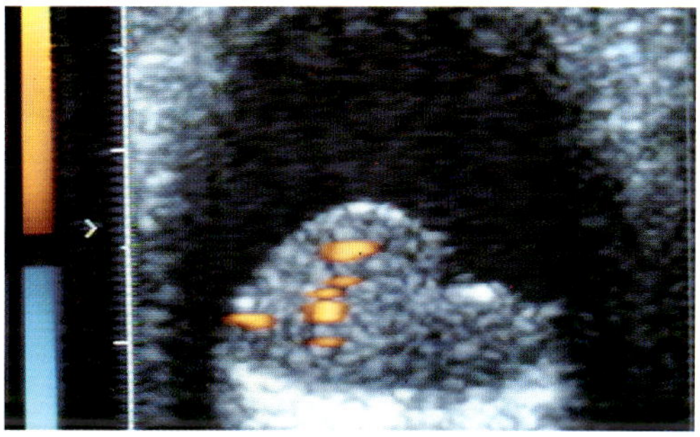

Fig. 4.**70h** Color-coded Doppler signal analysis shows that this area is the origin of frequency shifts toward the transducer

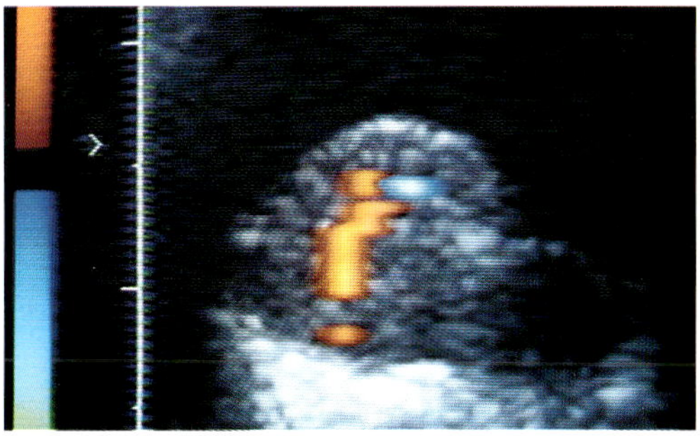

Fig. 4.**70i** Using highest sensitivity of the amplifier and decreasing the wall filter setting, we can differentiate between a structure of red color coding (vessels with the flow toward the transducer) and a circumscribed area close to the peak of the melanoma in which the blood flows away from the transducer (blue). This type of sonography may give us new clues as to planning and controlling the treatment of intraocular tumors

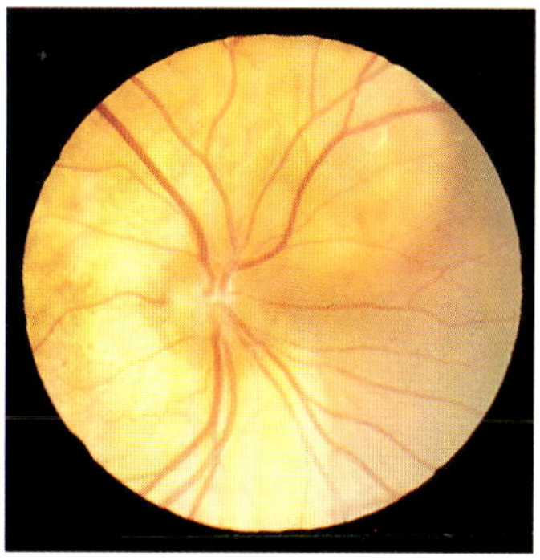

Fig. 4.**88a** Right fundus of a 9-year-old girl. Vision at the time the photo was taken 0.8. A yellow-brown, space-occupying lesion covers the posterior pole of the globe. Ophthalmoscopically, it is hardly elevated. It surrounds the optic nerve head like a pair of pincers

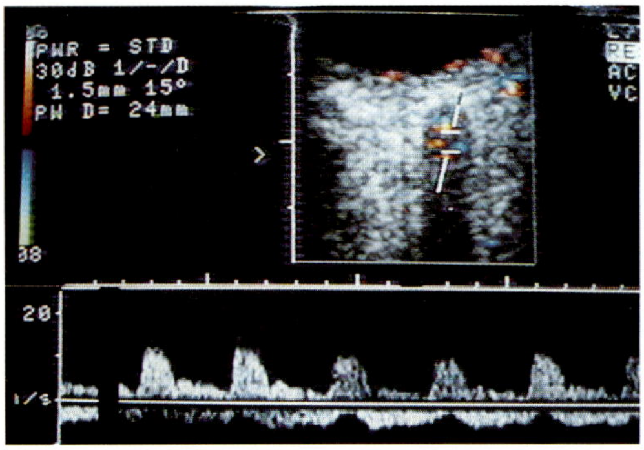


Fig. 5.**5c** Simultaneous documentation of color-coded Doppler sonography of the distal part of the optic nerve and of the frequency spectrum deduced from the region of interest.

**d**

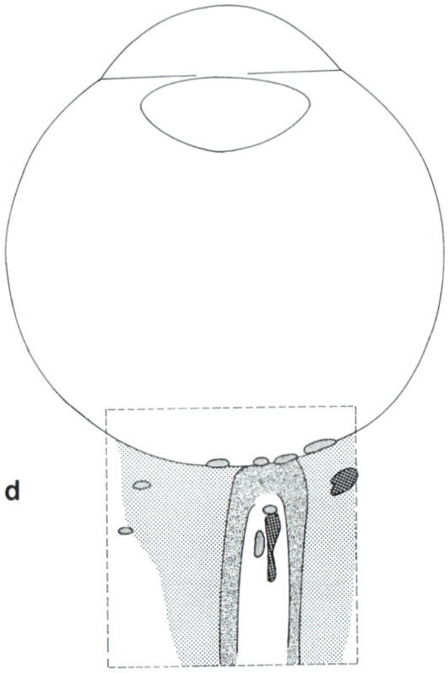

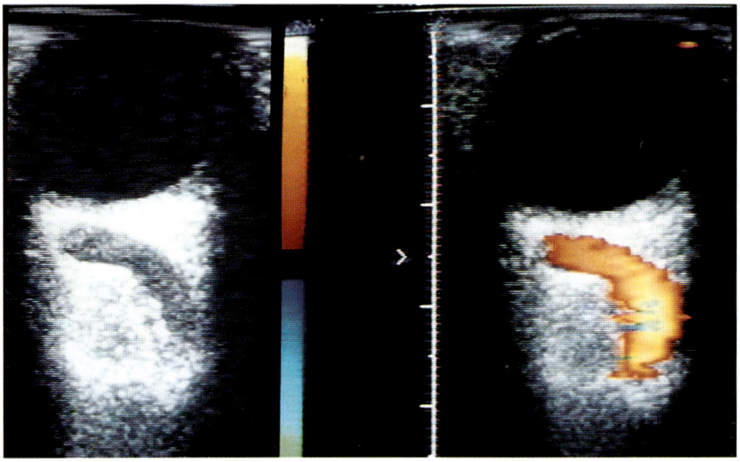

Fig. 6.**24d** Spontaneous fistula between dural arteries and the cavernous sinus. On the left, routine imaging; on the right, simultaneous Doppler analysis (color coding). The red color within the vascular lumen indicates that in this area the direction of flow is toward the transducer. The brighter color in the center of the vessel indicates higher velocity compared to the peripheral blood flow close to the vessel wall

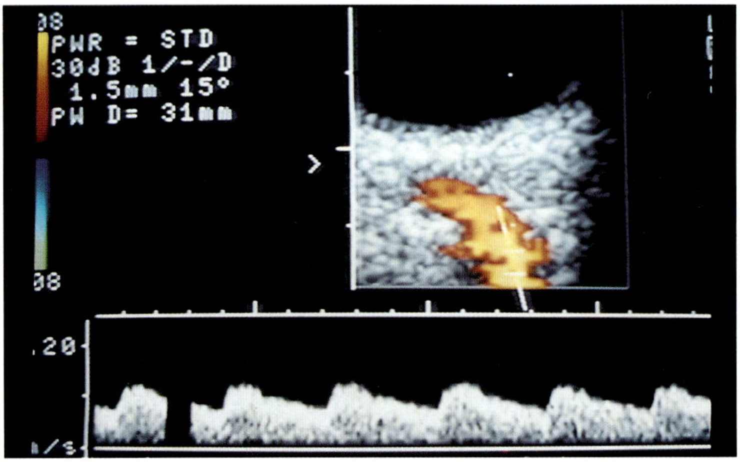


Fig. 6.**24e** A simultaneous frequency analysis reveals that in this example, the maximal systolic flow velocity is about 12 cm/s. The small differences between systolic and diastolic maximal velocity would indicate a high impedance by the peripheral vessels

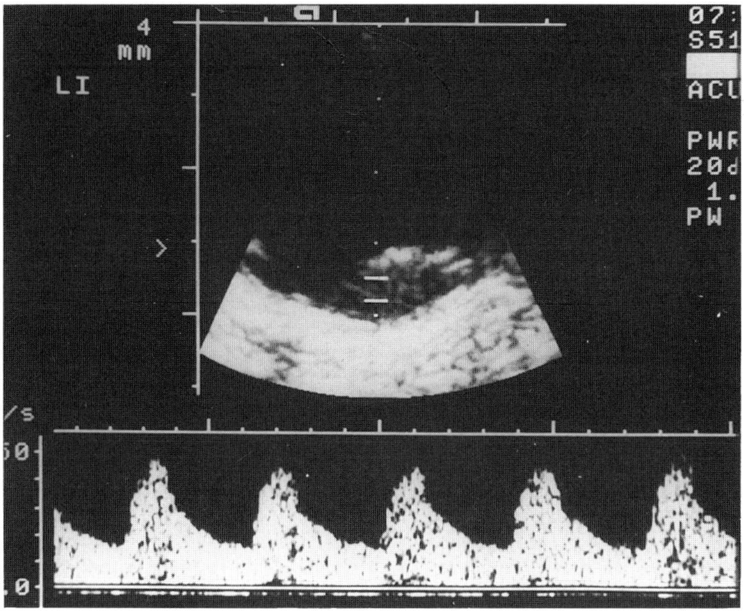


Fig. 4.**73** B-mode Doppler sonography (Duplex technique) of a choroidal melanoma of average size. In A-mode the occasionally observed flickering amplitudes are produced by the blood flow. They can be quantified when using a B-mode Doppler instrument of high resolution.

Table 4.**6** **A-mode echographic signs of a choroidal melanoma** (after Ossoinig) (1972)

1. Uniform internal structure.
   (Equal spike heights or continuous decay from the tumor surface to the sclera.)
2. Low to moderately high spikes from the interior of the tumor (10–60% of the scleral spike).
3. No aftermovements.
4. Signs of vascularization (flickering spikes).

velocities. In our own series, similar frequency shifts could also be observed within a choroidal hemangioma.

#### Possibilities and Limitations of Echographic-Histopathologic Correlations

In the development of echography it has been repeatedly attempted to correlate morphologic aspects of a tumor, especially of a choroidal melanoma, with its ultrasound image. The outer shape of a tumor may be imaged, independent of the quality of the optical media, by a B-mode echogram. However, the various grades of gray are less well quantified than the spikes of an A-mode tracing. Some authors (Rochels et al. 1983) believed that they could echographically differentiate between the various cell types of a choroidal melanoma with a high degree of probability by using certain examination procedures.

Stimulated by an unusual finding (Fig. 4.**74**), we have tried to compare echographic with histologic findings on our own material. We use the A-mode instrument 7200 MA in the examination technique recommended by Ossoinig. We evaluated 39 eyes with melanoma; they were examined echographically and histologically, considering the criteria listed in Table 4.**7**. The echographic measurements of the tumor were obtained with the help of a template for the B-mode. The base of the tumor was measured in the enucleated globe by transillumination after fixation; the elevation was measured in the histologic section.

The comparison (Tables 4.**7** and 4.**8**) showed no correlation between the pigment content and the degree of reflection, as could perhaps be suspected from the example in Fig. 4.**74**. In 32 out of 39 melanomas, however, we found other correlations. We divided the melanomas into one group which had a reflection of up to 45% of the scleral spike, and another group with a reflection up to 60%. The large majority of tumors with hemorrhages belongs to the first group; the same applies to tumors with extensive necroses. Tumors with

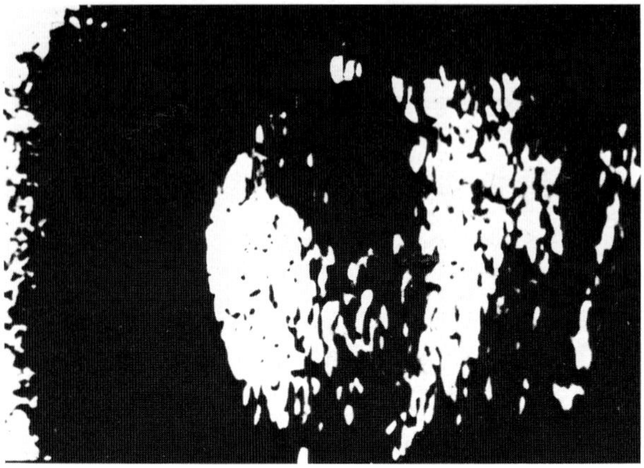

a

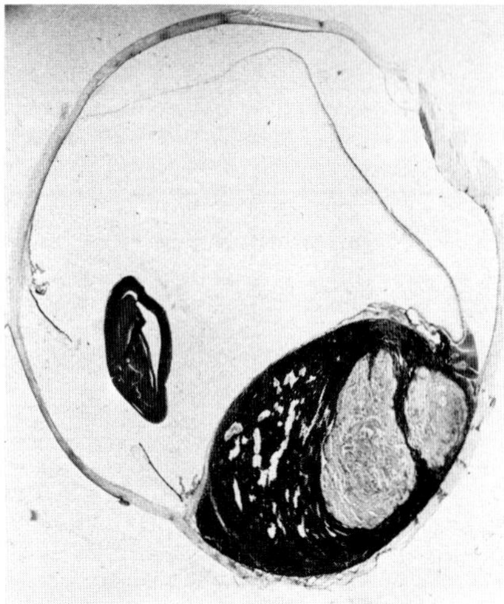

b

Fig. 4.**74 a, b** Cross sectional echogram and histologic specimen of a choroidal melanoma which consists of areas with varying pigmentation
**a** In the cross sectional echogram an area of low reflectivity can be sharply delineated from an area of high reflectivity
**b** Comparing this with the histologic picture we see that the zone of low reflectivity corresponds to an amelantoic part of the tumor; the zone of high reflectivity, to a deeply pigmented part. On the basis of this finding a correlation was suspected between the degree of pigmentation and the intensity of reflectivity. This could not be corroborated in a large series

Table 4.7 **Echographic and histologic parameters used to evaluate choroidal melanoma** (from Guthoff, v. Domarus, Schroeder: Gegenüberstellung klinischer, echographischer und histologischer Befunde beim malignen Melanom der Aderhaut. Klin. Mbl. Augenheilk. 179 [1981] 330)

| Echography | Histology |
|---|---|
| Tumor elevation (mm) | Tumor elevation (mm) |
| Tumor base (mm) | Tumor base (mm) |
| Amount of reflection (%) | Cell type |
| Effect of blood flow | Degree of pigmentation |
| Location (peripheral-posterior pole) | Vascularization (number of vessels, caliber) |
| | Necrosis |
| | Hemorrhages |
| | Connective tissue septa |

Table 4.8 **Choroidal melanoma** (from Guthoff, v. Domarus, Schroeder: Gegenüberstellung klinischer, echographischer und histologischer Befunde beim malignen Melanom der Aderhaut. Klin. Mbl. Augenheilk. 179 [1981] 330)

| Degree of Reflection | 0–45% | 50–60% |
|---|---|---|
| Histologic factors: | | |
| Hemorrhages | 7 | 1 |
| Necrosis | 6 | |
| Septa | 1 | 7 |
| Total | 22 | 17 |

pronounced connective tissue septa (with one exception) had a higher reflection and belonged to the second group. The other histologic characteristics, listed in Table 4.**8**, were evenly divided between the two groups and could not be correlated with a definite echographic feature. When comparing measurements on the size of the tumor, we distinguish between central and peripheral tumors.

Good correlation between histologic and echographic measurements was found for melanomas at the posterior pole; deviations up to 3 mm in tumor height and up to 5 mm in tumor base were observed in peripheral melanomas.

Measurements of the tumor size can therefore be echographically obtained with satisfactory results only for neoplasms at the posterior pole. In peripheral tumors we obtain only an estimate of tumor size.

If we now transfer these results of A-mode comparisons to the clinic, we can deduce that melanomas whith low reflection will probably harbor hemorrhages and/or necroses; a high degree of reflection, on the other hand, points toward an increased connective tissue framework inside the tumor mass. The same interpretation applies to blood-filled cavities in tumor areas in front of breaks in Bruch's membrane through which the tumor expanded. When following melanomas radiated with ruthenium, we also saw an increase in the amount of reflection. This could perhaps be explained as a postradiation increase in connective tissue contents of the tumor.

Compared to the discussions among histologists concerning the classification of various melanoma types, the visual evaluation of the A-mode echogram seems rather crude. Other authors have come to the same conclusion (Freyler et al. 1975, Mazzeo et al. 1988). Including a computerized analysis of the echographic signals (Coleman 1989, Trier 1979) opens new possibilities for tissue differentiation the limits of which cannot be anticipated.

According to our experience, the currently commercially available instruments with their routine echographic tracings cannot yet help us to clinically evaluate the prognosis or recommend a certain treatment modality. However, in about 50% of choroidal melanomas, histological characteristics influence the amount of reflection on the A-mode. This means that a tumor echogram still contains untapped information. For the interpretation of echographic data, loupe magnification corresponds best of the morphologic substrate of an echographic examination. Histopathologic diagnosis on the basis of echographic findings has to be regarded as questionable, purely on the basis of physical considerations. Figure 4.**75** schematically compares the A- and B-mode echographic criteria for a choroidal melanoma.

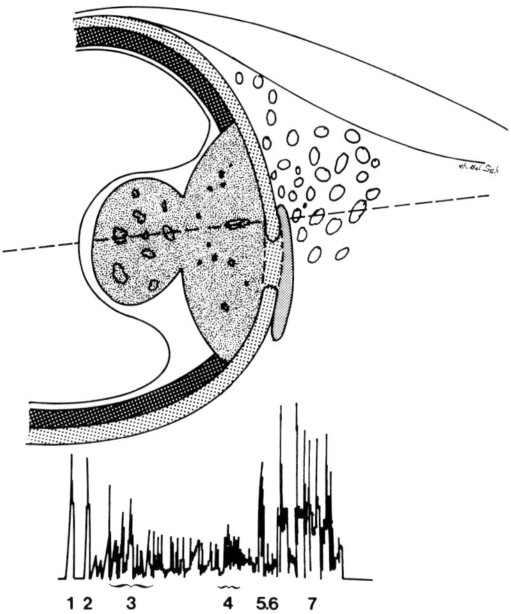


Fig. 4.**75** Schematic presentation of A- and B-mode echographic criteria for a choroidal melanoma
1 Strongly reflecting retinal surface
2 Spike with similar amplitude from the tumor surface
3–6 Signals from inside the tumor which can be used to characterize the type of neoplastic tissue
3 Strong reflectivity produced by the dilated vessels in the part of the tumor lying in front of Bruch's membrane
4 Flickering spikes on A-mode, produced by blood flow
5 Scleral spike
6 Extraocular tumor growth with low reflectivity
7 Orbital fat showing high reflectivity

#### Determining the Volume of a Choroidal Melanoma By Echography

A number of parameters have been evaluated which influence the prognosis of a choroidal melanoma. Among these are the cell type of the tumor, its rate of mitoses, its pigment content, its location and, above all, its size. The first-cited parameters are relatively equivocal and the reported survival rates calculated for each parameter are quite similar. On the other hand, there is no published and generally accepted exact and reproducible method to measure the volume or the size of a choroidal melanoma. It has been recommended that the size of the tumor be compared with the size of the lens (Coleman et a. 1977) or that the largest tumor diameter be measured in mm. Flocks et al. (1955) and Thomas, Green and Maumenee (1979) use the product of length, width and elevation of the tumor as a prognostic indicator. They obtain these measurements from the histologic section. Kramer and Lapiana (1976) published several mathematical equations which allow an exact volume calculation for all possible tumor shapes. The necessary measurements are difficult to determine, even from a histologic section, and are often inaccurate. The conservative treatment of melanomas

Table 4.9a **Correlation between tumor elevation, average tumor diameter and tumor volume in biconvex choroidal melanomas** (after Guthoff, R., D., Hallermann: Ruthenium Irradiation of Choroidal Melanomas – Methods of Planning and Controlling Therapy, in: P., K., Lommatzsch, F. C. Blodi (eds.), Fortschritte der Onkologie, 9, Intraocular Tumors. Akademie-Verlag, Berlin 1983, p. 302 ff.).
Tumor Elevation (mm)

| Tumor Base (mm) | 1.0 | 2.0 | 3.0 | 4.0 | 5.0 | 6.0 | 7.0 | 8.0 | 9.0 | 10.0 |
|---|---|---|---|---|---|---|---|---|---|---|
| 2.0 | 2.0 | 7.1 | 18.3 | 38.8 | 71.7 | 120.2 | 187.4 | 276.5 | 390.6 | 532.8 |
| 3.0 | 3.9 | 10.7 | 23.5 | 45.3 | 79.5 | 129.1 | 197.2 | 287.0 | 401.7 | 544.3 |
| 4.0 | 6.6 | 15.8 | 30.7 | 54.6 | 90.5 | 141.6 | 211.0 | 301.8 | 417.3 | 560.5 |
| 5.0 | 10.0 | 22.4 | 40.2 | 66.6 | 104.7 | 157.8 | 228.8 | 321.0 | 437.5 | 581.5 |
| 6.0 | 14.3 | 30.5 | 51.8 | 81.4 | 122.3 | 177.7 | 250.8 | 344.7 | 462.5 | 607.4 |
| 7.0 | 19.4 | 40.3 | 65.8 | 99.1 | 143.3 | 201.6 | 277.1 | 373.0 | 492.3 | 638.3 |
| 8.0 | 25.3 | 51.6 | 82.1 | 119.8 | 167.9 | 229.5 | 307.9 | 406.1 | 527.2 | 674.5 |
| 9.0 | 32.8 | 64.7 | 100.8 | 143.6 | 196.1 | 291.7 | 343.3 | 444.2 | 527.4 | 716.2 |
| 10.0 | 39.9 | 79.6 | 122.1 | 170.6 | 228.3 | 298.2 | 383.6 | 487.5 | 613.1 | 763.6 |
| 11.0 | 48.7 | 96.4 | 146.2 | 201.2 | 264.6 | 339.5 | 427.1 | 536.4 | 664.7 | 817.1 |
| 12.0 | 58.6 | 115.3 | 173.2 | 235.5 | 305.4 | 335.8 | 480.1 | 591.3 | 722.6 | 877.1 |
| 13.0 | 69.6 | 135.4 | 203.4 | 273.9 | 350.9 | 437.6 | 537.2 | 652.7 | 787.3 | 844.2 |
| 14.0 | 81.8 | 159.9 | 237.1 | 316.7 | 401.7 | 495.3 | 600.8 | 721.1 | 859.5 | 1019.1 |
| 15.0 | 95.6 | 136.1 | 274.7 | 364.3 | 458.3 | 559.7 | 671.7 | 797.4 | 939.0 | 1102.5 |
| 16.0 | 110.0 | 215.4 | 316.5 | 417.5 | 521.4 | 631.5 | 750.8 | 822.5 | 1029.7 | 1195.6 |
| 17.0 | 128.0 | 248.1 | 363.4 | 477.0 | 592.1 | 711.9 | 839.3 | 977.7 | 1130.2 | 1299.8 |
| 18.0 | 147.3 | 285.0 | 416.2 | 544.1 | 671.7 | 802.3 | 939.0 | 1084.9 | 1243.2 | 1417.0 |

Tumor Volume ($mm^3$)

Table 4.9b **Schematic drawing and mathematical approach to determine tumor volume** under the assumption that choroidal melanomas are biconvex in cross-section (Guthoff 1980)

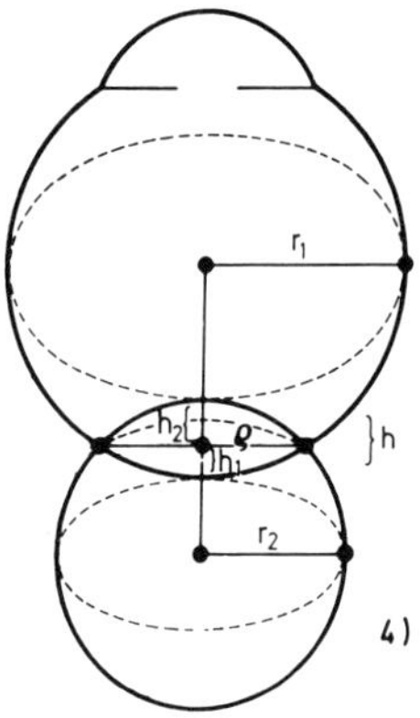


1) $V = \pi \cdot \frac{h^2}{3} \cdot (3r - h)$

2) $V = \pi \frac{h}{6} (3\varrho^2 + h^2)$

3) $V = \pi \frac{h_2}{6} (3\varrho^2 + h_2^2) + \pi \frac{h_1^2}{3} (3r - h_1)$

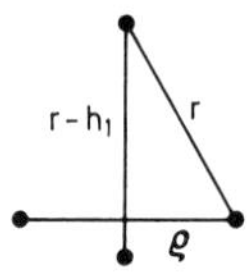


$h = r - \sqrt{r^2 - \varrho^2}$

$h_2 = h - h_1$

4) $V = \frac{\pi}{6} \left[ (h - r + \sqrt{r^2 - \varrho^2}) \cdot (3\varrho^2 + (h - r + \sqrt{r^2 - \varrho^2})^2) + 2 \cdot (r - \sqrt{r^2 - \varrho^2})^2 \cdot (3r - r + \sqrt{r^2 - \varrho^2}) \right]$

(brachyradiation, external radiation with protons or helium ions) do not provide us data from histologic specimens. Echography is capable of giving us precise measurements on tumor size as we need them for the conservative treatment of melanomas.

In this connection, we have to ask questions concerning the

- elevation of the tumor and
- extent of the tumor base.

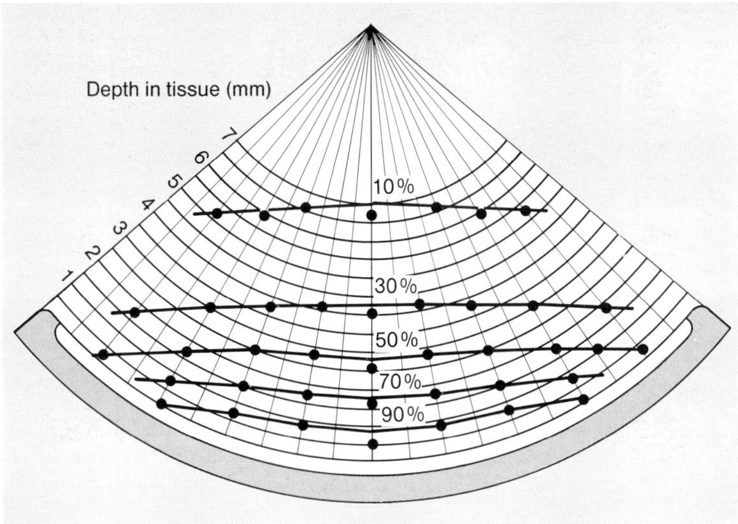


Fig. 4.**76** Measuring protocol for a Ruthenium Applicator Type CCC; diameter of the emitting plane, 21 mm. At 5 mm from the applicator surface, only 25% of the scleral contact dose is still available. Because of this steep decay of effective radiation it is indispensable to plan the treatment exactly

Both can be measured echographically. The precision with which we can determine these parameters depends upon a number of factors. When measuring the elevation of a tumor, we are dealing with the velocity of sound as we know it from other biometrical examinations (see oculometry in eyes with intraocular lens implants). We determine the time which the ultrasound beam needs from the tumor surface to the surface of the sclera. In order to obtain reliable values, we have to localize the tumor peak precisely. The sound velocity within the tumor has been determined as 1660 m/s (Coleman et al. 1964, Nover et al. 1965). In order to measure exactly the lateral extent of a tumor, the quality of electrical mechanical coupling with the B-mode transducer and amplifier is decisive. The lateral resolution power of a modern contact B-mode machine is around ± 2 mm (Guthoff et al. 1981). The reliability of such measurements becomes questionable when the peak of the tumor lies anterior to the equator.

Confining ourselves primarily to biconvex tumors (as these represent the majority of cases treated conservatively by radiation), we can calculate the tumor volume from the elevation of the tumor and the average between the largest and smallest diameter of the tumor base. Table 4.**9a** lists these tumor volumes by using a calculation (Table 4.**9b**) published in 1980 (Guthoff et al.). Newly developed equipment (Coleman et al. 1989) allows computer reconstructions of various acoustical sections for higher precision in tumor volume measurements.

## Brachyradiotherapy of Choroidal Melanomas

### The Role of Echography for Planning the Treatment and Following Its Results

#### Planning the Treatment

The aim of any radiation therapy is to destroy tumor tissue and to spare adjacent tissues as far as possible. Scleral contact radiotherapy using ruthenium-106, cobalt-90 or iodine-125 applicators, shows a relatively steep decay of radiation dosage. It is therefore important to determine the exact extent of the tumor to be treated. Figure 4.**76** shows the isodose curves for ruthenium-106 applicators. At a distance of about 8 mm from the radiation surface, only 10% of the energy is still available. In order to achieve complete tumor necrosis in this area, we therefore need an application

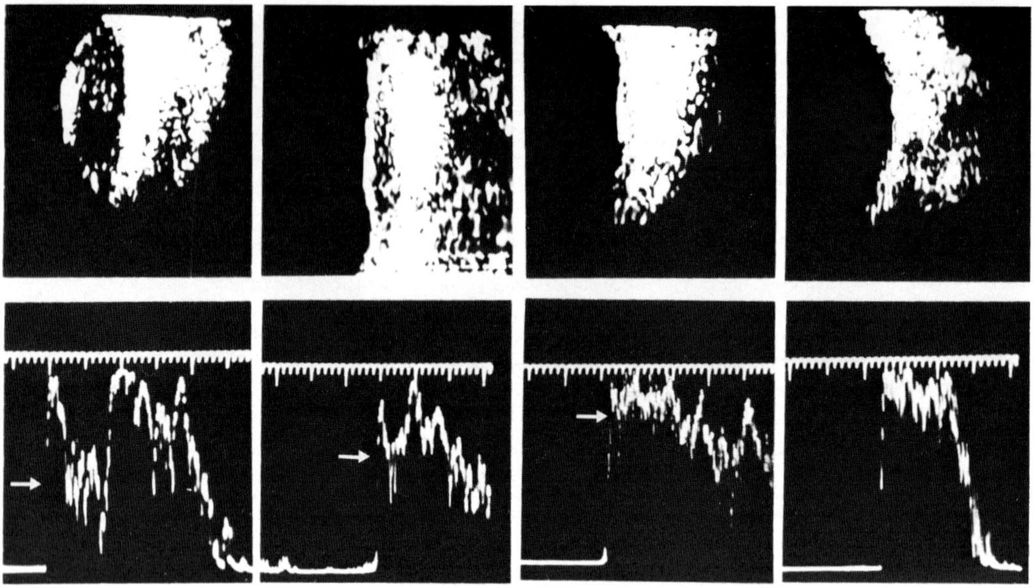

Before radiation
Vol. 380 mm$^3$
Refl. 40%

After 4 months
Vol. 230 mm$^3$
Refl. 80%

After 8 months
Vol. 100 mm$^3$
Refl. 90%

After 10 months
Vol. 0 mm$^3$

Fig. 4.**77** A- and B-mode echograms during follow-up controls of a successfully treated choroidal melanoma. The tumor volume was reduced from 380 t0 0 cmm within ten months. After eight months the spikes within the tumor increased from about 40% of the scleral spike to about 90% (white arrows) (from Guthoff et al.: 10 Jahre Erfahrung mit der Ruthenium-106/Rhodium-106-Behandlung des malignen Melanoms der Aderhaut. Klin. Mbl. Augenheilk. 188 [1986] 576)

time 10 times the duration of radiation treatment for a part of the tumor close to the sclera. It is important to take into account a retinal detachment over the peak of the tumor when calculating the total tumor elevation. In this way we avoid unnecessary side effects (Fig. 4.**66**).

## Treatment Control

It is advisable to check the position of the applicator in relation to the tumor and the sclera already on the first postoperative day. In a few cases a slit may be seen between the applicator surface and the scleral surface. In these cases the duration of application has to be correspondingly prolonged (Coleman 1987, Guthoff 1980) (Figs. 4.**79**, 4.**80**). If these changes are not considered, the tumor dosage may be too low.

In addition to a precise ophthalmoscopic control of the radiated tumor, the following echographic parameters have proven valuable in checking the treatment effect:

1. elevation of the tumor;
2. tumor base (these two factors determine the tumor volume);
3. reflectivity of the internal tumor structure.

Figure 4.**77** illustrates an echographically documented successful treatment of a choroidal melanoma. Within ten months the volume was reduced from 380 cmm to 0 cmm; already after four months there was a marked increase of reflectivity in the internal tumor structures.

In some cases (Fig. 4.**78**) the increased reflectivity within the tumor is the only echographic parameter which changes after radiotherapy. The A-mode echogram alone, however, does not allow us to correlate a possible complete tumor necrosis with the ultrasound image. In our own patient material, we have tumors which showed a similar echographic behavior, but still contained viable tumor cells though their malignant potential could not be estimated.

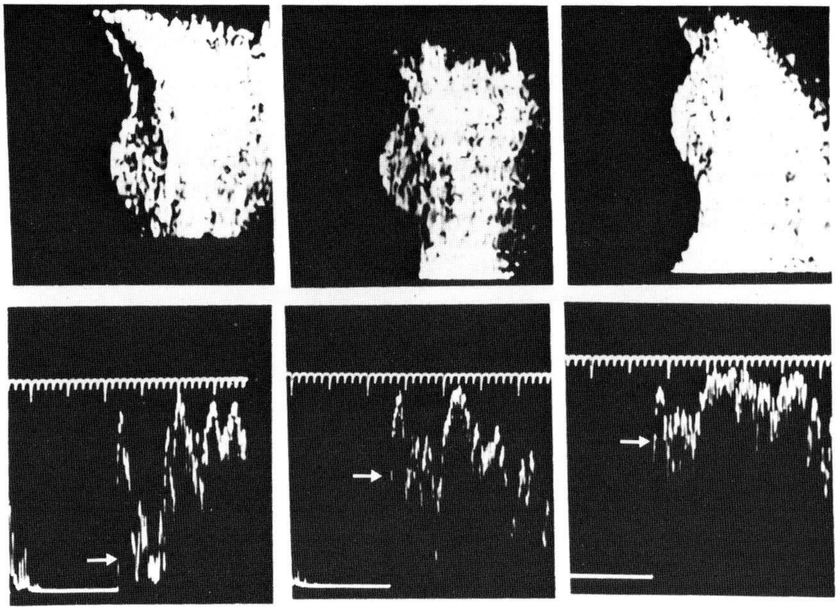

Befor radiation
Vol. 250 mm$^3$
Refl. 20%

8 months after radiation
Vol. 250 mm$^3$
Refl. 70%

36 months after 1st radiation
22 months after 2nd radiation
Vol. 250 mm$^3$, Refl. 80%

Fig. 4.**78** A- and B-mode echograms demonstrating the effect of brachyradiotherapy on a choroidal melanoma. The external shape of the tumor also remains unchanged after the second series of radiation; the reflectivity of the tumor increases from about 20% of the scleral spike before radiation to about 80% after radiation (white arrows) (Guthoff et al.: 10 Jahre Erfahrung mit der Ruthenium-106/Rhodium-106-Behandlung des malignen Melanoms der Aderhaut. Klin. Mbl. Augenheilk. 188 [1986] 576)

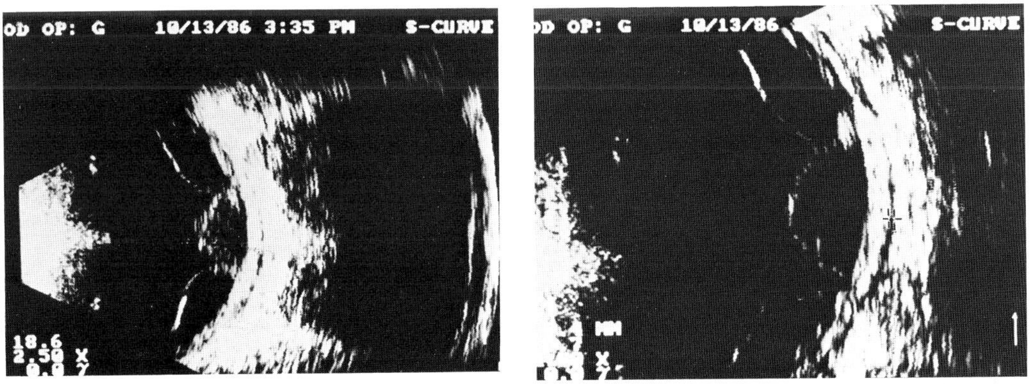


a b

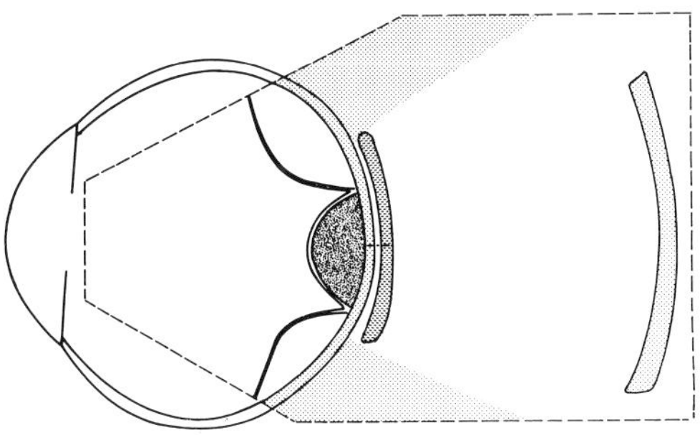

c

Fig. 4.**79a–c**
**a, b** Echogram of an eye with the Ruthenium-Beta applicator in place. The slit between the posterior scleral surface and the applicator is filled with fluid and is less than 0.5 mm wide (measuring marks shown). The lateral extent of the applicator is marked by the sound shadow
**c** Schematic drawing

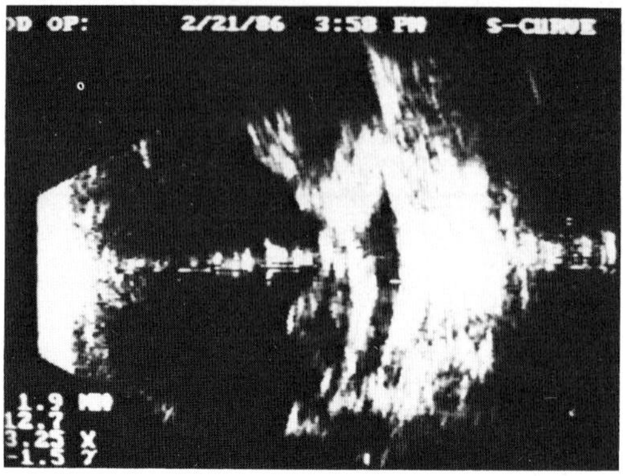

a

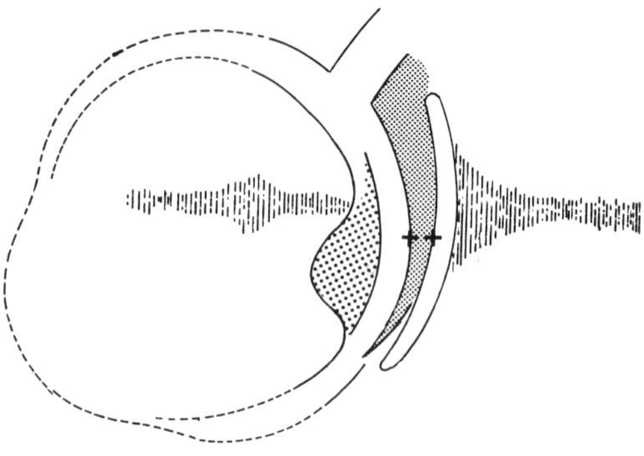
b

Fig. 4.**80** a, b
**a, b** Ruthenium-Beta applicator in place with a wide slit between the sclera and the applicator surface. On the basis of this echographic finding the position of the applicator should be changed or the duration of the treatment has to be prolonged. Distance of the measuring marks: 1.9 mm. **b** Schematic drawing

**Additional Information on Treatment Control Using B-Mode Doppler Instruments**

An essential aspect of the biological impact of radiotherapy is its effect on tumor vessels. We can expect that the blood flow in a highly vascularized choroidal melanoma will change under the influence of radiation. High-frequency ultrasound B-mode Doppler instruments will therefore provide additional information about the destruction produced in the tumor.

We examined 23 patients in our clinic before and after ruthenium radiotherapy with a Doppler sonographic instrument (Guthoff et al. 1989). In summary, we can state that two to three days after removing the applicator, an increase in maximal flow velocity in the tumor vessels was noted in some cases. Two to ten months postradiation, the volume of all tumors had decreased. A third of the eyes did not show a Doppler shift in the remaining tumefaction. In 3 of the 23 patients there was minimal remaining circulation, and in 7 eyes, the flow velocity in the tumor vessels remained unchanged though ophthalmoscopically, the melanoma showed definite radiation effects. In two patients no frequency shift could be detected in the remaining tumefactions, which, 1½ to 2 years after radiation, still had volumes of 150 and 400 $mm^3$. The interpretation of these findings is speculative.

Determining the blood flow by B-mode Doppler sonography provides us with an additional parameter which could indicate that these remaining tumefactions are actually necrotic masses which are not broken down and absorbed because the adjacent vessels have been damaged by the radiation (Fig. 4.**81 a**: elevated tumor before radiation; Fig. 4.**81 b**: elevated remaining tumefaction with biphasic Doppler sound, which is not synchronous with the pulse).

### 4.4.4 Metastatic Choroidal Tumors

In 12% of 230 patients who died from carcinoma, metastases could be found in the eye on pathologic examination (Bloch et al. 1971). According to these findings, many intraocular metastases certainly remain undetected. The average survival time after treatment is 7.4 months (Ferry et al. 1974). Many of these patients are therefore not followed ophthalmologically. The most frequent primary tumors are breast (40%) and lungs (29%). All types of carcinoma and sarcoma may metastasize to the choroid.

A typical carcinoma metastasis to the choroid presents a high-reflecting thickening of the ocular coat. The internal acoustic properties resemble a disciform macular degeneration or a choroidal hemangioma (Fig. 4.**82**). A metastatic adenocarcinoma (Fig. 4.**83**) may, because of its adenoid-like histologic structure, present strong acoustic interfaces.

During the last years different echographic patterns have been reported which do not fit into this definite picture (Manschot 1981, Verbeek 1981). In one instance, a metastasis from a small-cell bronchial carcinoma was echographically misin-

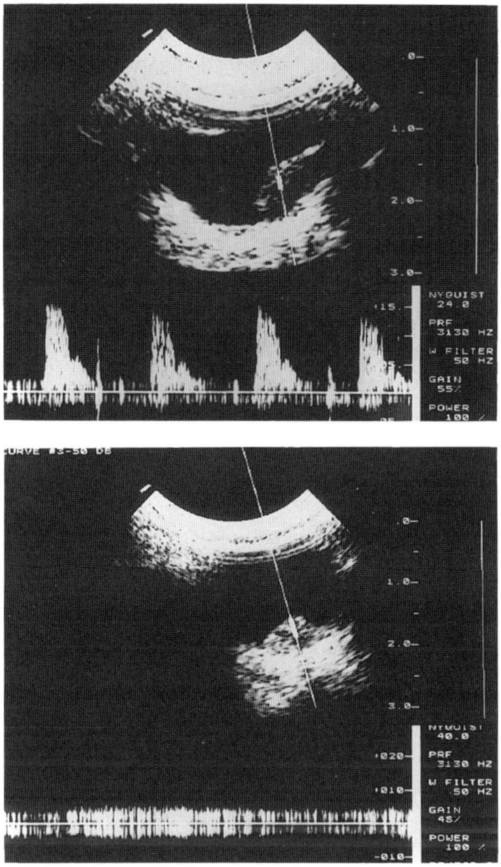


a

b

Fig. 4.**81 a** Choroidal melanoma with an elevation of 5 mm. Cross sectional echogram obtained with the Duplex instrument ATL MARK 8. The sample volume is identified by the marks on the aiming beam. In this area Doppler spectra are obtained indicating a high blood flow velocity (represented in the lower part of the illustration)
**b** Same patient as in **a**, four months after radiation treatment of the choroidal melanoma with ruthenium. There is still a considerable volume of tumor remaining (maximal elevation, about 3.5 mm). No frequency shift can be obtained from the interior of the tumor when using Duplex examination. The tissue lying in the guiding beam produces only a biphasic noise (illustrated in the lower part of the picture)

terpreted and the eye enucleated because a melanoma was suspected (Fig. 4.**84**) (Verbeek 1981).

Choroidal metastases from a cutaneous melanoma cannot be differentiated clinically or echographically from a primary choroidal melanoma (de Bustos et al. 1985). Some authors have claimed a high

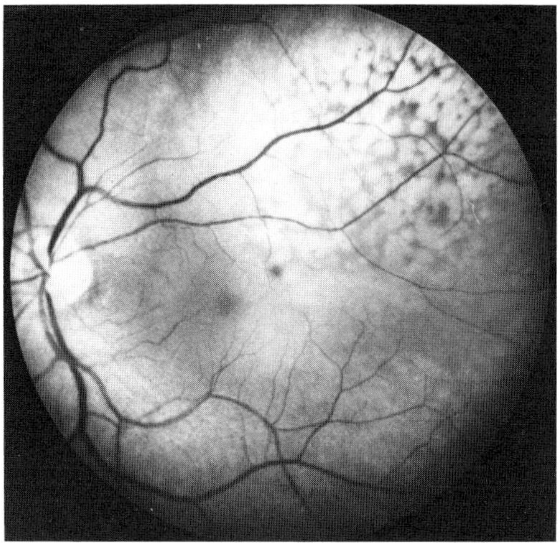

Fig. 4.**81** Choroidal metastasis from a breast carcinoma. Temporal from the disk is a subretinal space-occupying lesion with an exudative retinal detachment and a circumscribed reaction of the pigment epithelium

specificity of the echogram in metastatic carcinomas (Ossoinig 1979, Hauff et al. 1980). This statement should be modified on the basis of new experiences.

### 4.4.5 Choroidal Hemangioma

Choroidal hemangioma may be an isolated lesion or may be one of the signs of the Sturge-Weber syndrome (Font 1972). Isolated hemangiomas usually occur at the posterior pole. They are slightly elevated and associated with a retinal detachment and secondary changes of the pigment epithelium. They are rather diffuse, with blurred margins, and therefore barely recognizable with the ophthalmoscope (Fig. 4.**85**). Only the histologic examination of the enucleated globe will reveal the actual size (Witschel et al. 1976). Echographically, they appear as a strongly reflecting, nearly concentric widening of the ocular coats. The echogram of a choroidal hemangioma is similar to that of metastatic adenocarcinoma or disciform macular degeneration. In spite of the abundant vascularization, choroidal hemangiomas do not echographically show with conventional techniques circulating blood as we see it in choroidal melanomas. Due to the slow circulation, we might be dealing here with laminar flow in the cavities of dilated blood vessels,

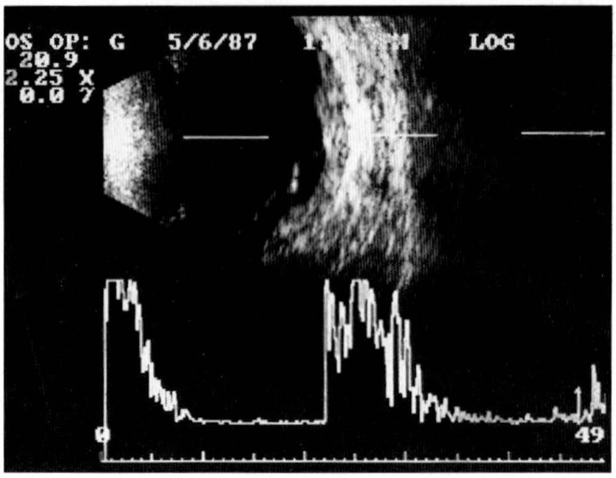


a

◀ Fig. 4.**83 a–c** Extensive choroidal metastatic tumor in the lower nasal quadrant
**a** On the echogram the choroid is widened to about 2.5 mm; the retina is partly detached by an exudate. The tissue inside the metastatic tumor shows high acoustic reflectivity
**b** Histologic section of a metastatic adenocarcinoma in the choroid. The gland-like structure provides good acoustic interfaces
**c** Schematic drawing

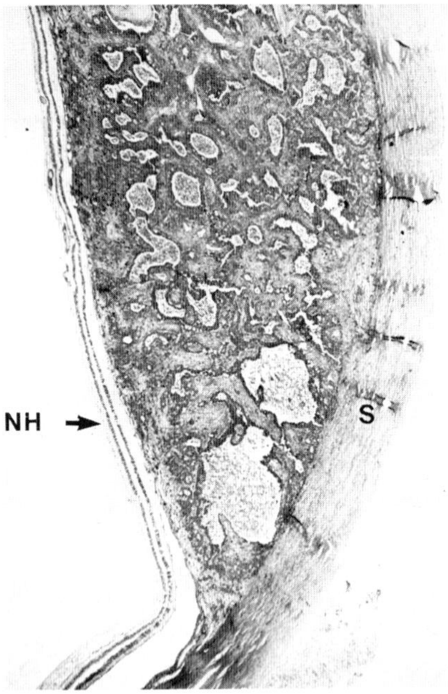


b

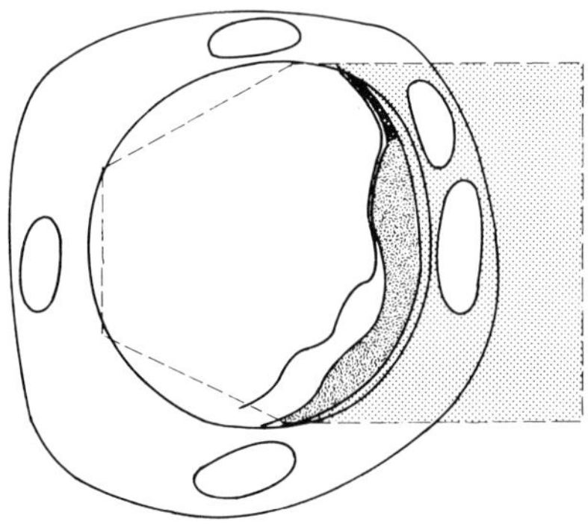

c

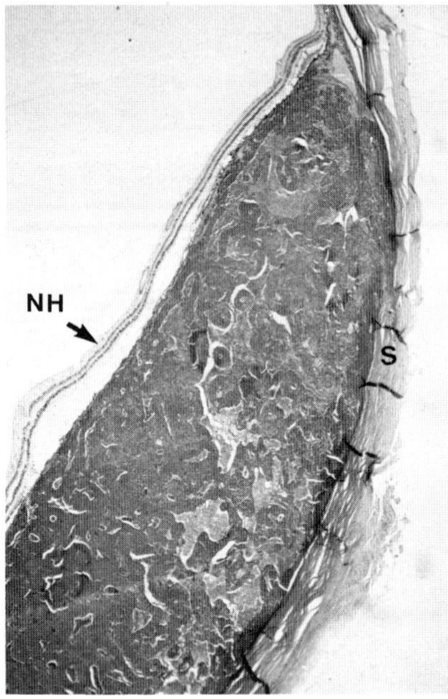


Fig. 4.**84** Metastatic tumor from a small-cell bronchial carcinoma. The echogram resembled that of a typical choroidal melanoma. Similar findings have been seen in choroidal metastases from cutaneous melanoma

Fig. 4.**85 a–d** Extensive choroidal hemangioma in Sturge-Weber syndrome (additional finding: total retinal detachment) ▶
**a** Cross sectional echogram through the area of the optic nerve head. In the lower quadrant the ocular coats are markedly thickend. (In spite of the associated retinal detachment, the intraocular pressure was 50 mmHg by applanation)
**b** With reduced sensitivity, the scleral surface can be delineated in spite of the high acoustic reflectivity within the tumor (distance of the measuring marks 3.1 mm)
**c** Histologic section through the tumor illustrated in **a** and **b**: The septa of the cavities are thin and lined with endothelium. They produce strong reflectivity within the lesion
**d** Schematic drawing

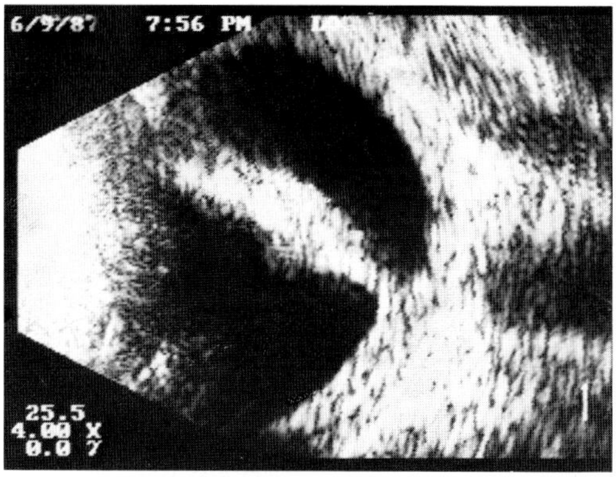


a

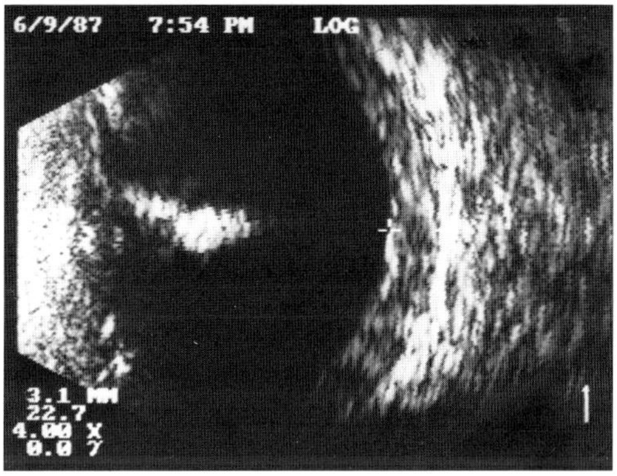


b

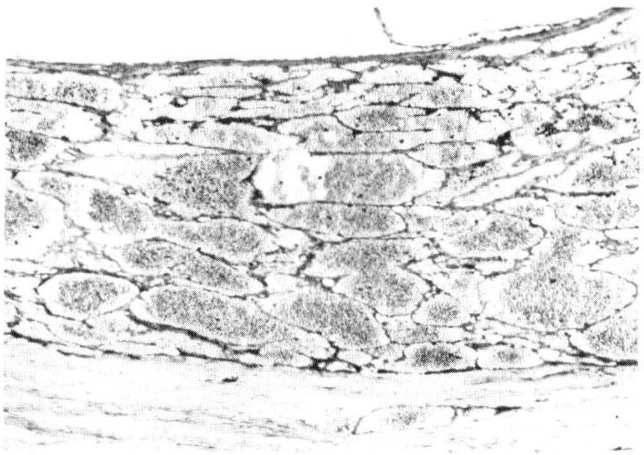

c

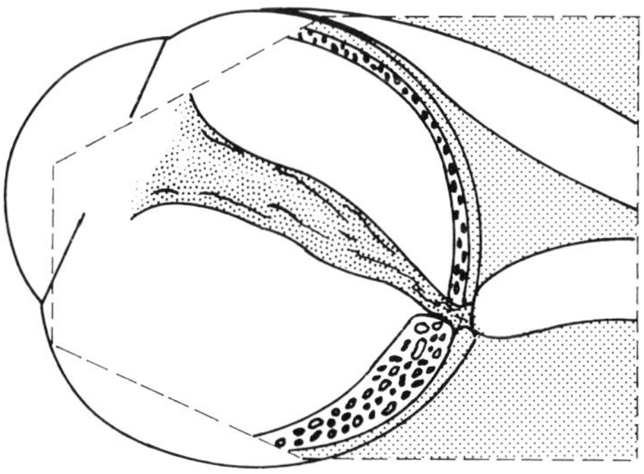

d

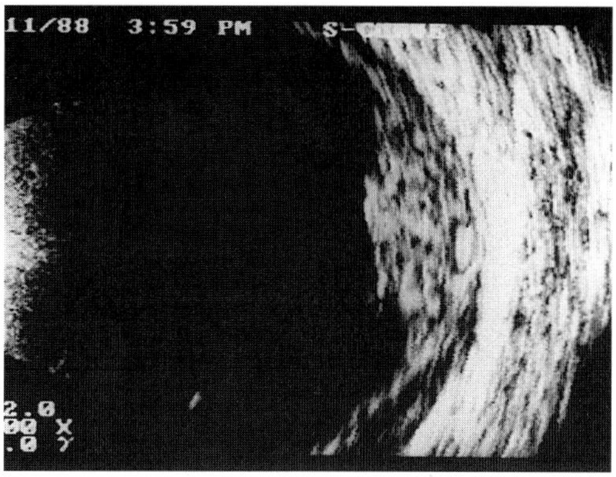


a

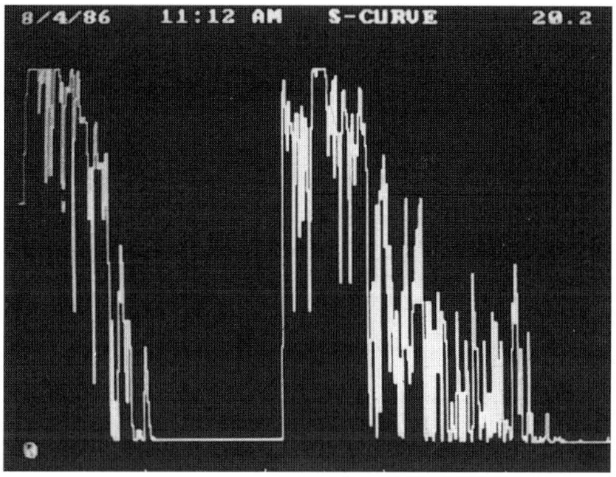


b

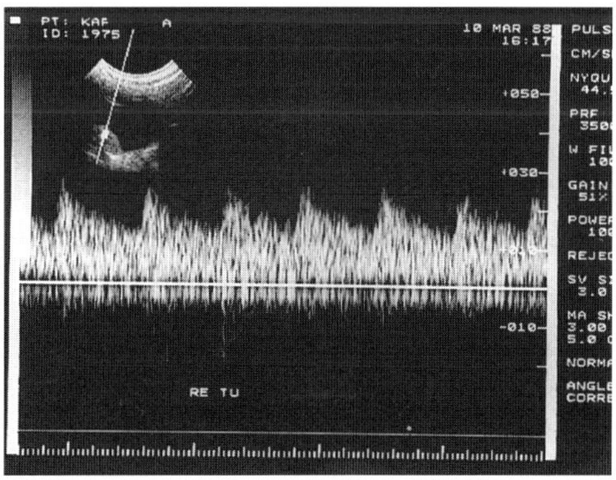


c

Fig. 4.**86a–c**

**a** Cross sectional echogram of a circumscribed choroidal hemangioma in a 12 year old boy. The tumor has an elevation of 4 mm

**b** In an A-mode echogram with S-shaped amplification the cross sectional picture corroborates the high reflectivity of the tumor

**c** On Doppler sonography (Duplex scanner ATL MARK 8), we see blood circulating within the tumor, synchronous with the pulse. The illustrated velocity profile speaks for a relatively low resistance by the blood vessels

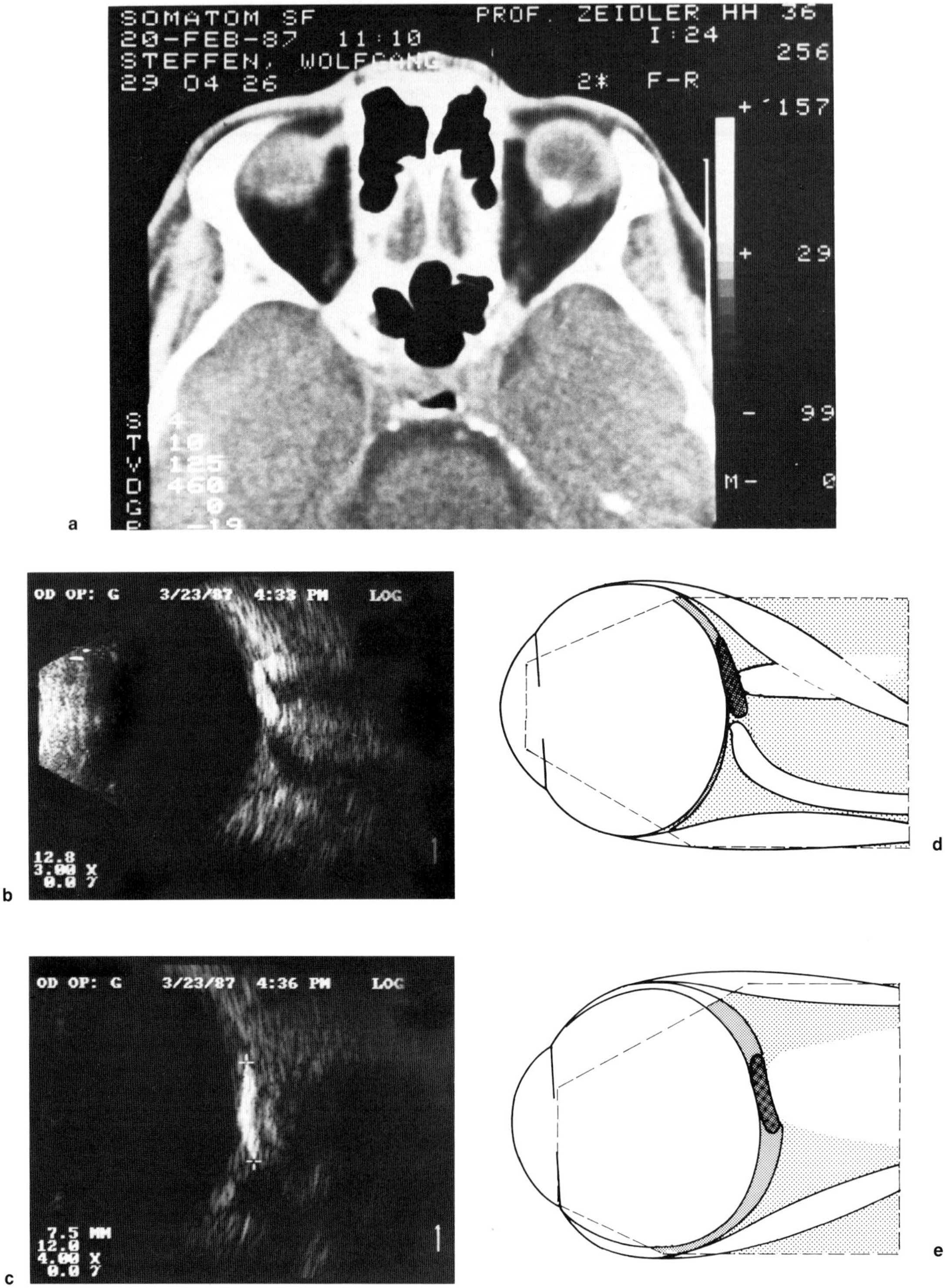
SOMATOM SF
PROF. ZEIDLER HH 36
20-FEB-87 11:10
I:24
STEFFEN, WOLFGANG
256
29 04 26
2* F-R
+157
+ 29
- 99
M- 0
a
OD OP: G 3/23/87 4:33 PM LOG
12.8
3.00 X
0.0 7
b
OD OP: G 3/23/87 4:36 PM LOG
7.5 MM
12.0
4.00 X
0.0 7
c
d
e

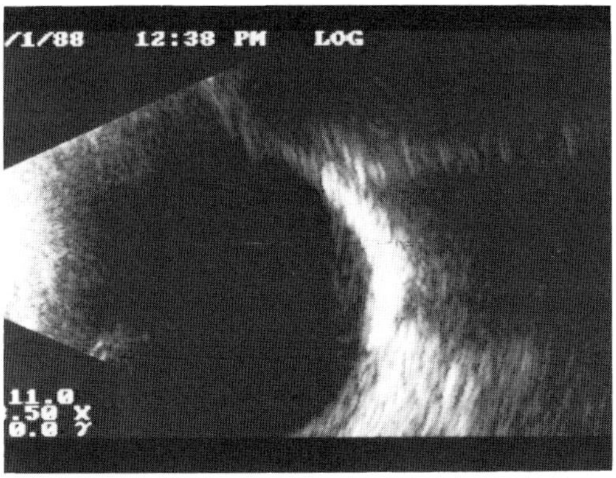

b

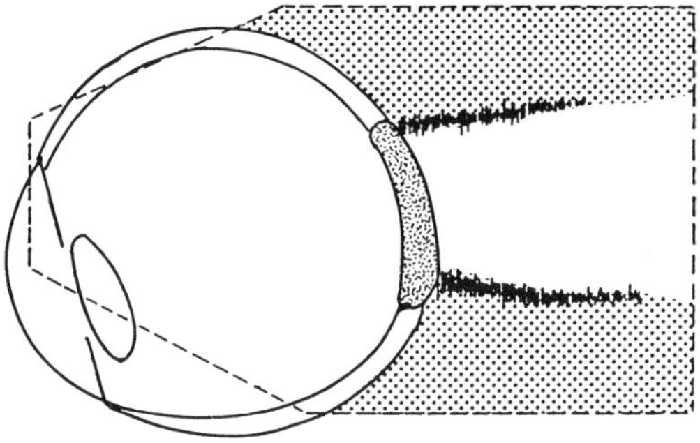
d

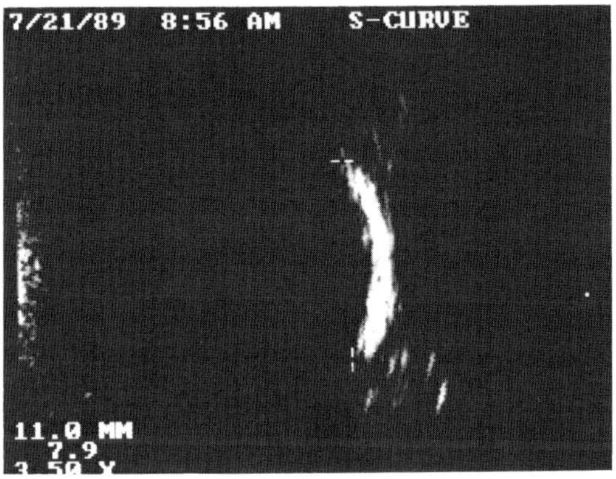

c

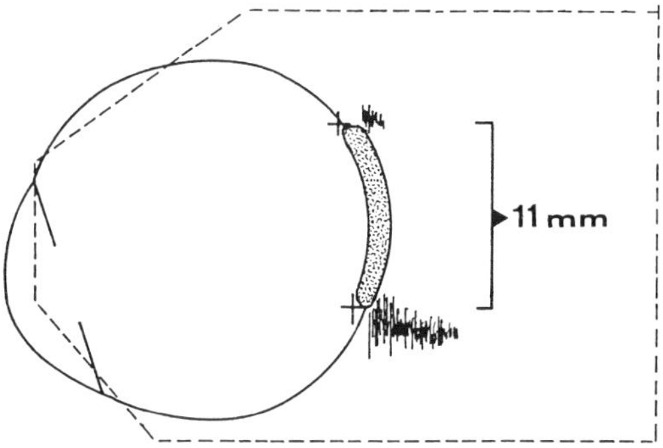

e

Fig. 4.**88a–e** Choroidal osteoma **a** See color plates
**b** Cross sectional echogram of the choroidal osteoma shown in **a**: in this echogram the lesion is characterized by total reflection of the ultrasound, and shadow formation. An elevation cannot be unequivocally documented
**c** Schematic drawing
**d** With reduced amplification it is possible to image the ossification as an isolated signal. The horizontal diameter is 11.0 mm
**e** Schematic drawing (Fig. 4.**88a–e** from Guthoff et al. Osteome der Bulbuswand. Erscheinungsformen in Abhängigkeit von Lage und Ausdehnung, Klin. Monatsbl. f. Augenhk., in press)

◀ Fig. 4.**87a–e** Metastatic calcification of the ocular coats of unknown etiology; differential diagnosis: choroidal osteoma
**a** A CT scan was obtained because of nonophthalmological problems. A circumscribed calcified structure within the ocular coats was found incidentally
**b** In cross sectional echograms, a lesion of the ocular coats above the optic nerve head showed total reflection of the ultrasound
**c** The lateral extension was about 7.5 mm
The fundus of this 52-year-old man was normal and so was his vision. A metastatic calcification of unknown etiology was assumed. We know from the literature that choroidal osteomas produce nearly identical echograms, but they are associated with ophthalmoscopically visible changes
**d, e** Schematic drawings

which could be shown by Doppler ultrasonography (Fig. 4.**86c**). The pronounced vascular supply of the tumor can occasionally be proven by tonography. The oscillations of intraocular pressure are synchronous with the pulse and can be demonstrated by the excursion of the tonogram (Jörgensen et al. 1987).

In long-standing cases the epichoroidal layer may ossify, producing sound shadows. In this stage a hemangioma cannot be differentiated from an osteoma or a metastatic calcification of the choroid (Shields et al. 1989, Wende et al. 1978).

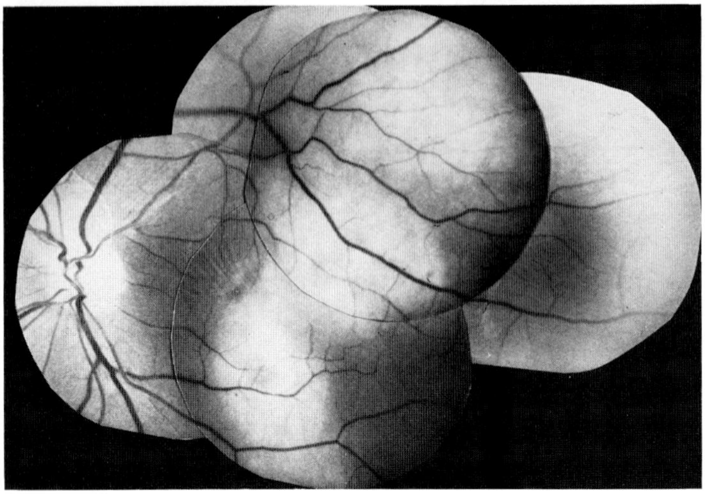

Fig. 4.**89** Fundus picture of a 52-year-old woman with active pulmonary tuberculosis. Vision: 0.1

### 4.4.6 Choroidal Osteoma – Metastatic Calcifications

Choroidal osteoma is a rare condition which has to be differentiated from a hemangioma or a metastatic carcinoma (Gass 1978, 1979, Wing et al. 1972). Echographically, the lesion is characterized by a localized area of high reflectivity at the ocular coats, manifesting all the signs of a dense calcium foreign body (Fig. 4.**87**). In order to differentiate this lesion from metastatic calcification of the choroid and the sclera, the calcium metabolism has to be checked (Shields et al. 1987, Zakov et al. 1987). The two conditions give identical clinical, echographic and CT scan images.

Ossification of the ocular coats may be caused by a number of etiologic factors. Morgagni described these changes for the first time, based on observations by Morand (1730). These were all bone formations in blind, phthisical eyes. Bone develops in tissue, due to altered metabolism, and is based on calcium deposition which acts as a stimulant for osteoblastic activity. Poniedel (1947) described uveal deposits of calcium salts in a patient with hyperparathyroidism. Bony tissue may also develop as a result of the activity of displaced osteoblasts, without any systemic or local metabolic disorder (Fig. 4.**88a–e**). This is the etiology of an osseous choristoma (Gass 1979) or of an episcleral plaque, which may be visible from the outside.

Clinically (Fig. 4.**88a**), choroidal hemangioma and a metastatic carcinoma have to be differentiated (Gass 1978, 1979; Wing 1982). Episcleral ossification (Fig. 4.**88**) is usually diagnosed incidentally when a CT scan reveals calcium densities in the ocular wall or when ultrasound is totally reflected by this scleral plaque, and a shadow is cast behind it (Guthoff 1990).

It has been recommended that the calcium metabolism be checked in order to differentiate a metastatic calcification from bone formed by displaced osteoblasts (Shields et al. 1990, Zakov et al. 1990). If the choroid is involved, these conditions will produce identical clinical, echographic and CT scan pictures.

### 4.4.7 Choroidal Tuberculoma

Choroidal tuberculomas are extremely rare (Blodi 1977). According to the literature, it is not possible to differentiate this lesion clinically from a choroidal melanoma. Ophthalmoscopy, fluorescein angiography, P32 uptake and echography do not provide us with unequivocal results. In our clinic we observed a woman (Figs. 4.**89**, 4.**90**) with acute pulmonary tuberculosis and a fundus lesion which improved within four months on antituberculous treatment. According to the literature (Blodi 1977), a comparable choroidal lesion may occur even years after the primary tuberculous complex has healed, without any other signs of a recurrence. Our single observation does not allow us to claim that the demonstration of Tenon's space is a characteristic finding here (Fig. 4.**90**).

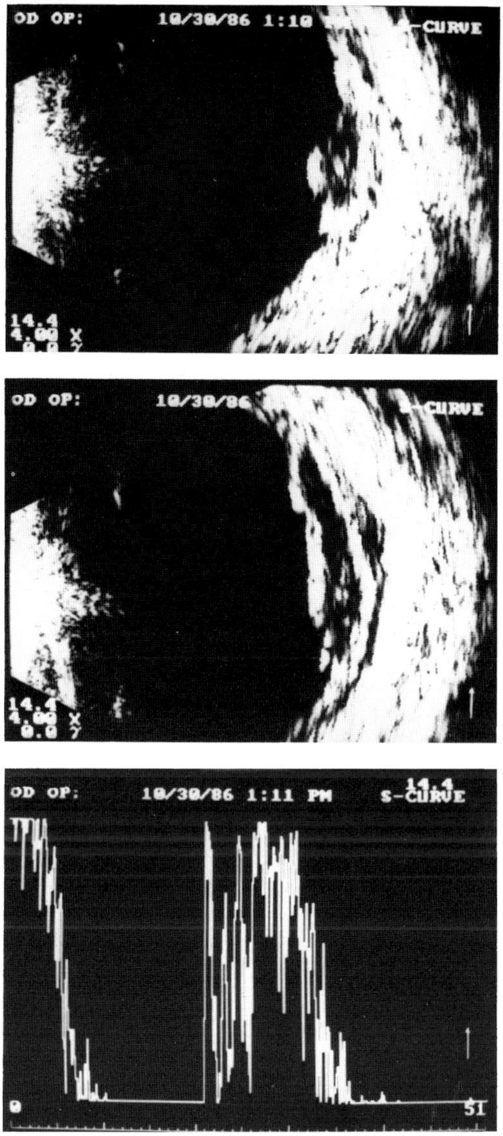


a
b
c

Fig. 4.**90** **a–c** Echogram of the fundus lesion shown in Fig. 4.**89**. The lesion is characterized by low acoustic reflectivity. Tenon's space can be well demonstrated. The reflectivity corresponds to that of a choroidal melanoma. The infiltration of Tenon's space points toward inflammatory etiology

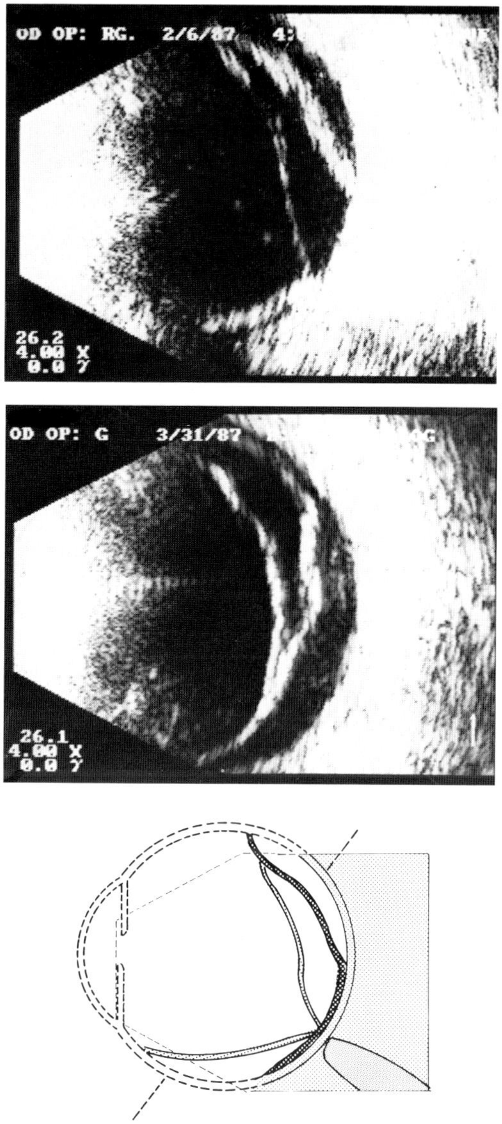


a
b
c

Fig. 4.**91** **a–c** Uveal effusion syndrome in a 55-year-old woman

**a** In the axial cross section, the retina is attached to the optic nerve head. There is an associated, strongly reflecting choroidal detachment

**b** Cross section at 90° to **a**

**c** Schematic drawing

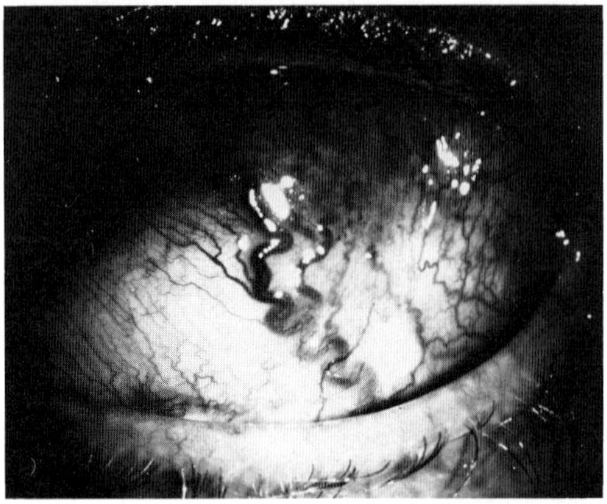

Fig. 4.**92** Conspicuous sectorial dilatation of conjunctival and episcleral vessels in an eye with brawny scleritis

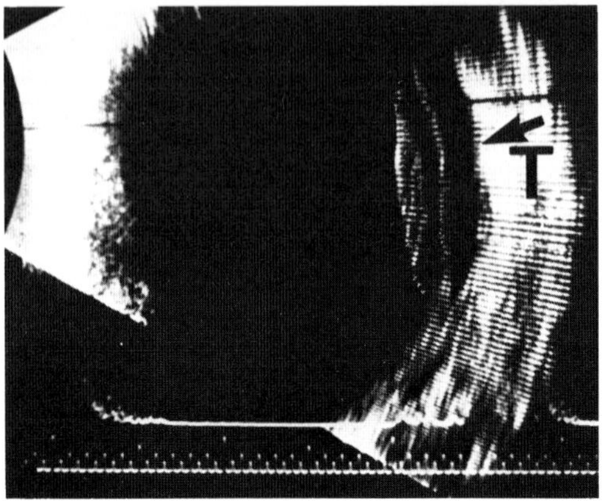


a

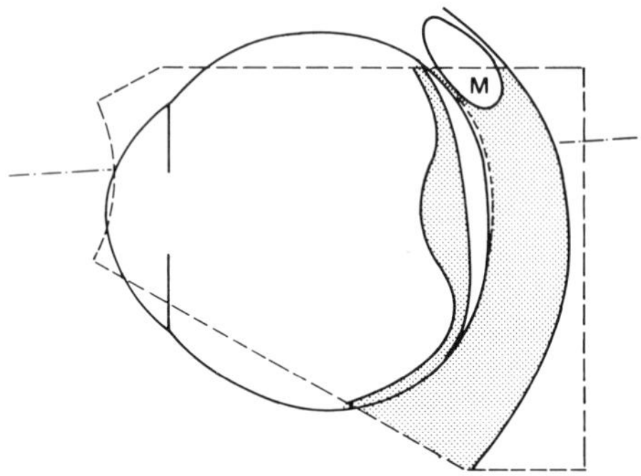


b

Fig. 4.**93 a, b**
**a** Brawny scleritis with inflammatory infiltration of Tenon's space. This disease entity can occasionally be neither clinically nor echographically differentiated from a choroidal melanoma (T = Tenon's space, M = cross section through a muscle)
**b** Schematic drawing

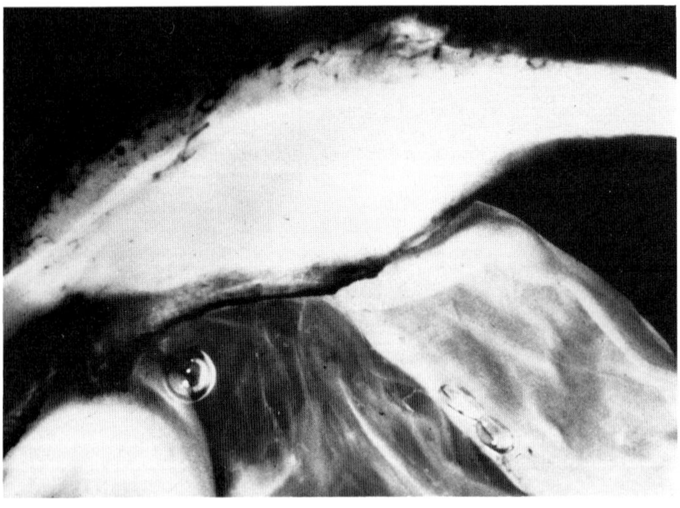

Fig. 4.**94** Macroscopic photo of a brawny scleritis. On the basis of the echographic findings and a positive P32 test, the eye was enucleated because a melanoma was suspected

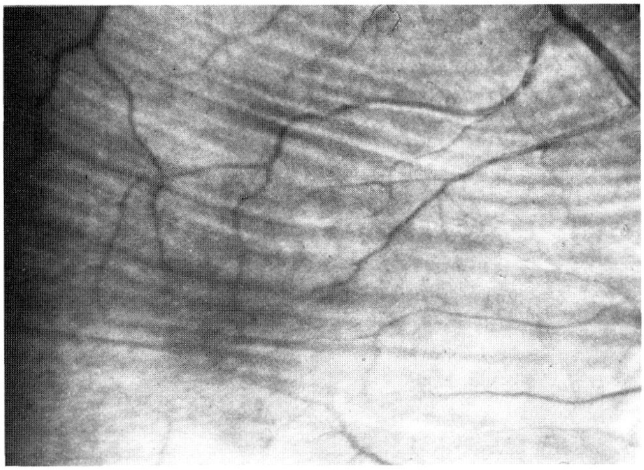
a

Fig. 4.**95** **a, b** Posterior scleritis
**a** Choroidal folds in the macular area. Best corrected vision: 0.4 with metamorphopsia (acute hyperopia of 3 diopters)
**b** Change of echographic findings with systemic corticosteroid treatment over four weeks. In spite of a clinically complete healing, the infiltration of Tenon's space could be documented over several months

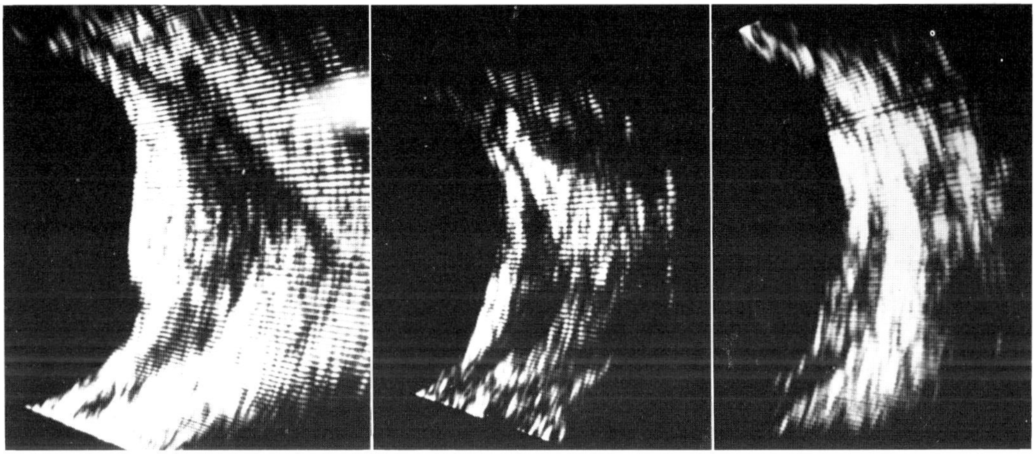
b

### 4.4.8 The Uveal Effusion Syndrome

It is claimed that outflow disturbances in the uveal circulation may lead to the **uveal effusion syndrome**; hypoplasia of the vorticose veins has been suggested. Clinically, we find a partial or circular choroidal detachment combined with an exudative retinal detachment (Fig. 4.**91**). The differential diagnosis against a space-occupying lesion in the choroid (tumor, metastasis, hemorrhage) can be established by proving the serous nature of the choroidal detachment (Witold et al. 1976, Verbeek 1981, Brockhurst 1987).

## 4.5 The Sclera

### 4.5.1 Scleritis

In a typical case of anterior scleritis, the diagnosis can be made on the basis of the clinical picture and the course of the disease, without requiring any further diagnostic methods.

The proliferative form of scleritis is difficult to differentiate from a choroidal or ciliary body melanoma and therefore requires the use of all kinds of diagnostic methods. Echography plays an important role here (Guthoff 1974, Feldon et al. 1978). The normal high reflectivity of the sclera will be decreased by the inflammatory swelling. This produces an image of a low-reflecting thickening of the ocular coats (Fig. 4.**93**). The signal intensity within the sclera corresponds to that of a choroidal melanoma so that a brawny scleritis can still be misdiagnosed and may lead to an enucleation because a melanoma was suspected (Feldon et al. 1978). In these cases an increased P32 uptake would also support the diagnosis of melanoma (Fig. 4.**94**). A differential diagnostic clue may be the fact that Tenon's space can be demonstrated on the echogram. Similar findings can be obtained when a choroidal melanoma breaks through the sclera. On the other hand, small and medium-sized tumors – and only these have to be considered from a differential diagnostic point of view – hardly ever break through the sclera. This sign therefore should, in cases of doubt, point toward an inflammatory etiology.

Echography is the diagnostic method of choice for posterior scleritis (Cappaert et al. 1977, Guthoff et al. 1983, Singh et al. 1986). The clinical picture is characterized by an acute loss of vision, and folds at the posterior pole. Choroid and vitreous may appear normal; occasionally, there is a slight exudation into the subretinal space with accompanying papilledema (Fig. 4.**95**). The loss of vision is usually due to increased hyperopia produced by the local inflammation. Echographically, we find a thickening of the ocular coats at the posterior pole, which shortens the axial length of the eye. In a cross sectional echogram, the posterior pole of the eye appears flattened (Hinzpeter et al. 1980, Unsöld et al. 1980, Singh et al. 1986). In 50% of the patients fluid accumulates in Tenon's space (Guthoff 1974) (Fig. 4.**95b**).

The course varies from spontaneous remissions within a few days (Guthoff et al. 1983) to an induced hyperopia, sometimes lasting for years and interpreted by some authors as a post inflammatory scleral shrinking at the posterior pole (Kalina et al. 1980, Cennamo et al. 1981).

# 5 Echographically Demonstrable Anatomical Features of the Orbit

The orbit is an anatomically clearly defined space. It is surrounded by the bones of the skull and by the lids. It can be compared to a pyramid and has a volume of about 35 ccm. It contains a variety of tissues, e.g., smooth and striated muscles, sensory and motor nerves, the optic nerve, excretory glands and the eyeball.

The main acoustic interfaces extend in an anteroposterior direction. The desirable direction for echographic examination is at right angles to these interfaces and therefore, even a pronounced tilting of the transducer will allow an echographic examination of only the anterior part of the orbit.

## 5.1 Methodology of the Examination – Evaluation of the Findings

So far the literature on the recommended methodology for examining the orbit has been influenced by the extensive experience which some examiners (Ossoinig et al. 1975) have gained with A-mode echography. The results obtained with B-mode technique (Coleman et al. 1977) were gathered mainly with instruments that needed fluid coupling, but which, in clinical practice, were of limited use. Only the introduction of contact B-mode devices (Bronson 1972) facilitated the spatial orientation during examination. This method makes it possible to describe disease processes within the orbit on the basis of topographical criteria (Schroeder 1978). During the last years, instruments with excellent temporal resolution power have been developed. These are capable of digitally producing up to 30 images per second. They allow us to incorporate all motions of the orbital soft tissue into the examination process. The following methodology of examining patients with orbital diseases has proven useful:

**Recommendations for a rational echographic examination of the orbit:**

1. searching for the normal orbital anatomical features with the contact B-mode technique;
2. topographic localization of pathologic findings – attempt to describe the topographic relation of the lesion to the main orbital structures as precisely as possible.
3. evaluation of the echogram produced by the lesion.
4. measuring the echo time (distance measurements) for affections of the optic nerve and the extraocular muscles.

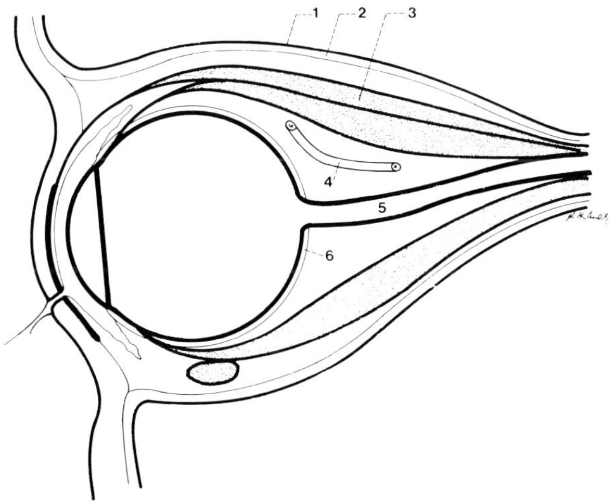


Fig. 5.1 Schematic drawing of the echographically demonstrable orbital structures under physiologic and pathologic conditions
1 Bony orbital wall
2 Periosteum of the orbit
3 Extraocular muscles, including the levator
4 Orbital veins
5 Optic nerve
6 Tenon's space

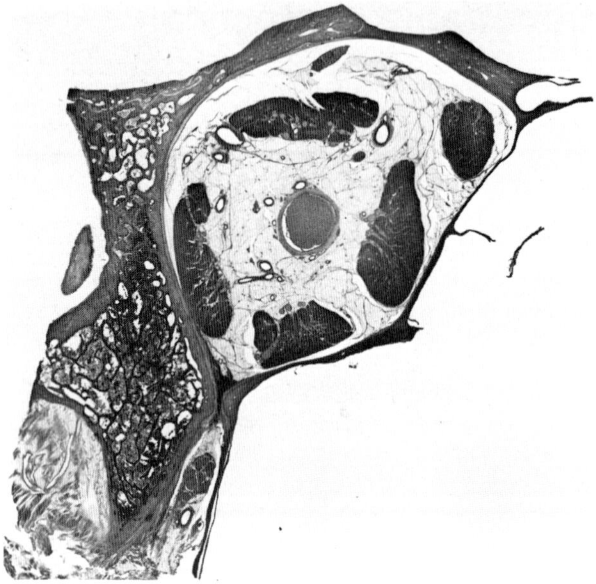

Fig. 5.**2** Frontal section through the right orbit by Koorneef. The main acoustic interfaces of the orbit can be seen under loupe magnification: bony orbital wall plus periosteum, muscle sheaths (transition to orbital fat, muscle belly), connective tissue septa within the orbital fat, vascular walls, meninges of the optic nerve (transition of dura to subarachnoidal space) (from Koorneeff, L.: Spatial Aspects of Orbital Musculo Fibrosis Tissue in Man. Swets & Zeitinger, Amsterdam 1976)

In the following chapters we attempt to describe the echographic findings of anatomical structures in the normal orbit. We present the spatial orientation in relationship to the main orbital structures (Figs. 4.**1**, 5.**2**).

## 5.2 Tenon's Space

Tenon's space is the connection between the outer scleral surface and the orbital contents. It is transversed by elastic fibers which contribute to a stabilized position of the globe. It functions like a slit space in a ball joint.

> Under normal conditions, Tenon's space cannot be imaged echographically.

The highly reflecting sclera borders directly on the orbital fat, which is also highly reflecting.

In order to investigate the conditions under which Tenon's space can be imaged, we performed a few experiments. On autopsy material, 5 ml of physiologic saline solution was injected 12–16 hours after death into the orbital apex. Fifteen minutes later an echo-free zone was created, lying directly in the tissue adjacent to the sclera (Fig. 5.**3**). This area corresponds to Tenon's space, dilated by the injected fluid. It continues into the optic nerve sheaths at the orbital apex.

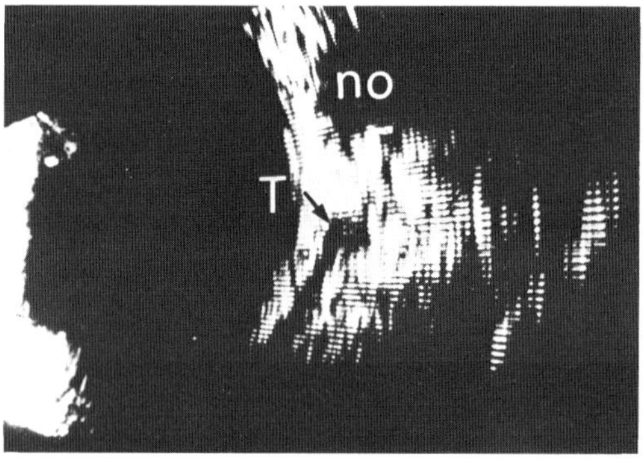


Fig. 5.**3** Fluid has been injected into the retrobulbar adipose tissue in this anatomical specimen. Tenon's space can be appreciated. When physiologic saline solution is injected, Tenon's space appears as an echo-free zone between sclera and orbital fat. The space extends toward the globe between dural sheath and orbital adipose tissue

This **potential slit-like space** is of great importance for echographic diagnosis.

> Whenever Tenon's space can be imaged echographically, we are dealing with a pathologic condition.

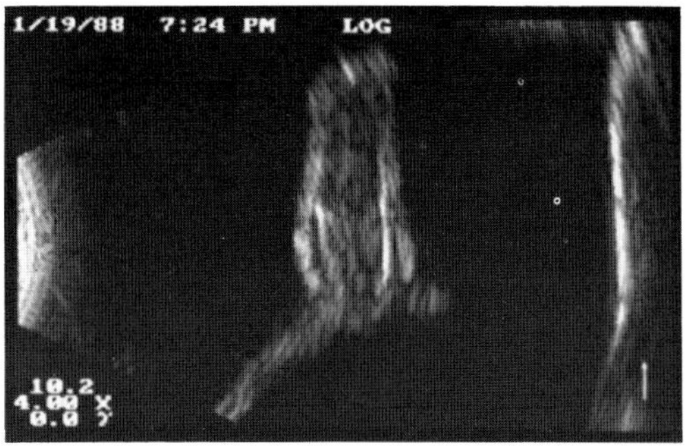

a

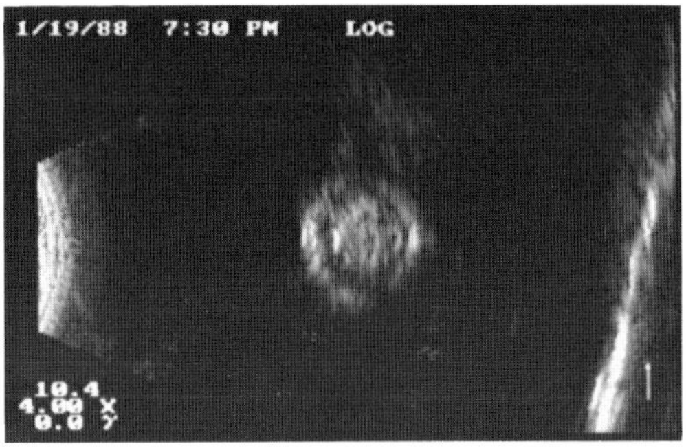

b

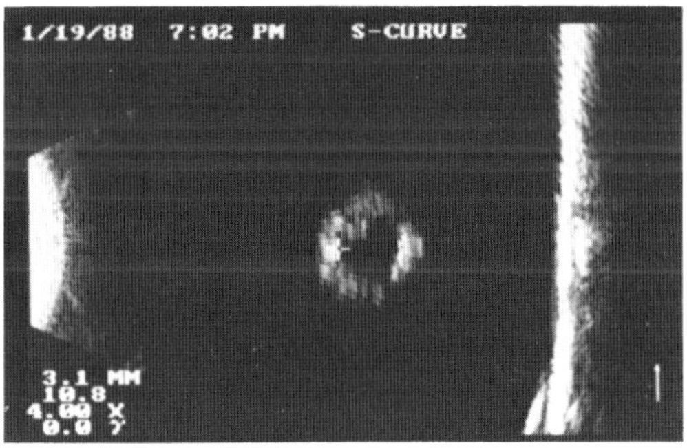

c

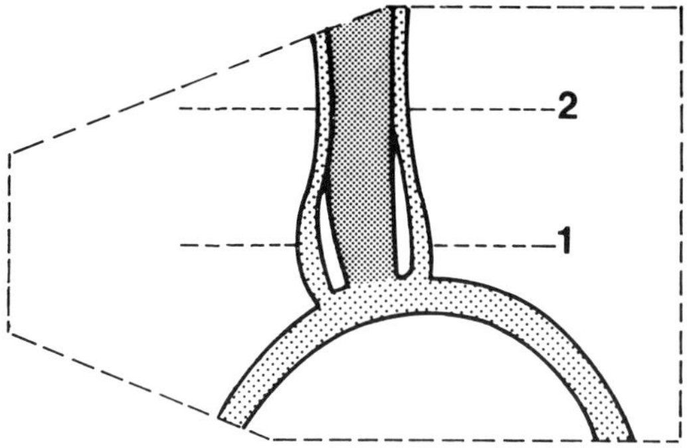

d

Fig. 5.4 **a–d** Demonstration of the anterior part of the optic nerve on an anatomical specimen in a water bath
**a** Longitudinal section through the optic nerve, including the dural sheaths. Toward the globe there is a slight dilatation of the subarachnoidal space
**b** Frontal section through the optic nerve near the ocular wall. Under these ideal experimental conditions, it is possible to differentiate dura, subarachnoidal space and optic nerve
**c** About 10 mm behind the optic nerve head the dura lies directly on the optic nerve, and a subarachnoidal space cannot be demonstrated. The most important difference in acoustic impedance occurs, according to the experiments by Schroeder, where the dura and the subarachnoidal space meet. The measuring marks at the anterior dural surface are separated by 3.1 mm
**d** Schematic drawing

## 5.3 The Optic Nerve

The optic nerve is surrounded by strongly reflecting orbital adipose tissue, and images as a nearly echo-free space (Fig. 4.**8a**). The area of the optic nerve head, where the optic nerve merges with the globe, can be precisely localized echographically. This landmark is an important aid for the topographic correlation of intraocular processes.

Under experimental conditions the optic nerve and the dura appear on cross section as two concentric circles (Fig. 5.**4**). Under ideal experimental conditions the A-mode echogram provides spikes from the external surface of the dura, from the internal surface of the dura and from the surface of the optic nerve. For identification of these interfaces, three spikes should be available in order to make an exact anatomical correlation possible (Schroeder et al. 1969). The strongest signal is created at the transition of the dural sheath to the subarachnoidal space. Schroeder calls the distance to the opposite internal dural surface the "internal dural diameter" (Schroeder 1976). We have used this term or the expression "dural diameter" in the following chapters (Fig. 5.**5**).

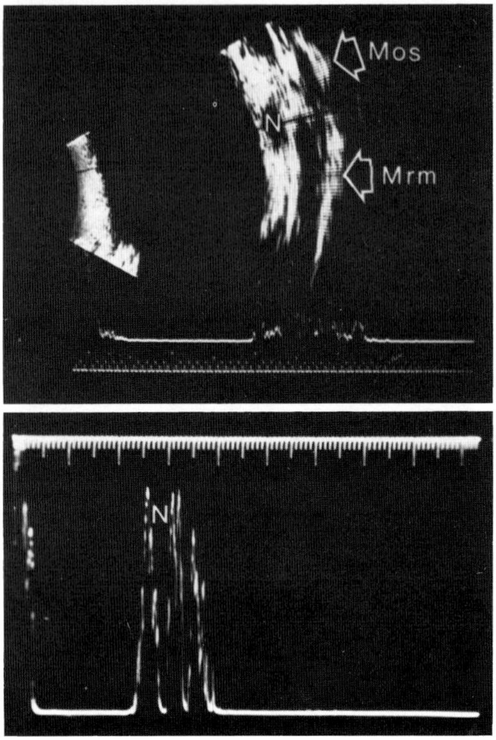


a

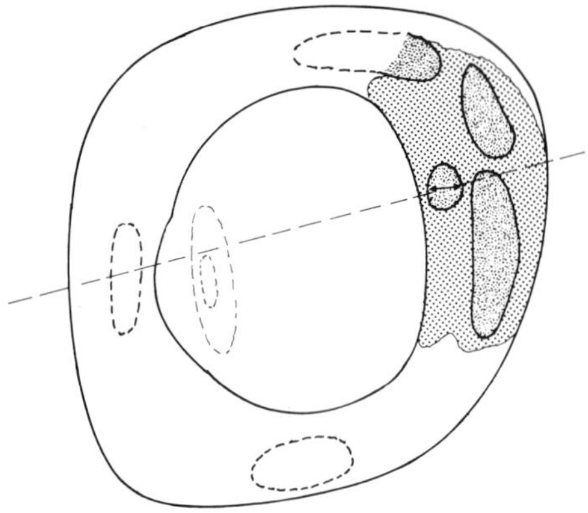

b

Fig. 5.**5** **a, b**
**a** Frontal section through the nasal orbit. The globe is maximally abducted in order to show the optic nerve in cross section. The normal dural diameter is, according to the method of Schroeder, up to 4 mm wide. The dotted line in the schematic drawing indicates the direction of examination of the A-mode shown in the lower part of the picture. MOS = superior oblique muscle, MRM = medial rectus muscle, N = optic nerve
**b** Schematic drawing
**c, d** See color plates

In order to measure this diameter in vivo, we have to direct the ultrasound waves vertical to the optic nerve. For anatomical reasons, this prerequisite cannot be fulfilled. We come closest to an ideal situation by placing the transducer over the outer canthus while at the same time abducting the globe (Figs. 5.**5** and 5.**6**). Using this method of examination, reliable normal values were obtained without claiming that they correspond to exact anatomical measurements. Ossoinig (1976) recommends measuring in primary position of the globe; in our experience, measurements in abduction have proven technically easier (Schroeder, 1979, 1976) (Table 5.**1**). The same values have been gained with contact B-mode technique. We recommend reducing the amplifier sensitivity to such a degree that the most strongly reflecting inner dural surface can be well identified (Fig. 6.**30**).

Table 5.**1**

| µs | mm | |
|---|---|---|
| 2.5 | 2.0 | |
| 3 | 2.4 | |
| 3.5 | 2.8 | |
| 4 | 3.2 | |
| 4.5 | 3.6 | Normal area |
| 5 | 4.0 | |
| 5.5 | 4.4 | |
| 6 | 4.8 | |
| 6.5 | 5.2 | |
| 7 | 5.6 | |
| 7.5 | 6.0 | |
| 8.0 | 6.4 | |
| 8.5 | 6.8 | |
| 9 | 7.2 | |
| 9.5 | 7.6 | |
| 10 | 8.0 | |

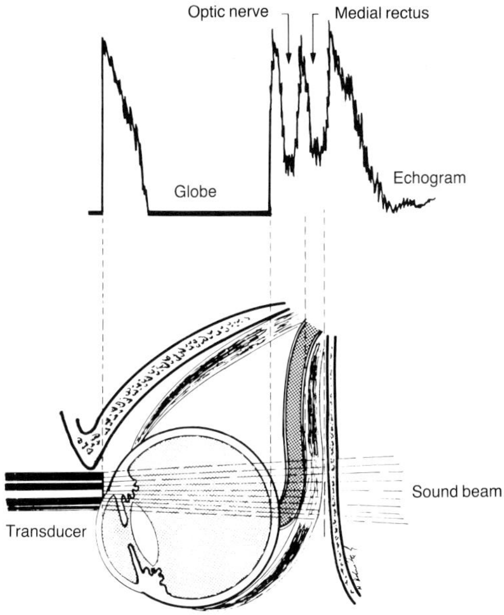


Fig. 5.**6** Schematic presentation of measuring the optic nerve according to Schroeder (from Schroeder 1976)

Color-coded Doppler sonography allows us to document frequency shifts in the distal part of the optic nerve. Figures 5.**5c** and **d** (see color plates) demonstrate the flow spectrum of the central retinal artery and vein as we can deduce it from the cross sectional echography, which is imaged simultaneously. The red color indicates shifts toward the transducer (maximal flow velocity in the example is here 12 cm/s); the blue color indicates shifts away from the transducer (maximal flow velocity of the central retinal vein in the illustrated example is about 5 cm/s).

## 5.4 The Orbital Adipose Tissue

The lobular structure of the orbital fat is characterized by connective tissue septa described by Koorneeff (1971). It presents a number of good acoustic interfaces so that this area shows high acoustic reflectivity. The border between adipose tissue to other, less reflecting orbital structures produces differences in impedance, and facilitates orientiation during the examination. The strong attenuation produced by scatter causes a marked sound attenuation of the spikes in A-mode, with a decrease of about 15 dB/cm (Thijssen 1973).

## 5.5 The Orbital Vessels

The cross sections of orbital veins, as we know them from phlebographic examinations (Lloyd 1970), and their anatomical structure should be visible on echography. This assumption can also be supported by the fact that in about 20% of the patients, a normal superior ophthalmic vein can be seen on a CT scan (Unsöld 1979, Jacobs et al. 1980). No echographic examinations of normal orbital veins have been published. In our experience, a slightly increased venous pressure will make these vessels visible on echography. We could perhaps deduce that the application of the transducer will exceed the physiologic venous pressure in the adjacent tissue. Thus, a collapse or at least a decrease in vascular lumen could change the acoustic interfaces in such a way that they could not be seen on echography. An exception would be the veins of a crying infant in whom the intrathoracic pressure increase apparently extends the vessel wall of the valveless orbital veins. In this manner, these vessels become echographically demonstrable (Fig. 5.**7**).

> Echographically demonstrable orbital vessels in young patients or adults have to be regarded as pathologic findings.

## 5.6 The Extraocular Muscles

The four rectus muscles and the belly of the superior oblique can be shown on B-mode echography. They can be delineated from adjacent tissue because the distance among the fibers within a specific muscle is smaller than the echographic resolution power. The muscle tissue produces significantly lower ultrasound signals than the adjacent adipose tissue or the orbital walls (Fig. 5.**8**).

Cross sections exactly at 90° to the course of the muscle fibers cannot be obtained, because of interference by the bony orbital wall. Therefore, the thickness of an extraocular muscle can be evaluated only with reservations. The A-mode measurements recommended by McNutt et al. (1977) seem time consuming and expensive. These authors need at least three polaroid photos to document measurements for each muscle. Their measurements, on the other hand, give thickness values down to a few tenths of a millimeter. The spindle shape of the

a

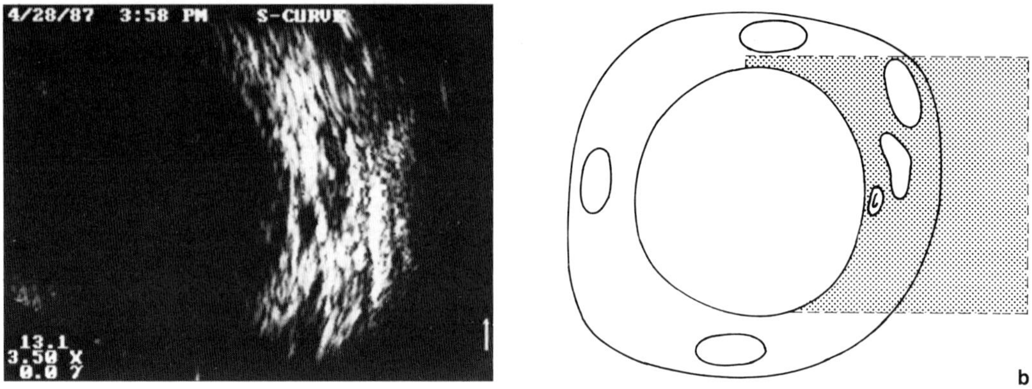


b

Fig. 5.**7 a, b**

**a** Frontal section through the nasal orbit in a crying infant. Between the globe and the medial rectus, a cross section of a branch of the superior ophthalmic vein can be demonstrated. This vessel cannot be imaged echographically in an adult, even if a Valsalva maneuver is undertaken. **b** Schematic drawing

a

b

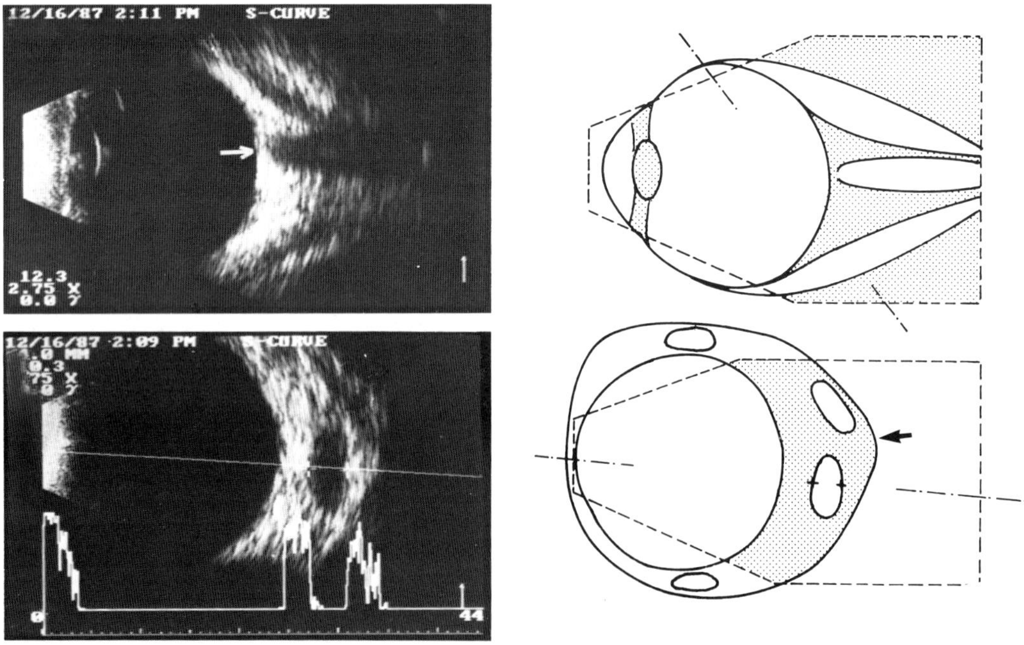


c

d

Fig. 5.**8 a–d** Sagittal and frontal sections through the globe and the orbit

**a** Sagittal section: in this section using a horizontal examination plane, the medial and lateral rectus muscles appear as spindle-shaped structures. The optic nerve is a nearly echo-free space. The white arrow indicates the area of the optic nerve head

**b** In frontal section the muscle thickness can be evaluated in A- and in B-mode echography. The electronic measuring marks are here placed at a distance of 4 mm. The arrow marks the border between the frontal and the ethmoidal bones, where the ethmoidal vessels enter

**c, d** Schematic drawings

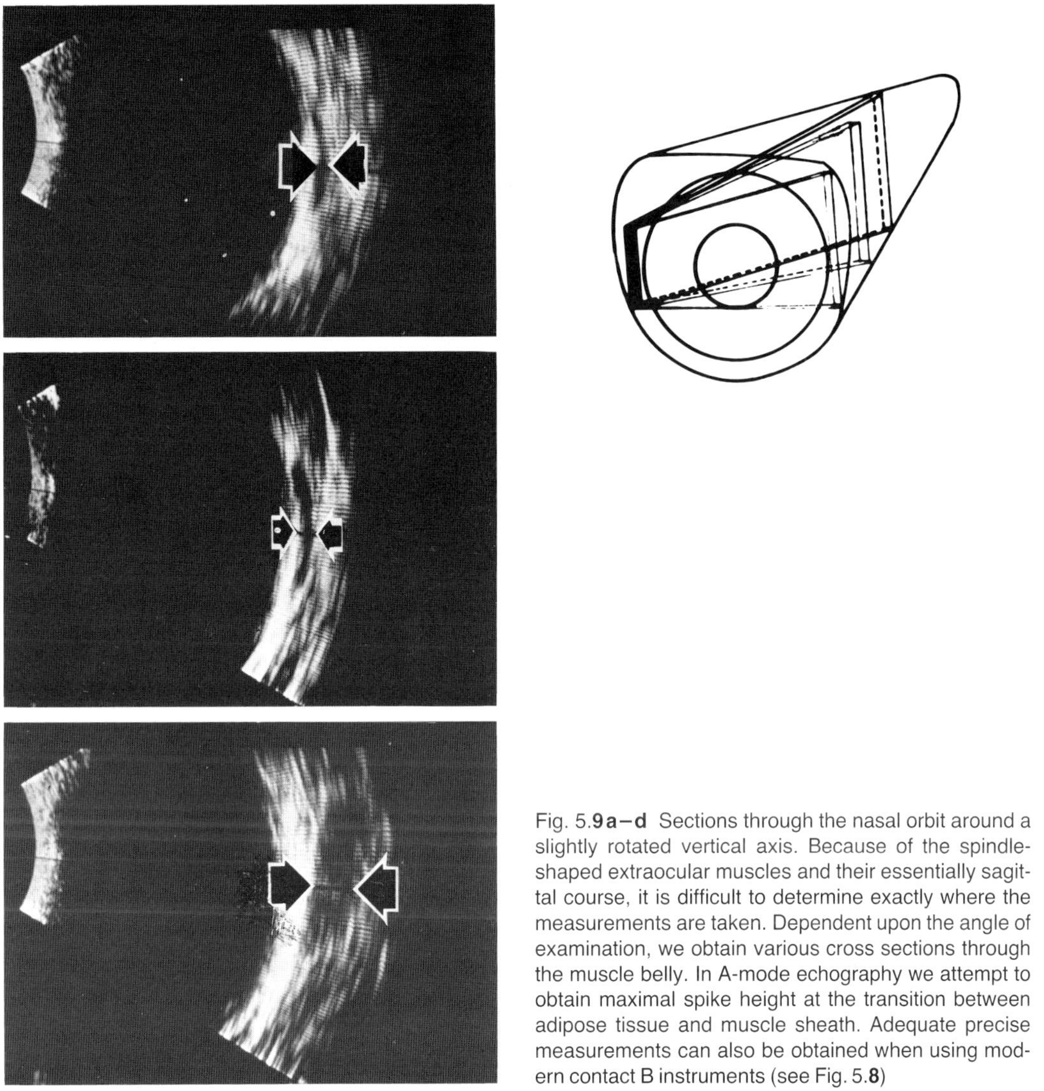

a b c d

Fig. 5.**9a–d** Sections through the nasal orbit around a slightly rotated vertical axis. Because of the spindle-shaped extraocular muscles and their essentially sagittal course, it is difficult to determine exactly where the measurements are taken. Dependent upon the angle of examination, we obtain various cross sections through the muscle belly. In A-mode echography we attempt to obtain maximal spike height at the transition between adipose tissue and muscle sheath. Adequate precise measurements can also be obtained when using modern contact B instruments (see Fig. 5.**8**)

extraocular muscles and the not precisely defined examination directions make the precision of such measurements somewhat questionable. Contact B-mode echographic examinations show that even slight tilting of the transducer will cause an apparent change in the muscle diameter (Fig. 5.**9**). This phenomenon is even more accentuated when dealing with pathologically thickened extraocular muscles, because the volume increases in direct relationship to the muscle belly present. The difference in thickness between the insertion and the belly is here considerably widened (Sect. 6.3). In our experience, cases of myogenic exophthalmus echographically show such an obvious thickening of the muscle, even at a time when the first signs appear, that the precision measurements proposed by Ossoinig are superfluous. Following the data of

Table 5.2 **Muscle thickness** Upper limit of norm

| | |
|---|---|
| Recti muscles and superior oblique | 3.5 mm |
| Interior oblique | If echographically demonstrable, already pathologic |

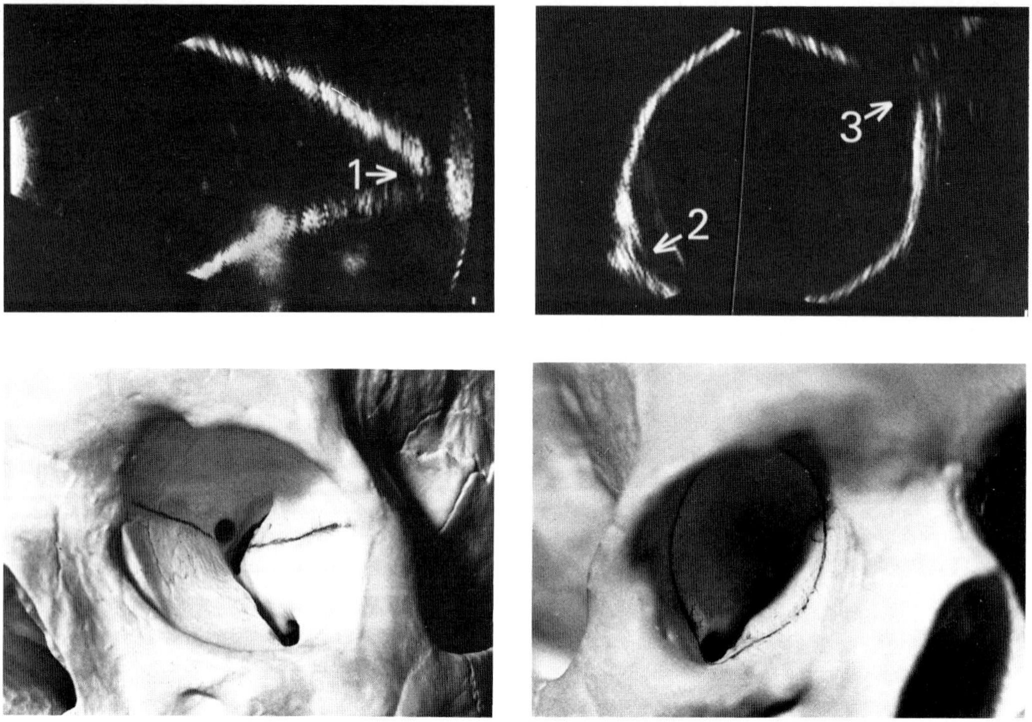


a b c d

Fig. 5.**10a–d** Examination of a plastic skull model in a water bath
**a, c** Sagittal-horizontal section
**b, d** Frontal section

1 Optic canal
2 Inferior orbital fissure
3 Entrance area of the ethmoidal foramina

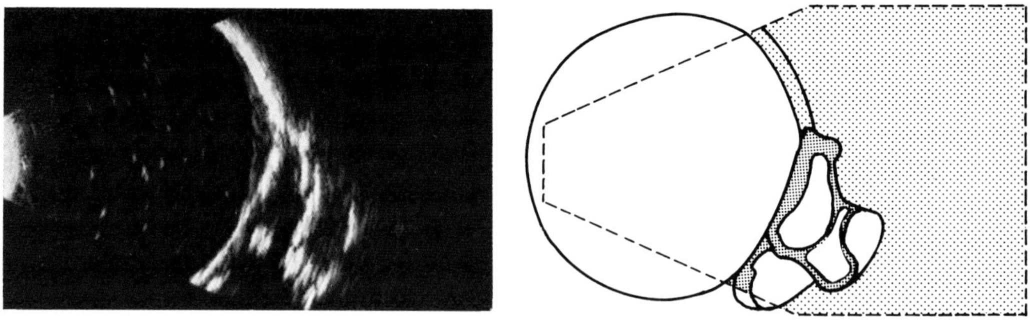

a b

Fig. 5.**11a, b**
**a** Examination of a skull model in a water bath. Approximately coronary section of the nasal orbit imaged from the temporal side (see Fig. 5.**10b, d**). The ethmoidal cells are filled with water, and sound can be propagated through the thin nasal orbital wall. Therefore, the ethmoidal cells can be demonstrated echographically. Similar findings are obtained in an empyema of the ethmoidal cells or in a mucocele
**b** Schematic drawing

McNutt et al., we find the values shown in Table 5.**2** adequate for clinical purposes. These values can be determined by A- or B-mode echography.

#### Evaluating the Intensity of Reflection From Muscle Tissue

The acoustic reflectivity of extraocular muscles is low. In order to quantify these reflections, we compare them with signals from the interface muscle sheath-orbital adipose tissue. For this purpose a definite transducer-amplifier combination is necessary (Ossoinig 1971) (the quantitative evaluation of signals from the muscle fibers is discussed in Sect. 6.3).

## 5.7 The Lacrimal Gland

A normal lacrimal gland cannot be visualized echographically. In order to delineate this organ from surrounding adipose tissue, the gland would have to be enlarged. According to our experience, this would lead to a widening of the upper temporal orbital space with few signals from that area (Sect. 6.2).

> Any lacrimal gland that can be visualized echographically has to be considered a pathologic organ.

## 5.8 The Orbital Wall

The orbital wall consists of bone and periosteum. Under normal circumstances these two structures cannot be differentiated echographically and will, as a unit, reflect ultrasound totally. This is due not only to the thickness of the bone, but also to the air filling in the adjacent sinuses (see Sect. 6.1).

The orbital contents, especially the adipose tissue, absorb and reflect the ultrasound signal to that images from the deeper or apical part of the orbit are inadequate for a clinical examination. As a basis for evaluating changes of the orbital walls, we use echograms which were obtained under ideal circumstances from a skull model placed in a water bath (Fig. 5.**10**). The inferior orbital fissure and the ethmoidal foramina present well demonstrable landmarks during a clinical examination.

## 5.9 The Paranasal Sinuses

The interface between paranasal mucosa and air reflects ultrasound totally. The sound can only be propagated if air has been replaced by fluid or by a tumor. Therefore:

> Propagation of sound into the paranasal sinuses or their echographic representation has to be regarded as a pathologic finding.

This situation can be simulated by examining a skull in a water bath (Fig. 5.**11**).

# 6 Ultrasound Diagnosis of Orbital Diseases

Table 6.1 **Diseases of the orbital wall which can be echographically demonstrated**

| |
|---|
| Mucocele |
| Sphenoidal meningioma |
| Fibrous dysplasia |
| Transmitted infection |
| Periorbital neoplasms |
| Fractures |

## 6.1 The Orbital Walls

A **mucocele** is a cystoid extension of a sinus with a capsule-like border. The echogram gives a clearly defined structure (Figs. 6.**1**, 6.**2**). Interior echos may occasionally be produced by septa or heterogenous mucous material. However, these are always separated by acoustically empty spaces. The border, consisting of mucosa and periosteum, may occasionally appear as a double spike on A-mode or as a double contour in a cross sectional echogram. In about half of the cases, we can echographically demonstrate the communication to a paranasal sinus, which would further corroborate the presumptive diagnosis. According to our ex-

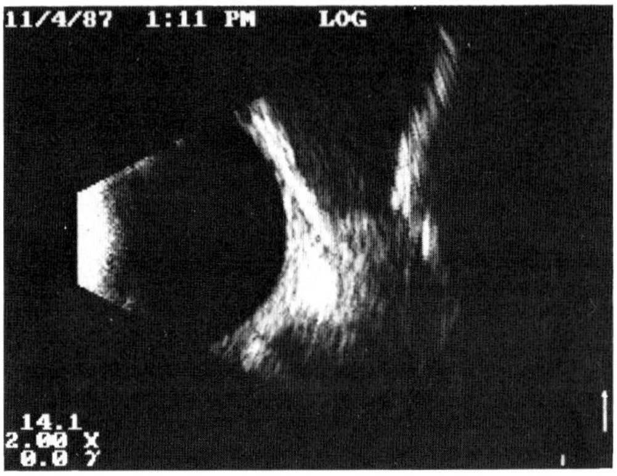

a

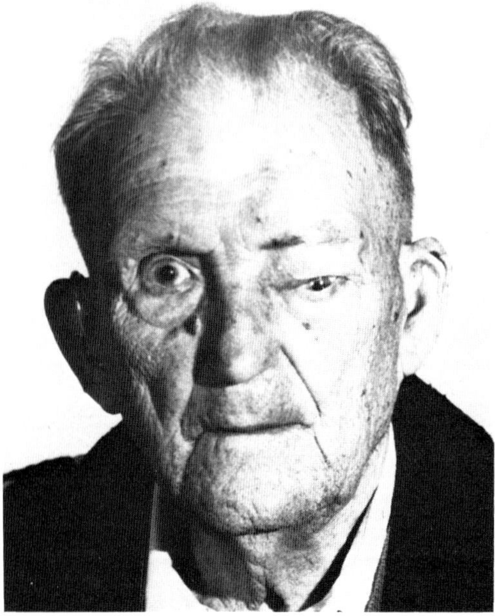
b

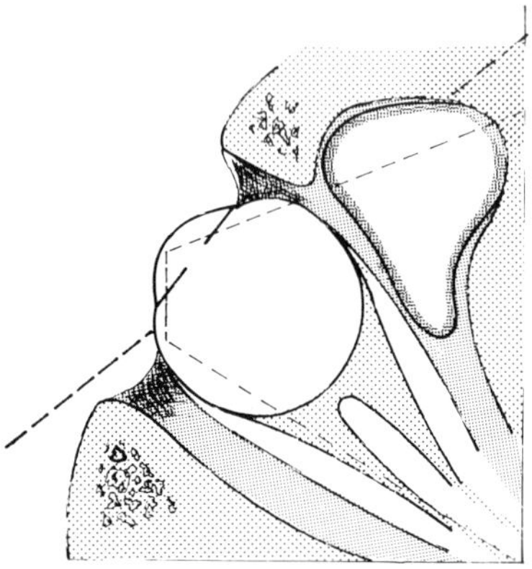
c

Fig. 6.**1 a–c** Mucocele of the frontal sinus in a 72-year-old man, eight years after an impression fracture of the frontal bone. Echographically, this condition is characterized by a smooth protrusion of the orbital roof with sound propagation into the frontal sinus, which is filled with secretion. Frequently, we can obtain a slight deformation of the tumor by pressing on it with the transducer

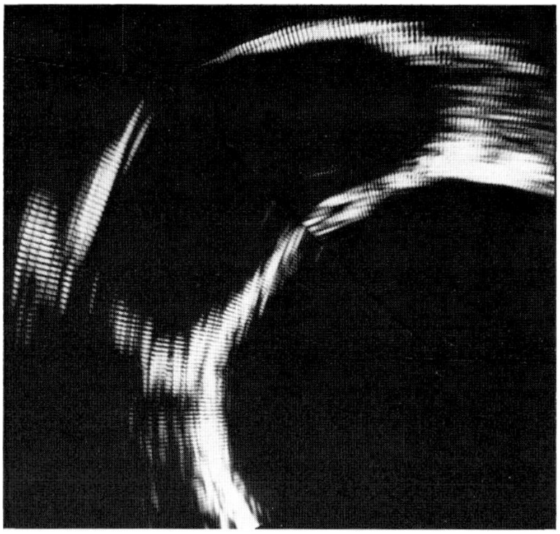

a

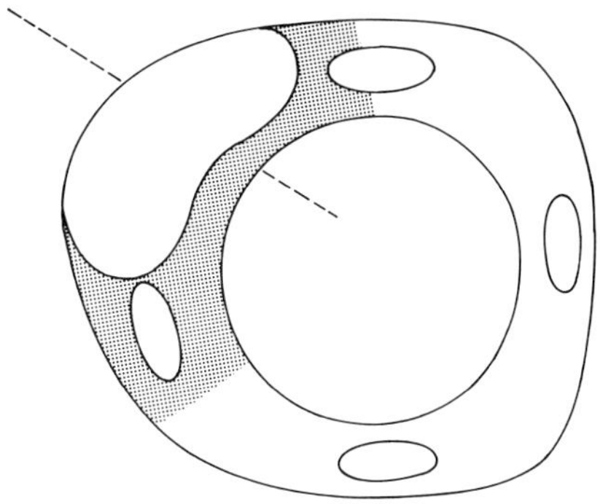

b

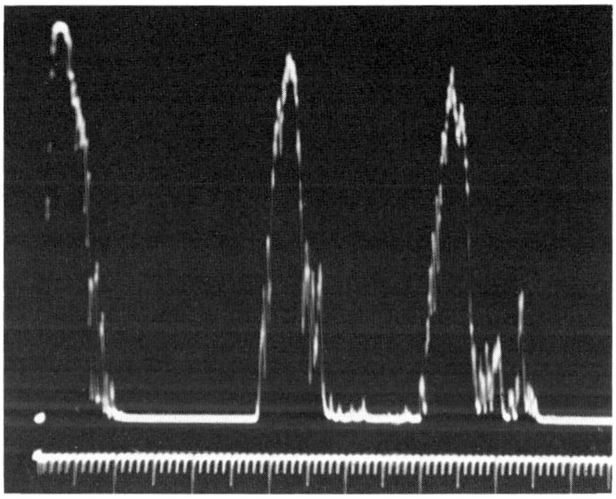

c

Fig. 6.**2 a–c** Mucocele extending from the anterior ethmoidal cells. Echographically, the tumefaction appears as a cystoid cavity without definite acoustic borders. In A-mode with maximal amplification, small spikes can be demonstrated within the tumefaction. In contrast to this case, more pronounced heterogenous structures may be imaged with heterogenous material, e.g., various consistencies of mucus or mucosal septa

perience, which corresponds to the literature (Till et al. 1979, Hasenfratz et al. 1983, Nasr et al. 1984, Rochels et al. 1985), echography gives here reliable results. In spite of the accuracy with which the diagnosis can be made, we have to keep in mind that a typical mucocele may be caused by a malignant, space-occupying lesion or may be associated with one. Guerry et al. (1975) reported on three patients in whom the final diagnosis of a sinus carcinoma was only established after the recurrence of a presumed mucocele could be examined histologically. Accumulation of mucus within the water-filled cavity may simulate mucous polyps (Fig. 6.**3**).

**Meningiomas** of the sphenoidal wing may also alter the contour of the orbital walls. Occasionally, this may produce a mucocele-like echographic image due to displacement of orbital contents (Fig. 6.**4**). A differential diagnosis can usually be made because the meningioma may show high reflectivity due to calcifications within the neoplasm (Ossoinig 1975) and because there will not be any sound propagation into the sinus. A definite identification of the lesion is here, as with all orbital tumors, echographically impossible. The CT scan will exactly demonstrate the extent of the lesion outside the orbit and will provide indispensable information (Wende et al. 1978).

Table 6.2 **Echographic charakteristics of a mucocele**

| |
|---|
| Smoothly outlined, cystoid cavity |
| Double contour of the cyst wall |
| Communication to a perinasal sinus can be demonstrated |
| Slightly compressible with strong pressure |
| Changes in the relief of the orbital wall |

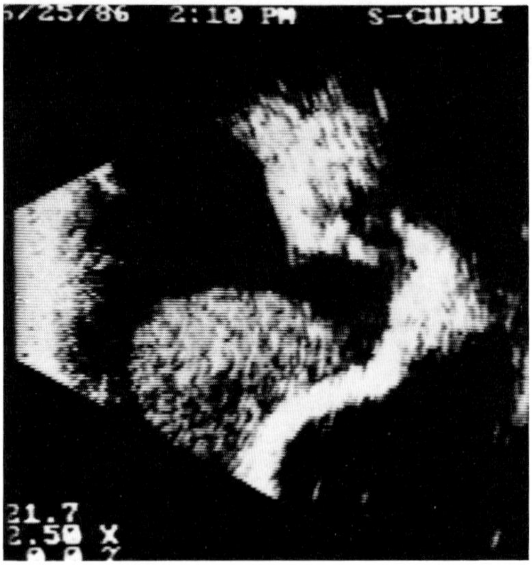


a

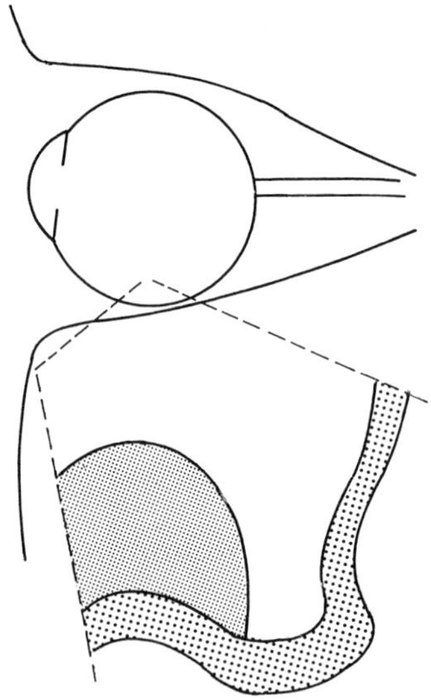

Fig. 6.3 **a, b**
**a** Mucocele of the sphenoidal sinus with an atypical mucous plug. The fluid-filled sphenoidal sinus allows propagation of sound beyond the orbital wall so that the entire sphenoidal sinus can be examined echographically. The transducer is placed over the lower lid. During the operation the lesion seen in the lower part of the illustration proved to be a mucous plug of considerable consistency. **b** Schematic drawing

**Fibrous dysplasia** has to be differentiated from meningiomas of the sphenoidal wing. The dysplasia will also cause a bulging of the lateral orbital wall. Reliable echographic patterns are not available.

**Orbital cellulitis** usually shows a typical clinical picture. Echography will help us to localize the seat of the cellulitis or an abscess. We have to determine whether there is a diffuse infiltration of the tissues, whether only certain structures are involved and whether there is tissue necrosis. Infiltrations usually decrease the amount of reflection and are therefore easily delineated in the strongly reflecting orbital fat (Fig. 6.**5**). If we find a strongly reflecting membrane close to the orbital wall, we have to assume that the periosteum is detached and that a subperiosteal abscess is developing. This complication is a direct precursor of an orbital abscess (Harris 1983) and requires immediate surgical intervention. The echogram does not give us any definite information as to whether the homogenous acoustic behavior of the adjacent soft tissues is due to an inflammatory infiltration or whether necrosis has already taken place. In any case, the detachment of the periosteum, which cannot be misinterpreted echographically, should be regarded as an accumulation of pus. It is absolutely necessary to drain the lesion and open the sinus. Echography offers a decisive examination method of this condition, as Damasty already recommended in 1980 (Fig. 6.**5**). Occasionally, Tenon's space may become visible early in the disease process as a sign of a disturbed vascular permeability involving the entire orbit (Fig. 6.**6**).

The phenomenon of sound propagation through the thin medial orbital wall is especially important for lesions of the ethmoidal bone. According to our experience, a diagnosis of even a subclinical orbital involvement can be made by imaging ethmoidal cells filled with secretion (Fig. 6.**7**). A traumatic orbital hematoma proves the precision with which fluid-filled cavities can be delineated in the orbital adipose tissue. In spite of the short distance between the optic nerve and the hematoma (about 2 mm), the suspected diagnosis of optic nerve sheath hematoma, based on a CT scan, could be eliminated (Fig. 6.**8**).

In our experience, **defects in the orbital wall** must reach a certain size before they can be demonstrated unequivocally. The limited lateral resolution power of the B-mode echogram is a hindrance here. The diagnosis is also uncertain with A-mode

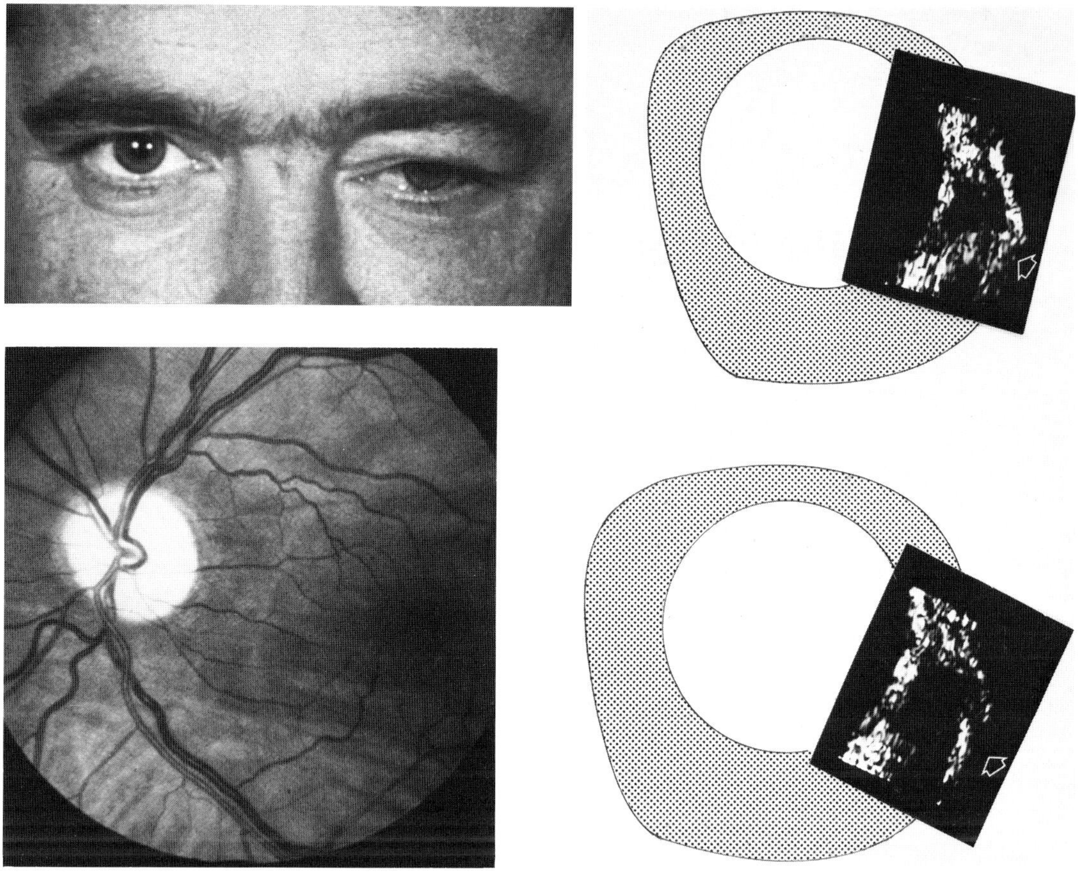

Fig. 6.4 **a–d** Sphenoidal meningioma on the left with destruction of the orbital wall in a 46-year-old man. There is a 3 mm proptosis and the globe is displaced 2 mm downward. Fundus picture: optic atrophy, choroidal folds. A frontal cross sectional echogram of the left orbit shows few echoes in the area of the inferior orbital fissure (**c**, **d**: white arrow)

echography because of the unfocused transducer (see Sect. 1.5). The first diagnostic indication of malignancies which infiltrate the orbit from a perinasal sinus is the sound propagation. Only when there is an extensive erosion of the orbital wall will we be capable of demonstrating the bone margins replaced by tumor (Fig. 6.**9**).

Changes of the orbital floor in **blow-out fractures** are extremely difficult to demonstrate echographically. Some authors (Nover et al. 1986) recommend specific echographic examinations for elucidation. We could not corroborate these findings on our patients with a sufficient degree of reliability. It should be remembered that lesions of the orbital floor will not allow vertical sections because of the unfavorable examination direction. If there is a discrepancy between the clinical findings and the echographic results and if an orbital floor fracture is suspected, other examination methods should be used, e.g., coronary sections of a CT scan, so that the situation can be clarified.

## 6.2 Lacrimal Gland and Peripheral Orbit

Diseases of the lacrimal gland are rare. In a series of 1000 patients seen at the orbital clinic of Moorfields Eye Hospital in London, only about 5% had a pathologic process of the lacrimal gland (Krohel et al. 1981). Few characteristic signs are known for a preoperative differential diagnosis. Radiological-

a
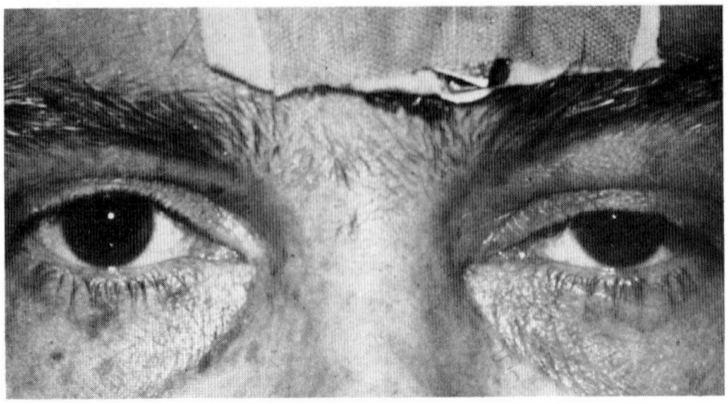

b
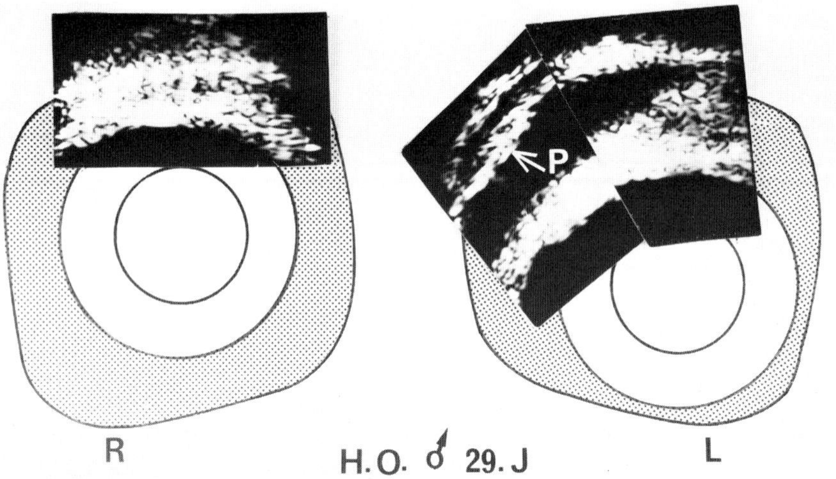


Fig. 6.**5a, b** Detachment of the periosteum in a 29-year-old man with orbital cellulitis due to a sinusitis. There is a double contour of the orbital wall in the nasal upper quadrant, which is produced by the detached periosteum surrounded by necrotic tissue

a
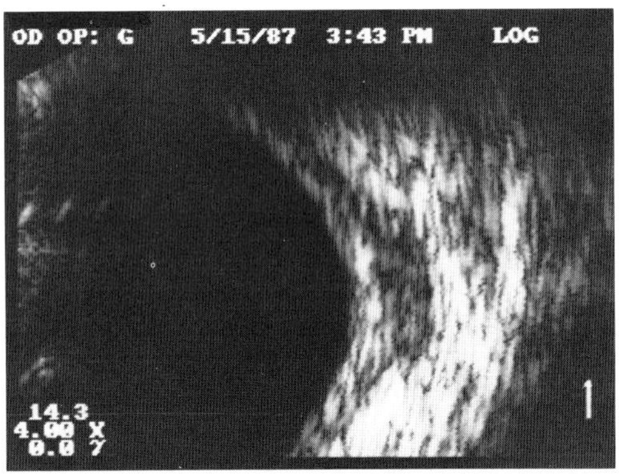


b
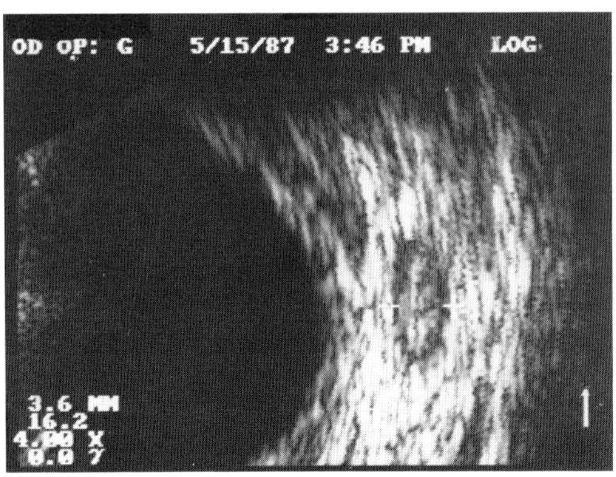


c
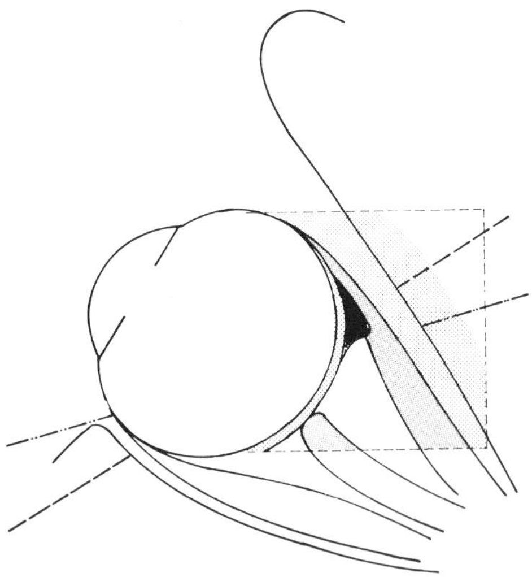

Fig. 6.**6a–c**
**a, b** Orbital cellulitis with Tenon's space demonstrable. In frontal sections we see, in addition to Tenon's space, a thickening of the medial rectus muscle close to its insertion
**c** Schematic drawing

a 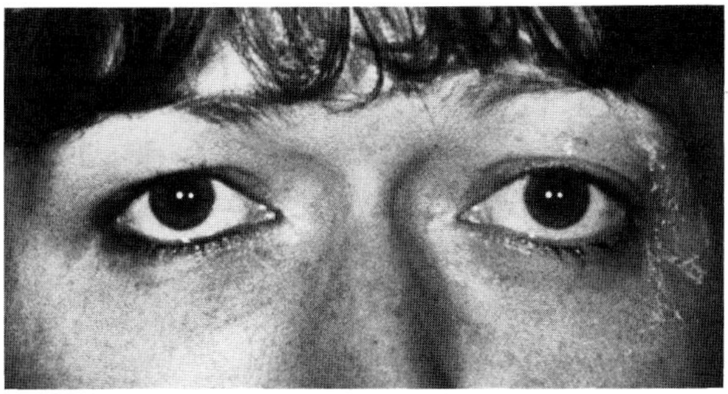

Fig. 6.7 **a, b** Sound propagation into the ethmoidal cells in a patient with empyema. Thirty-year-old woman, 3-mm exophthalmus, slight pain in the left orbit on pressure or with ocular motions. Nasally from the globe is a circumscribed homogeneous area of the peripheral orbit, and the sound is propagated into the ethmoidal cells. A transnasal ethmoidectomy was performed on the same day and a great deal of pus could be evacuated from this cavity

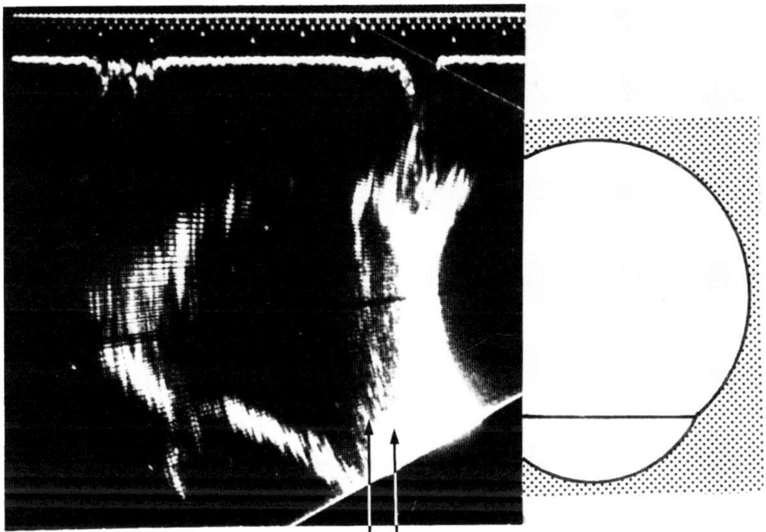


ly visible calcifications and enlargement of the lacrimal fossa are not definite signs of a malignant process, nor is the absence of such changes a reliable indication for a benign space-occupying lesion (Newton 1962, Steward et al. 1979, Wright et al. 1979).

The normal lacrimal gland cannot be imaged echographically with great reliability. In order to delineate the gland from the adjacent adipose tissue, the gland has to be enlarged. This will lead to a widening of the upper temporal aspect of the orbit. Only few echoes will be obtained from this area (Fig. 6.**10**). Some authors have attempted to correlate the A-mode echogram with histologic findings of the tumor, based on a series of benign and malignant lacrimal gland neoplasms. Retrospectively, the correlation was correct in a large percentage of cases. According to Wright (1979), X-ray pictures and history are the most decisive factors determing whether the entire gland should be excised or whether, after opening the capsule, a biopsy should be performed so that the assumed diagnosis can be confirmed or rejected.

The echographic pattern of affected adjacent structures can occasionally give us an indication as to whether the lesion is benign or malignant: malignant lesions usually confine themselves to the temporal upper orbital quadrant, though the neoplasm may be quite extensive. Pseudotumors and lymphomas, on the other hand, involve other orbital

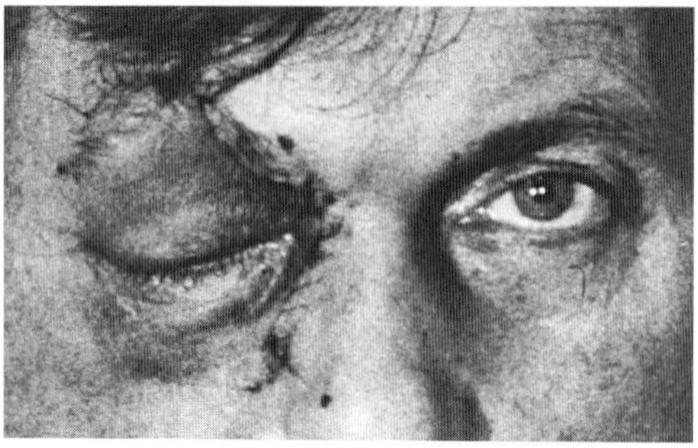

a

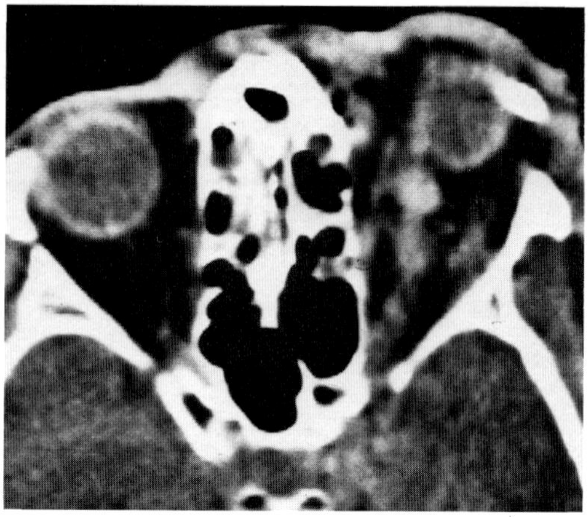

b

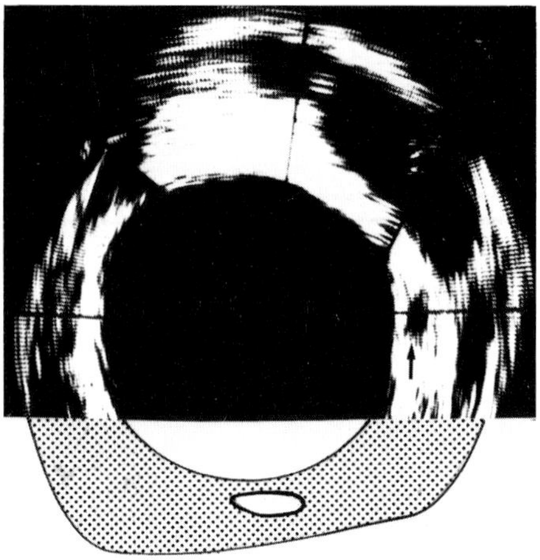

c

Fig. 6.**8a–c** Traumatic orbital hematoma. A CT scan was obtained immediately after the trauma, and a hematoma of the optic nerve sheath was suspected. Echographically, on maximal abduction of the globe, the optic nerve could be clearly separated from the hematoma (arrow)

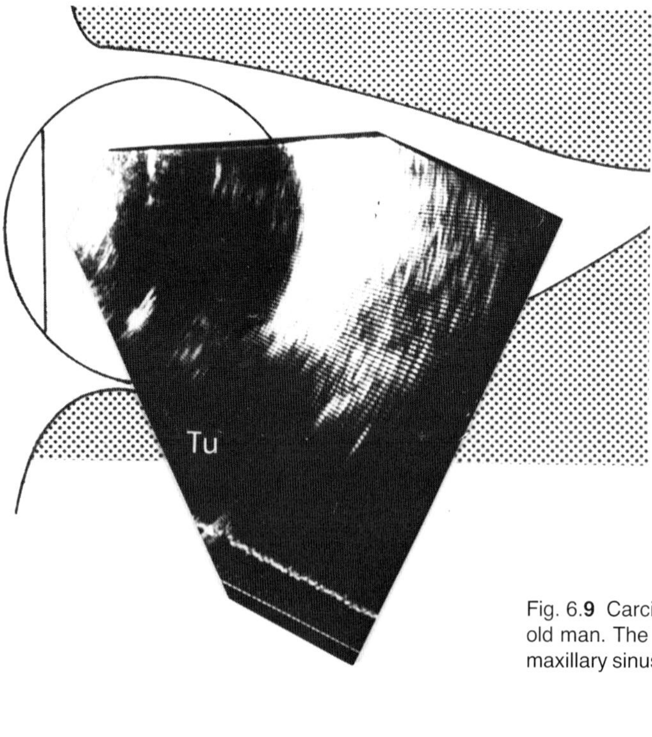


Fig. 6.**9** Carcinoma of the maxillary sinus in an 82-year-old man. The tumor allows sound propagation into the maxillary sinus

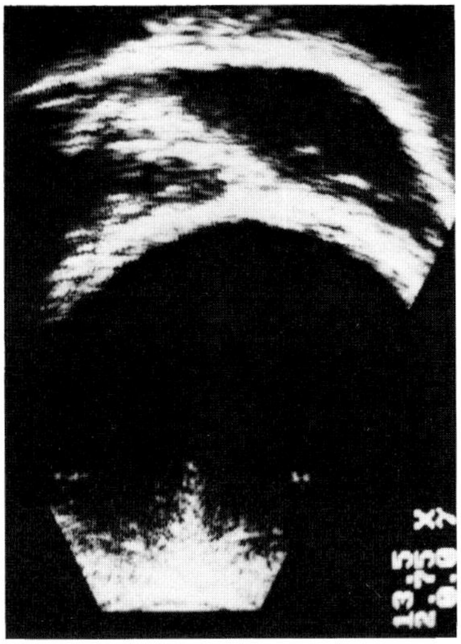

a

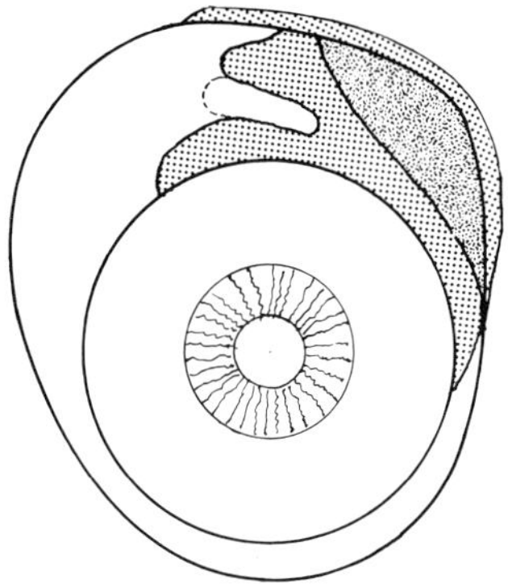

b

Fig. 6.**10 a, b**
**a** Histologically proven lymphoma of the lacrimal gland. A mass with reduced echogenicity adjoining the periosteum is spreading in the lacrimal fossa
**b** Diagram

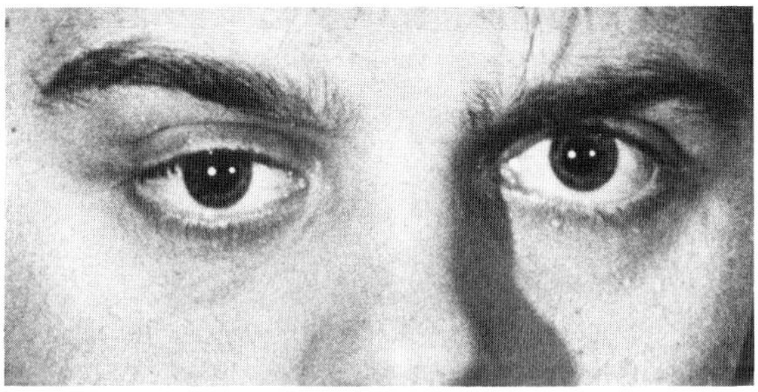

a

Fig. 6.**11 a, b**
**a** Carcinoma of the right lacrimal gland in a 21-year-old man. The history revealed occasional pain for the previous three months. The globe is displaced 7 mm downward and 3 mm nasally

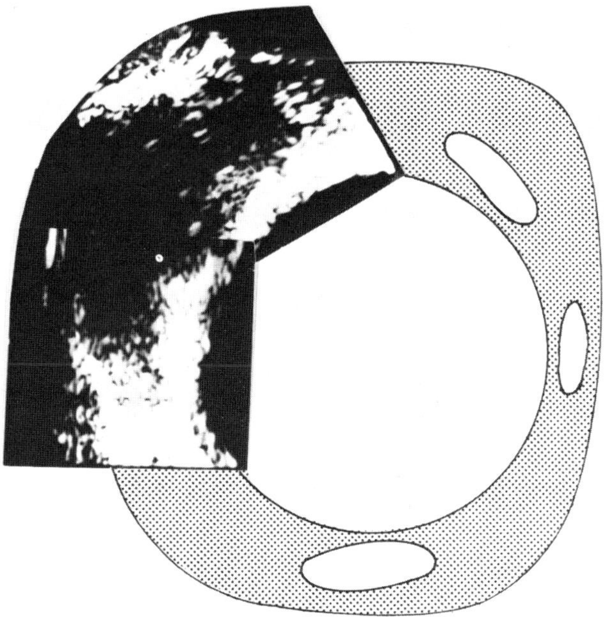

b

**b** Frontal section toward the upper temporal quadrant: echographically, heterogenous lesion in the lacrimal fossa with blurred margin toward the periosteum

Table 6.3 **Echographically demonstrable diseases of the lacrimal gland and of the peripheral orbit**

| |
|---|
| Dermoid |
| Inflammations and Neoplasms of the Lacrimal Gland |
| Rhabdomyosarcoma |
| Lymphoma |

structures, especially Tenon's space and the extraocular muscles (Figs. 6.**10**, 6.**20**). The involvement of other orbital structures makes the diagnosis of pseudotumor or lymphoma more likely and may therefore occasionally justify an attempt for a conservative treatment. If a malignant lesion is suspected and cannot be excluded by any examination method, histologic verification cannot be avoided (Fig. 6.**11**).

#### Lymphoma

*Lymphomas* are infiltrative growths which may occur in any area of the orbit. The differential diagnosis lies between a monoclonal lymphoid neoplasm, reactive lymphoid hyperplasia and an inflammatory pseudotumor. This differentiation may be difficult, even on histologic examination (see Sect. 6.4). Immunohistochemical methods are now increasingly used for classification. Echographically, these pathologic changes show a relatively uniform picture. An increasing inflammatory character of the pathologic change will nearly always reveal an involvement of Tenon's space and of the lacrimal gland area. Echographically, these lesions are characterized by low reflectivity in the affected orbital segment. The pathologic process usually extends into pre-existing structures, e.g., the lacrimal gland, extraocular muscles or Tenon's space (Figs. 6.**12**, 6.**13** and 6.**14**).

Echographic localization of the lesion will usually suffice for planning a biopsy, which is nearly always necessary in addition to a thorough systemic workup.

#### Rhabdomyosarcoma

*Rhabdomyosarcoma* does not affect any part of the orbit preferentially. On the basis of four personal observations, it can be said that these neoplasms extend into the outer orbital areas and are characterized by a homogenous echographic pattern. The tumor is well delineated from the adipose tissue (Fig. 6.**12**) and can be imaged echographically without any difficulty. We occasionally also see areas of average or high reflectivity, especially when the growing tumor infiltrates and destroys normal orbital structures. According to Ossoinig (1974), rhabdomyosarcoma, together with lymphoma and pseudotumor of the orbit represents, the so-called "low-reflecting orbital lesions". The echogram alone cannot give us unequivocal information and, in suspicious cases, a biopsy is necessary to ascertain the correct diagnosis. During the last years the treatment of these lesions has shifted from radical operation to a combined radio- and chemotherapy. Echography can be useful for follow-up examinations in order to avoid unnecessary radiation exposure by repeated CT scans (Rochels 1980, Bluth et al. 1981).

## 6.3 The Extraocular Muscles

In a number of orbital diseases the muscle volume will increase. In order to evaluate the role of echography, it is important to appreciate the manifold clinical appearances of such diseases (see Table 6.**4**).

We can expect an overlap of clinical signs, histopathologic findings and pathogenetic factors. This discussion aims to incorporate the echographic findings into a concept which will facilitate further diagnostic and therapeutic endeavors.

#### Dysthyroid

Independently from each other Graves (1835) and von Basedow (1840) described an orbitopathy which is usually associated with hyperthyroid goiter. It was soon recognized that this condition may also occur without goiter and without any signs of hyperthyroidism. The original definition therefore had to be enlarged. Recently, cases have been included in which the orbital signs were precursors of an endocrine imbalance which occurred years later (Werner 1955, Ullerich et al. 1976, Mornix et al. 1987). Older authors probably described these cases as pseudotumors.

Table 6.4 **Echographically demonstrable Diseases of extraocular muscles**

| |
|---|
| Graves' orbitopathy |
| Orbital pseudotumor |
| Infections |
| Metastatic tumors to the orbit |
| Lymphoma |

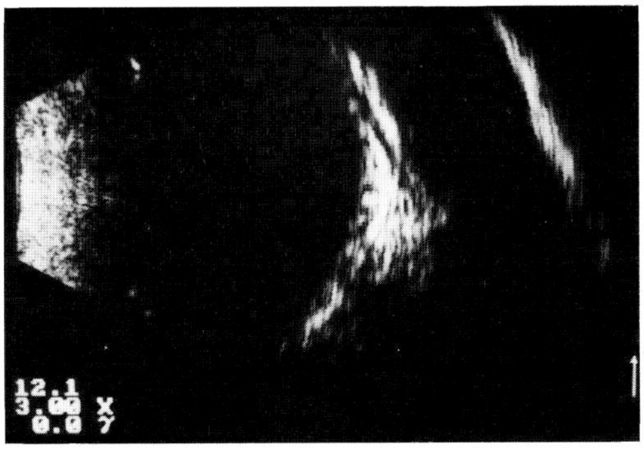


a

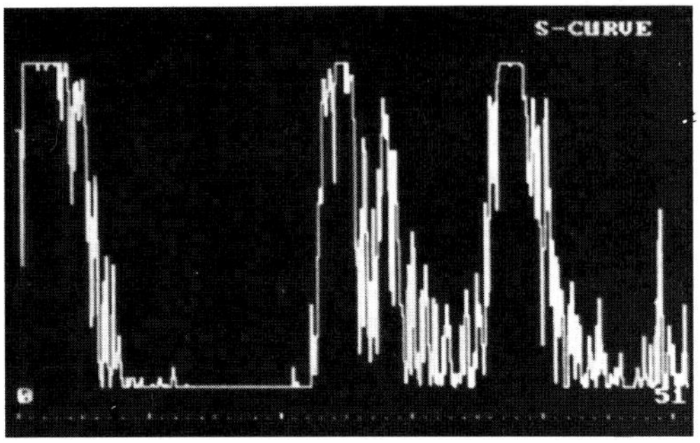


d

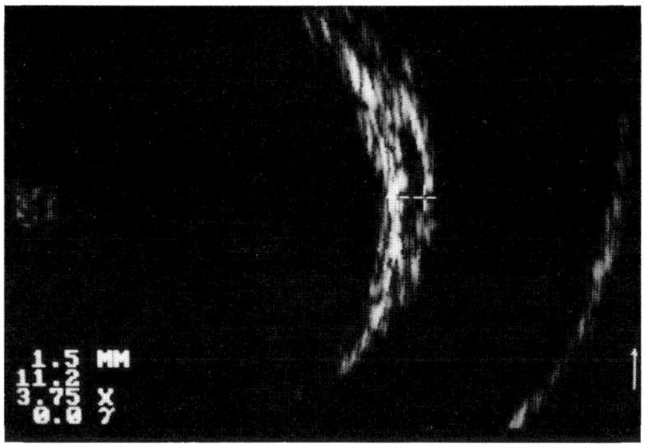


b

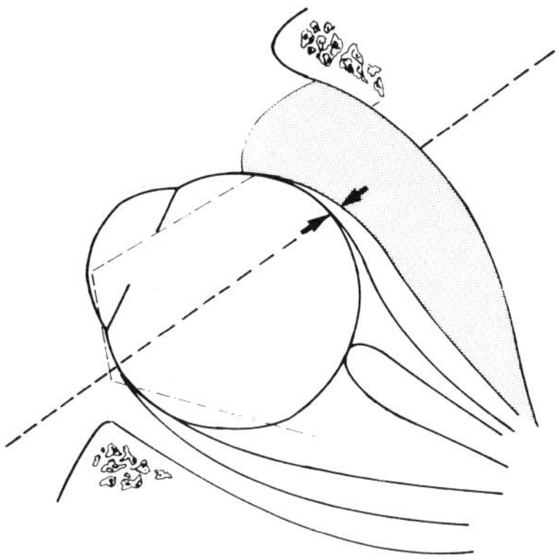

e

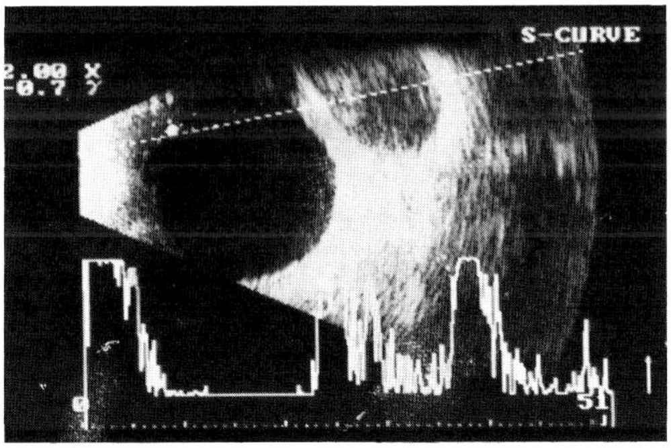


c

Fig. 6.**12a–e** Rhabdomyosarcoma of the temporal orbital space
**a** In a cross sectional echogram the tumor, which shows low reflectivity, can be clearly delineated from the superior rectus muscle
**b** At its insertion the muscle has a diameter of 1.5 mm
**c, d** With increasing tissue sensitivity, the lesion is characterized by low internal echoes of about 20% of the scleral spike
**e** Schematic drawing

Dysthyroid eye disease is a frequent condition; in most cases the question will be asked whether a bi- or unilateral exophthalmus shows echographic signs which are compatible with a presumptive clinical diagnosis of Graves' orbitopathy or whether there are other causes for the exophthalmus.

In the initial stages of the disease the patient complains about a dry eye. There may be a slight retraction of the upper lid. In these instances a measurable thickening of the extraocular muscles is only rarely found. It is important to keep in mind here that there are clinical forms in which only the lacrimal gland or exclusively the orbital adipose tissue is affected. In the large majority of patients, however, the exophthalmus is caused by an increase in muscle volume.

Echographically, the superior and the medial rectus muscles are preferentially involved (Shammas et al. 1980, Skalka, 1980, Guthoff et al. 1981). This does not correspond to the CT scans reported by Trokel et al. (1979) and by Langenbruch (1981). In both studies the inferior rectus muscle was most often affected. The radiologic findings

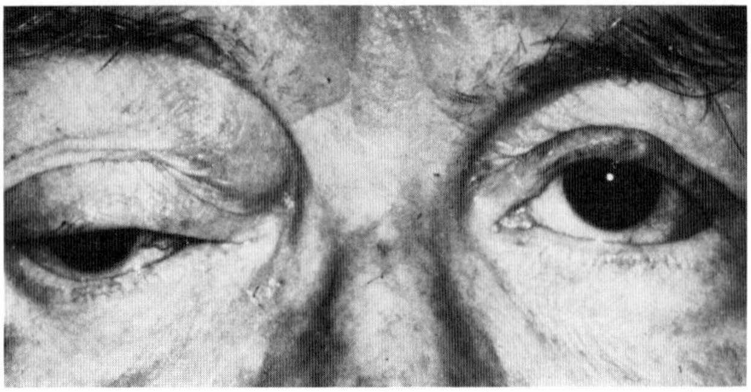

a

Fig. 6.**13 a–c** Eighty-three-year-old woman with lymphoma in the upper outer orbital segment, also involving the levator muscle (**a, b** from Schroeder 1978)
**b** In cross sectional echogram (compare with the other side) the lesion (L) has low acoustic reflectivity and can be clearly delineated from the superior rectus muscle (M). Functional deficits: ptosis, slightly decreased elevation of the right eye
**c** Under loupe magnification the lymphoma is characterized by densely packed cells without any definite stroma. The acoustic interfaces are separated by a distance which is less than the wavelength of the ultrasound; therefore, they produce only minimal reflections (L = lymphoma, BG = adjacent connective tissue) (**a, b** from: Schroeder, W.: Topographische Orbitadiagnostik mit der Kontakt-B-Bild-Echographie. Klin. Mbl. Augenheilk. 172 (1978) 12.)

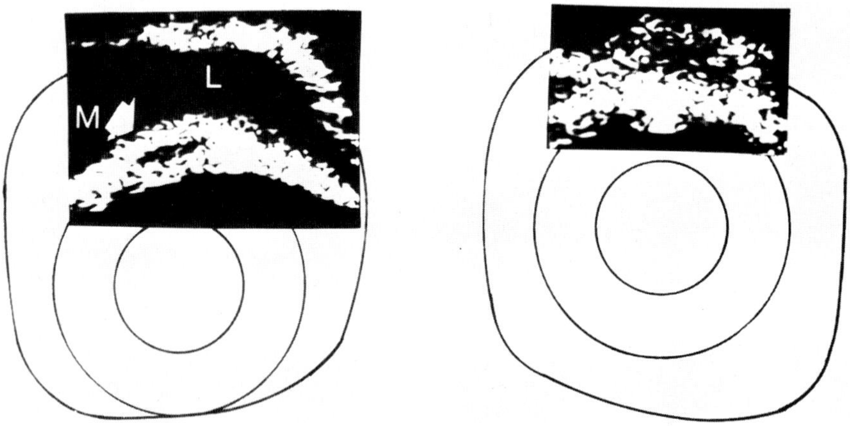


b

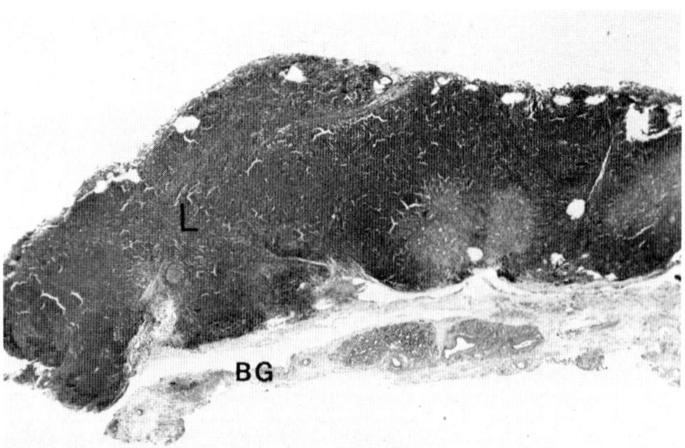


c

a

b

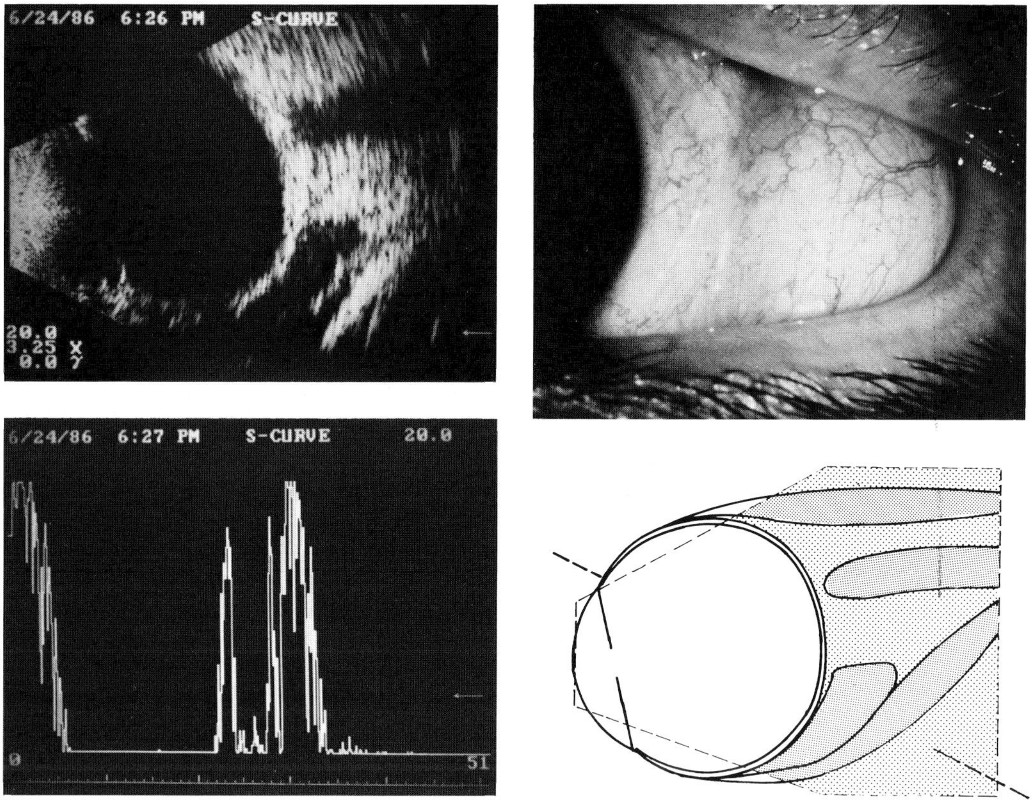


c

d

Fig. 6.**14a–d** Lymphoma of the orbit, involving Tenon's space. The tumor can be seen beneath the conjunctiva extending into the muscle cone

were obtained by combining axial and coronary cuts; therefore, there can be no doubt that they reflect the anatomical situation reliably. The inferior rectus muscle cannot be measured adequately echographically, because the anterior upper orbital margin impedes the motions of the transducer and therefore a widening of the echo can easily be overlooked.

Measuring the amount of reflection within a muscle (Fig. 6.**15**) represents an additional diagnostic factor which depends upon the method used and which was first described by Ossoinig (1982) in an extensive paper. He wrote that "increased reflection and a heterogenous internal structure of the muscle belly represent a new acoustic characteristic of Graves' orbitopathy". In our patient material we find these typical changes mainly in chronic cases. During the initial stage of the disease, i.e., a few months after the first symptoms have appeared, the reflection characteristics of the extraocular muscles do not differ significantly from normal findings. These acoustic phenomena within the muscle belly can be explained by the histopathologic changes during Graves' orbitopathy (Daiker 1979): the predominantly round cell infiltration of the initial stages pushes the muscle fibers aside, but does not create new acoustic interfaces.

During the further course of the disease, connective tissue septa develop and some muscle fibers are replaced by fat tissue (Unsöld 1980). These metaplastic changes create a substrate which produces high internal echos; we find them especially in long-standing cases of Graves' orbitopathy (Fig. 6.**16**). Whenever definite changes in the acoustic reflectivity of extraocular muscles develop, we have to assume that such patients will respond poorly to conservative treatment, e.g., systemic corticosteroids or radiation. At this point, the associated motility defects are probably irreversible so that it will be necessary to operate on

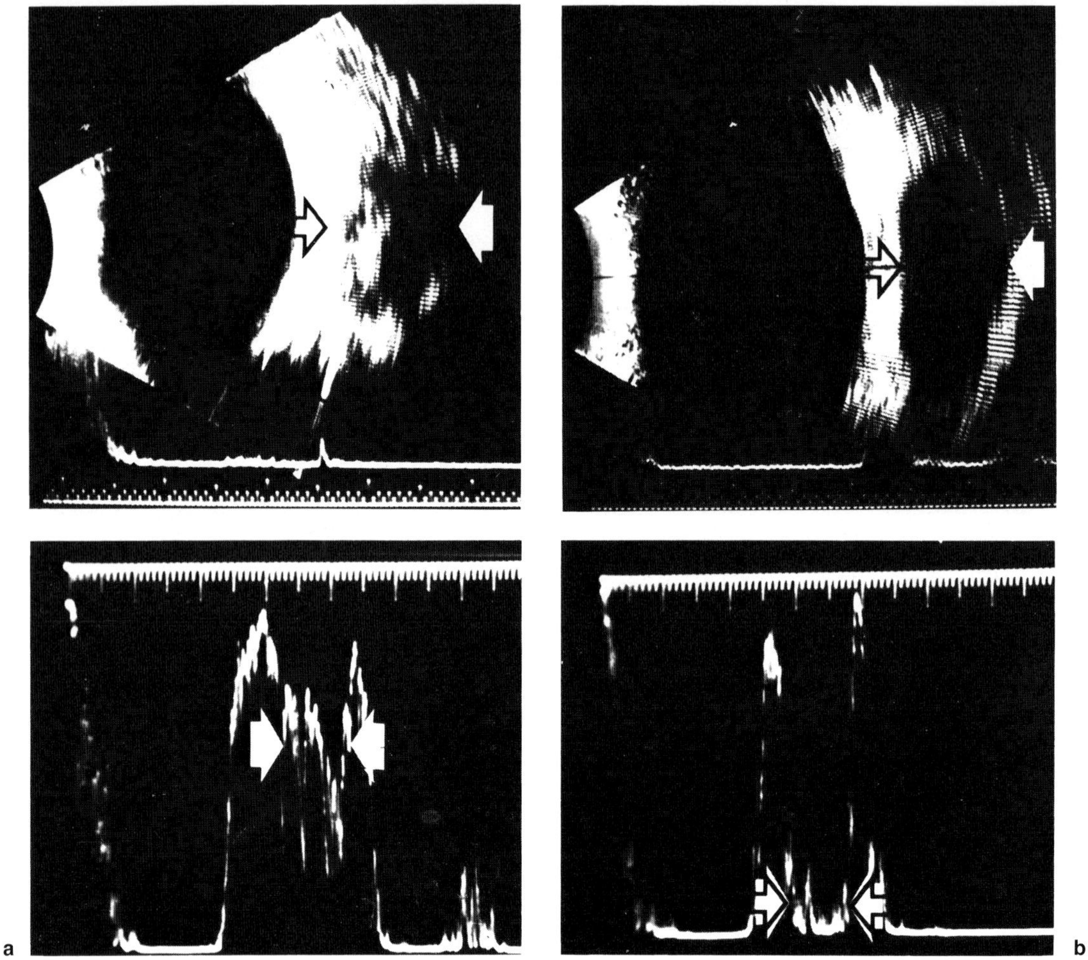

Fig. 6.**15a, b** Comparison of typical findings in chronic myositis (**a**) and in a case of chronic Graves' orbitopathy (**b**). Chronic myositis: the thickened muscle is characterized by low reflectivity. In the standardized A-echogram (lower picture) the amount of reflection from the muscle stroma is about 10% of the echo from the muscle sheath (arrows). In chronic Graves' orbitopathy the increased muscle volume is of about the same degree, but the widening of the muscle shows high acoustic reflectivity. The average amplitude in a standardized echogram is here about 70% of the echo from the muscle sheath

the affected extraocular muscles; otherwise, we may attempt to compensate for the deviation by using prisms (Fig. 6.**16**).

A main echographic sign of Graves' orbitopathy is a widening of the muscle echo. Other changes of the orbital tissues are rarely recognized echographically (Guthoff 1985) (only in 6% of our patients). In the further course of the disease, orbital edema will develop due to impedance of venous outflow. This will cause an echographical widening of the peripheral orbital space, which appears homogenous on ultrasound. At the same time the superior ophthalmic vein may be dilated so that it can be demonstrated echographically (Fig. 6.**17**). Trokel (1978, 1981) and Unsöld (1980) described an enlargement of the lacrimal gland. We could not

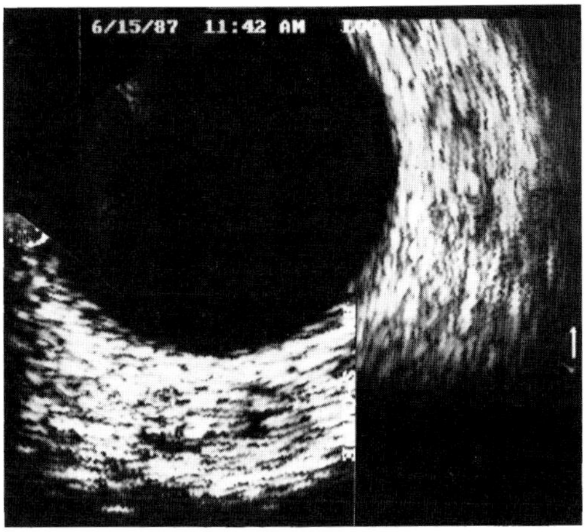


a

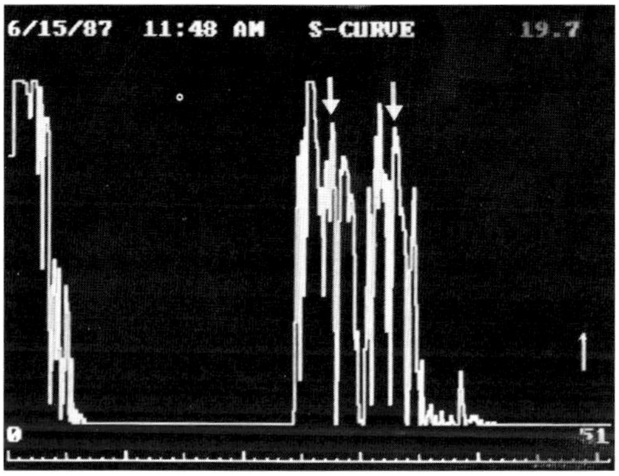


b

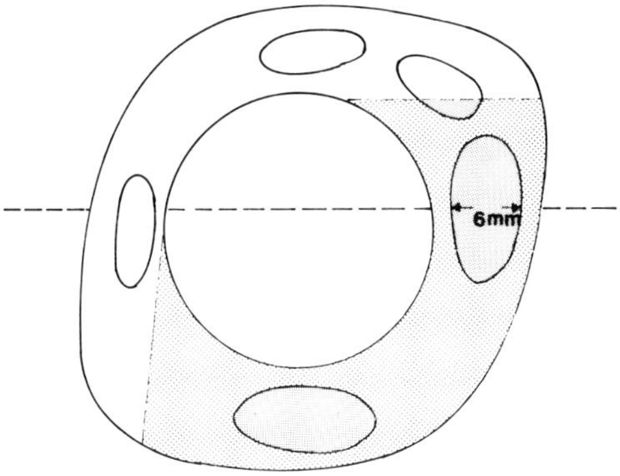


c

Fig. 6.**16 a–c**
**a, b** Pronounced Graves' orbitopathy with symptoms for the preceding 12 months. The muscle can be delineated from the orbital fat only with difficulty; the muscle thickness is about 6.0 mm (medial rectus) and 7.8 mm (inferior rectus)
**c** Schematic drawing

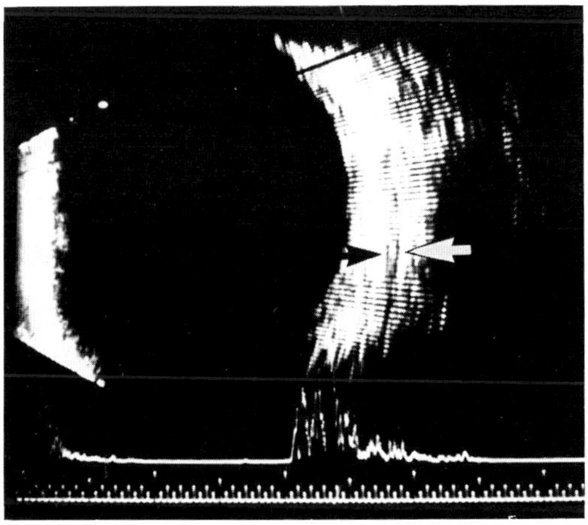

Fig. 6.**17** Echographically demonstrable orbital vein in a patient with progressive Graves' orbitopathy. The increased volume at the orbital apex may lead to venous stasis so that the orbital veins are echographically demonstrable. This is a pathologic finding. Under these conditions the coupling pressure of the transistor does not suffice to collapse the vessels and thereby make them disappear on the echogram

demonstrate this in our patients, though such an enlargement should be appreciated on echography.

Previously there was a controversy regarding the involvement of extraocular muscles and the defects of ocular motility (Esslen et al. 1961). It now seems certain that in the large majority of cases, the thickened extraocular muscle gives a normal or only minimally changed electromyogram (Jensen

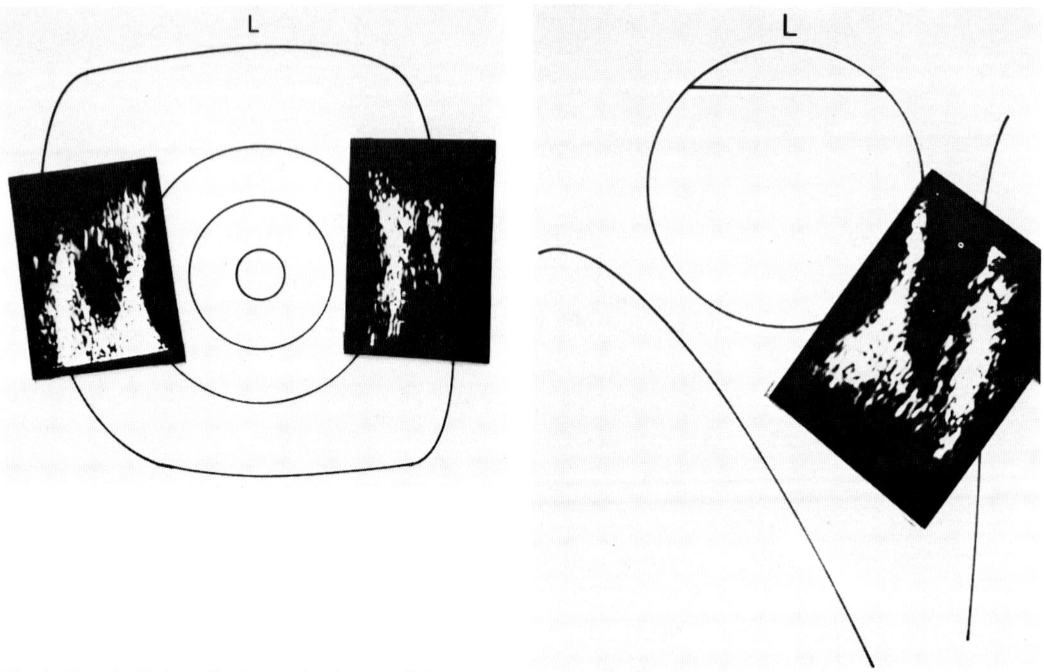


a b

Fig. 6.**18a, b** Metastatic tumor in the medial rectus muscle and its sheath in an 83-year-old woman who was suffering from metastasizing breast carcinoma. In frontal and sagittal cross sectional echograms, the widening of the muscle can be demonstrated. The tumefaction temporal and above the muscle could be interpreted as an infiltration of the muscle sheaths. Decreased ocular motility (adduction extent, 7 mm; abduction extent, 4 mm) indicates that there is decreased stretchability of the muscle infiltrated by metastatic tumor

1971). The resulting motility loss is apparently due to a decreased stretchability of the affected muscle, and appears clinically as a so-called "pseudoparesis" of the antagonist. This also explains the abnormal findings on tonometry in different directions of gaze: if the patient attempts to move his eye toward the side of the pseudoparetic muscle (in the direction in which the globe can be least rotated), there will be an increase in intraocular pressure due to squeezing of the globe caused by increased tension in the muscle (Draeger 1960, 1963).

In our experience it is not too difficult to echographically differentiate Graves' orbitopathy from an inflammatory orbital pseudotumor and its subdivision, acute and chronic myositis. It seems important to us that in Graves' orbitopathy the muscles alone are affected. The reflectivity of the muscles is unchanged or markedly increased. This is of additional diagnostic significance in delineating this orbitopathy from chronic myositis. Only in severe cases of Graves' orbitopathy will the increased orbital volume lead to an extracellular fluid accumulation which widens Tenon's space. This sign is therefore an important differential diagnostic characteristic against inflammatory changes (see below). These small areas of edema are caused by hydrostatic pressure only. The same applies to arteriovenous fistules in which large shunt volumes will produce fluid exudations around the dilated vessels (see Fig. 6.**23**). Vascular permeability is apparently not increased in either condition; in this respect they differ from the inflammatory orbital pseudotumor.

*Metastatic carcinoma to the extraocular muscles* has so far been only rarely reported. Bedford and Daniel (1960) and Ashton (1974) have published six histologically confirmed cases. Trokel (1979) reported metastatic carcinoma which, on CT scan, mimicked a widening of the muscle and led to a passive constriction of ocular motility. Ossoinig (1972) reported a histologically proven metastasis confined to the muscle sheaths which invaded neither the muscle fibers nor the adjacent orbital tissues. We also found in our patients a uniformly homogenous echographic widening of the muscle belly associated with passive restriction of ocular motility. In a patient with metastases from a breast carcinoma (Fig. 6.**18**), an isolated paramuscular mass could have been indicating an infiltration of the muscle sheaths as described by Ossoinig. However, frontal and horizontal sections showed that the muscle itself was also involved. Hasenfratz and Riedel (1987) reported a similar case. Such metastases are relatively rare. In Ashton's (1974) report, the orbital involvement occurred years before the primary tumor was found. The uniform clinical and echographic signs are remarkable; we should consider a metastatic lesion, in addition to myositis, whenever there is a homogenous echographic pattern from a widened muscle associated with a mainly passive restriction of ocular motility. The primary lesion may still be undetected. An isolated involvement of the muscle sheath is, according to the published reports, a pathognomonic sign. Figure 6.**19** shows an echographic cross section of a metastatic tumor in the region of the superior oblique muscle. The increased volume of the muscle belly central to the trochlea apparently decreased the stretchability of the muscle and inhibited elevation of the eye in adduction.

Echography can reliably prove the presence of thickened extraocular muscles and therefore represents the method of choice for this diagnostic problem.

> **Note:** Widening of the extraocular muscles is usually quite pronounced if it produces clinical signs and symptoms. If the widening is equivocal, then it is not present. In advanced Graves' orbitopathy, the echographic documentation may be difficult or even impossible because the reflectivity of the widened muscle resembles that of the adipose tissue.

## 6.4 Orbital Pseudotumor As a Working Diagnosis

Birch Hirschfeld introduced the term "pseudotumor orbitae" in 1905 for a special kind of exophthalmus which either regressed spontaneously or showed on biopsy only nonspecific inflammatory tissue. Blodi and Gass (1968) summarized and delineated the concept of an orbital pseudotumor as "a nonspecific inflammation of orbital tissue without any obvious systemic or local cause". The concept of an orbital pseudotumor is clinically useful, but should always be considered as a "working diagnosis" because, in principle, even a histologic examination cannot unequivocally prove the diagnosis. Nonspecific inflammatory tissue may also be found around malignant lesions, and a careless interpretation could delay the final diagnosis.

In our experience, echography, in connection with the clinical picture, is capable of clarifying the situation. The correlations of morphologic changes and function in the frequently affected extraocular muscles appear to be especially interesting. Jacobs et al. (1980) divide the pseudotumor into a myositic and a nonmyositic type on the basis of CT findings. Shibata et al. (1981) corroborate these concepts on the basis of echographic findings.

Echographically, the orbital pseudotumor is characterized by decreased reflectivity of the involved orbital segments (Fig. 6.**20**). The lesion could be described as an "infiltrative space-occupying process" which widens pre-existing orbital structures (Schroeder 1978). Orbital lymphomas may lead to practically identical signs, though the externally visible inflammatory reaction is here minimal or absent.

#### Orbital Myositis

If the extraocular muscles are involved in the inflammatory process, they appear as spindle-shaped structures of remarkably low acoustic reflectivity and can easily be delineated from the surrounding fat. They may be moderately or extremely widened, occasionally three times as wide as normal (Fig. 6.**21**). In our own series (Guthoff et al. 1988), 8 out of 15 patients showed loss of stretchability of the involved muscle, and in 4 out of 15 patients, no unequivocal diagnosis could be made because the muscles were affected repeatedly.

The disease process begins acutely with chemosis, pain and exophthalmus. An orbital cellulitis from a paranasal sinus or due to an embolus has to be excluded. According to the experiences of Mottow-Lippa (1981), inflamed dermoids also have to be considered from a differential diagnostic point of view. Henderson (1980) reported similar symptoms in orbital embryonal rhabdomyosarcoma.

If it is possible to localize the lesion accurately, histologic confirmation of the diagnosis seems to be reasonable. Echography can reliably demonstrate these nonspecific inflammatory lesions and

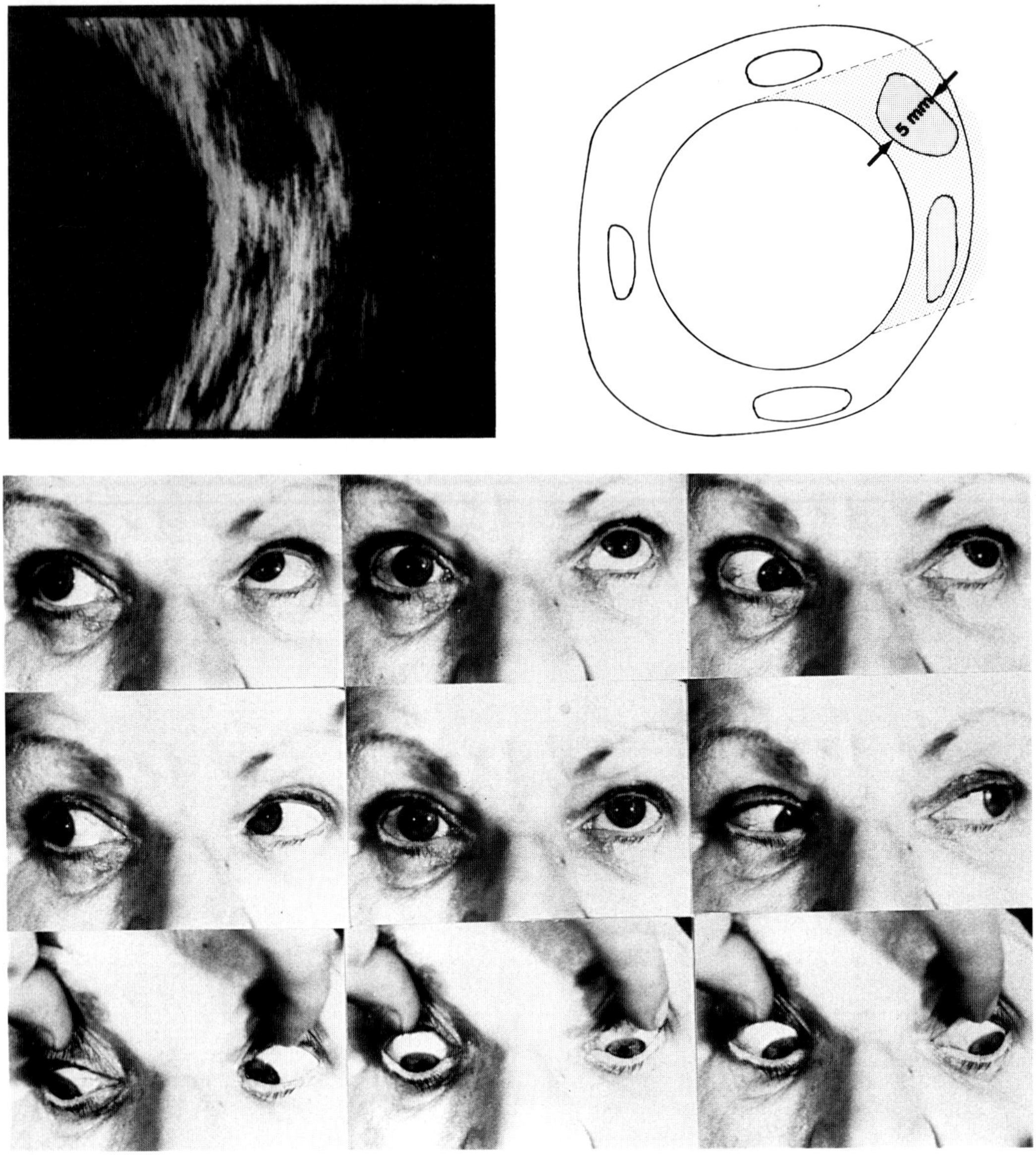


a b c

Fig. 6.**19a–c** Frontal cross sectional echogram and ocular motility in various directions of gaze in a 68-year-old woman with metastasizing carcinoma. The right superior oblique is widened to about 5 mm, and the motility deficit is characterized by a decreased elevation in adduction (acquired Brown syndrome)

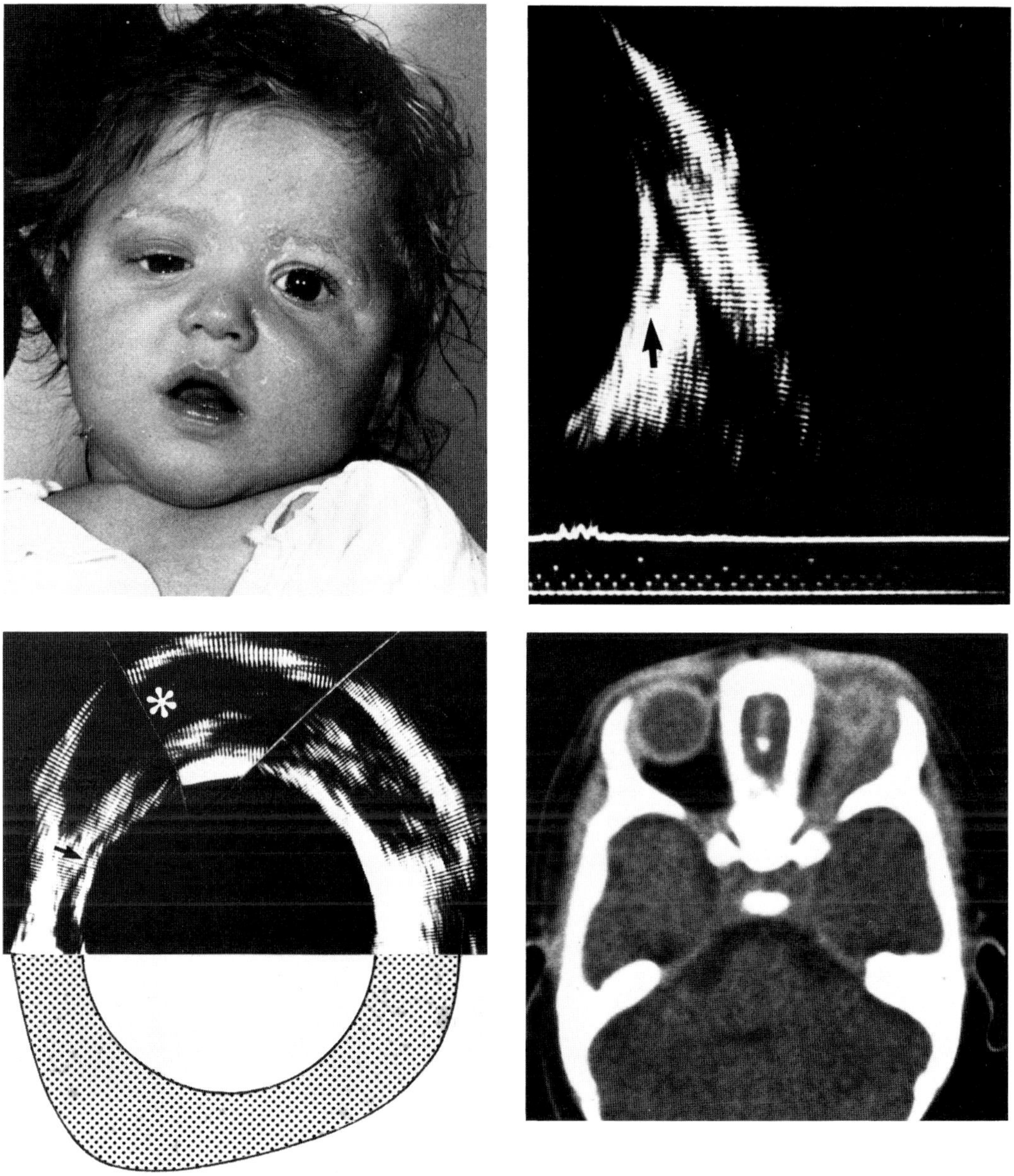

a c

d

b

Fig. 6.**20 a–d**
**a–d** Inflammatory pseudotumor with infiltration of the lacrimal gland, the temporal orbital segment and Tenon's space
**a** Nine-month-old girl: for four weeks, "conjunctivitis not responding to treatment"; for two weeks, elevated temperature
**b** In cross sectional echogram a widening of the upper temporal orbital segment involving the area of the lacrimal gland (*) (frontal section) with homogenous acoustic reflectivity
**c** Infiltration of Tenon's space (black arrow)
**d** Axial CT scan (obtained under general anesthesia): increased density in the upper orbital segment. The widening of Tenon's space could not be demonstrated on any CT section

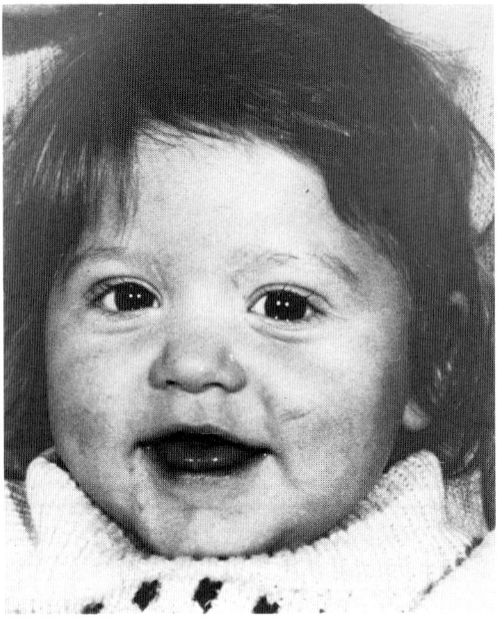

e

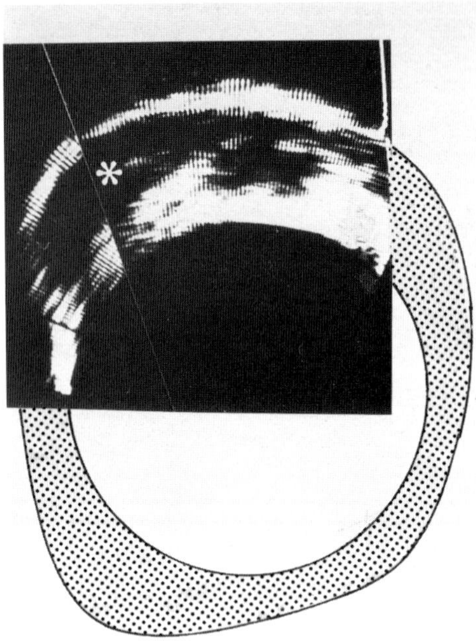


f

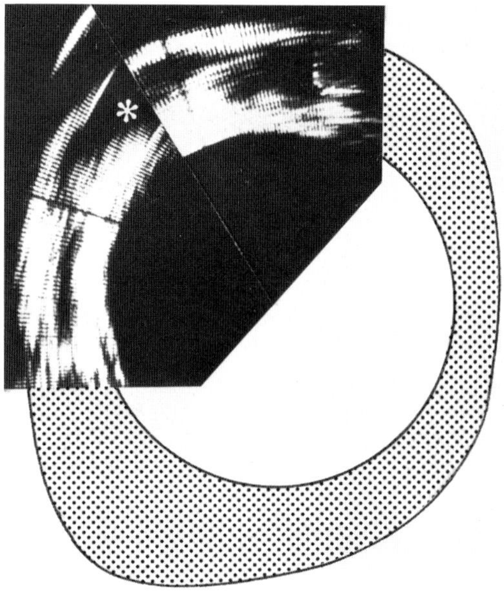


g

Fig. 6.**20e–g** The condition regressed clinically within two weeks, but the pathologic changes of the echogram could still be demonstrated. Four weeks after the first examination (**f**), the child was free of symptoms, but there was still a minimal enlargement of the lacrimal gland (**g**)

therefore, an attempt at treatment with corticosteroids seems justified. If the diagnosis was correct, the lesion should regress within a few days. Other disease processes, especially malignant lesions, may also respond to corticosteroids, but only the inflammatory pseudotumor will respond with such characteristic speed. Echography is also frequently used for controlling the course of the condition, as this method of examination does not carry any risks.

The CT scan is certainly necessary when we suspect that the process extends outside of the orbit. This

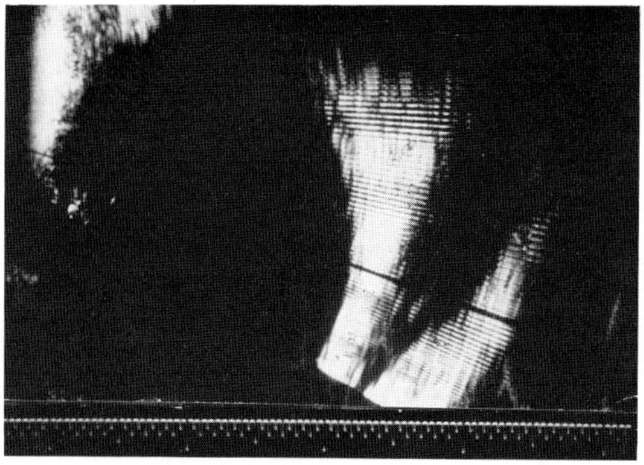
a

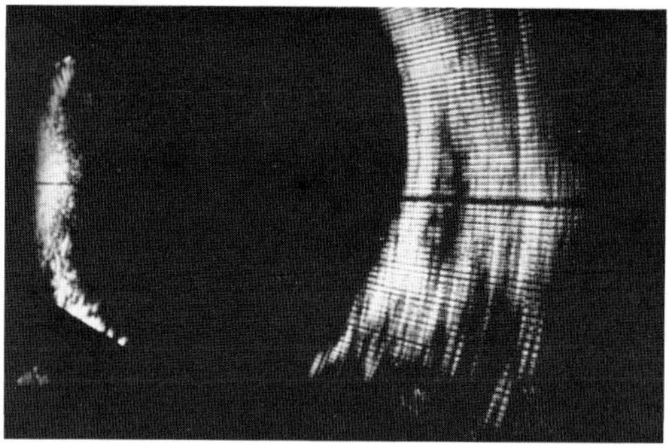
b

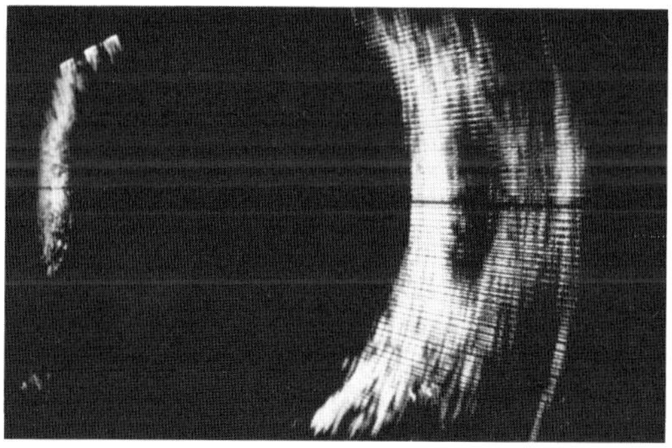
c

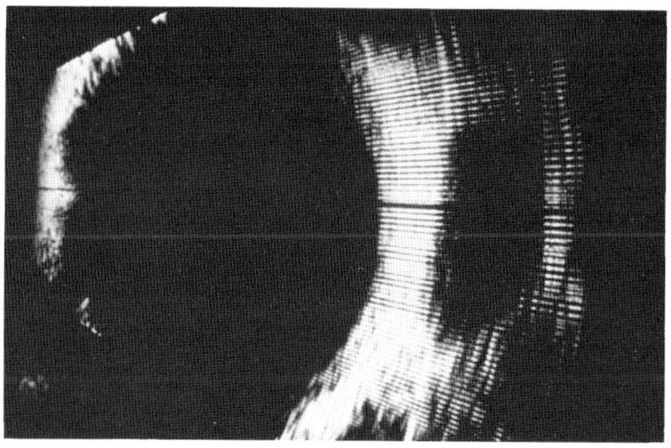
d

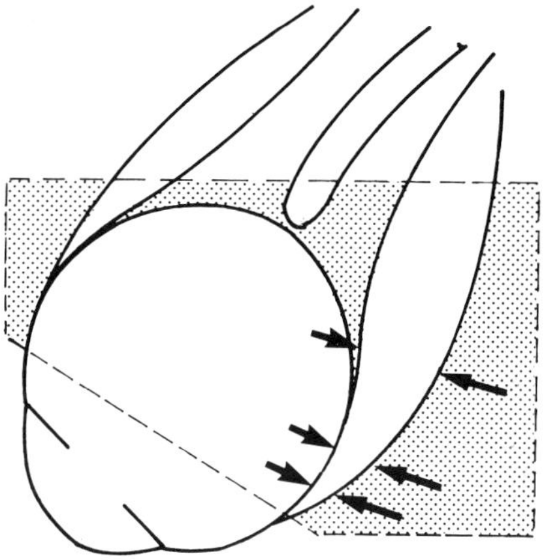
e

Fig. 6.**21 a–e** Chronic orbital myositis of the medial rectus muscle (myositic pseudotumor)
**a** The spindle-shaped widening of the muscle is best seen on a horizontal cross sectional echogram
**b–d** An exact measurement in the frontal plane is not possible because appropriate landmarks are missing
**e** Schematic drawing. The arrows correspond to the cross sectional echograms in **b–d**

radiologic method may not be necessary in infants and children. The time required to obtain a CT scan requires exact fixation, which frequently can only be achieved in deep sedation or under general anesthesia. Repeated follow-up examinations should only exceptionally be performed in children, in order to avoid the effects of radiation on growing organs (Bluth et al. 1981).

## 6.5 The Central Orbital Space

Table 6.5 **Diseases of the central orbital space echographically demonstrable**

| |
|---|
| Vascular exophthalmus |
| Spontaneous and traumatic fistules |
| Cavernous hemangioma |
| Thrombosis of orbital vein |
| Orbital varix |
| Lymphangioma |
| Metastatic neoplasms |
| Space-occupying lesions of the optic nerve and its sheaths |

### Vascular Exophthalmus

Disturbances of orbital circulation play an important role among the diseases which echographically seem to be located in the central orbital space. We classify as **vascular exophthalmus**: traumatic and spontaneous cavernous sinus fistulas, thrombosis of the orbital veins, orbital varix and cavernous hemangioma.

### Acquired Arteriovenous Fistula

Arteriovenous fistulas of the cavernous sinus have long been recognized as the most frequent cause of pulsating exophthalmus. In the majority of patients a cranial trauma is responsible for this condition. Fractures of the bony wall or shearing effects in a severe contusion may damage the arterial wall. Only during the last years, due to improved diagnostic methods, can we diagnose a spontaneous carotid-cavernous sinus fistula more easily.

The cavernous sinus is the only intracranial area in which an artery passes through a venous sinus. Here, arterial bleeding will not expand in the subarachnoidal or subdural space, but will overload the cerebral venous circulation. The blood will be drained through the ipsilateral ophthalmic vein and perhaps through an intercavernous shunt on the other side as well.

### Traumatic Carotid-Cavernous Sinus Fistula

The classical sign and symptom, in addition to pulsating exophthalmus, is a bruit heard by the patient or by the examiner. This will, in most cases, lead to the correct diagnosis before an echographic examination has been done (Fig. 6.**22**). In these patients the diagnosis can be corroborated echographically within seconds by finding in the muscle cone a vessel which pulsates on pressure. This vessel can be imaged on B-mode without difficulties (Guthoff et al. 1987) with A-mode it may take some practice to find the fast flickering spikes (Ossoinig et al. 1975).

### The Spontaneous Carotid-Cavernous Sinus Fistula (Red Eye Shunt Syndrome)

In the majority of our patients with acquired arteriovenous orbital fistula, the signs and symptoms were less dramatic and there was no trauma in the history. The pulsating and therefore arterialized vessel was found by chance. An exact analysis, occasionally complemented later by a carotid angiogram (Guthoff et al. 1987), led us to conclude that these were spontaneous fistulas between dural vessels and the cavernous sinus, i.e., ruptures of small vessels which branch from the internal or external carotid and course in the cavernous sinus (Peeters et al. 1979). These shunts with rather small volume and minimally increased venous pressure are not capable of producing pulsation and bruits. The ophthalmologic signs frequently lead to an erroneous diagnosis, e.g., myositis, episcleritis, orbital pseudotumor or unilateral glaucoma of undetermined etiology.

> The key to a diagnosis of an arteriovenous fistula is the echographic documentation of an intraconal blood vessel pulsating on pressure.

Most frequently affected is the anterior communicating vein, which courses between the medial rectus muscle and the optic nerve and connects the superior and inferior orbital veins. By applying the transducer temporally on the globe, the vessel can be imaged on a cross section, when using a horizontal examination plane, and on a longitudinal section, when using a frontal examination plane (Fig. 6.**23**).

Pulsations as a sign of arterialization will only be visible when the tissue pressure exceeds the diastolic intravascular pressure. We can achieve this in

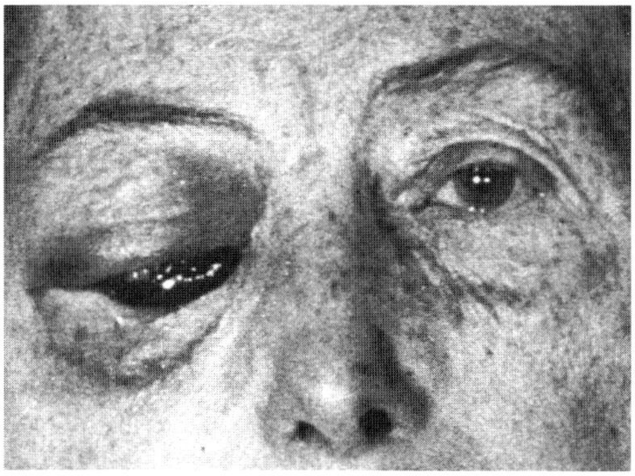
a

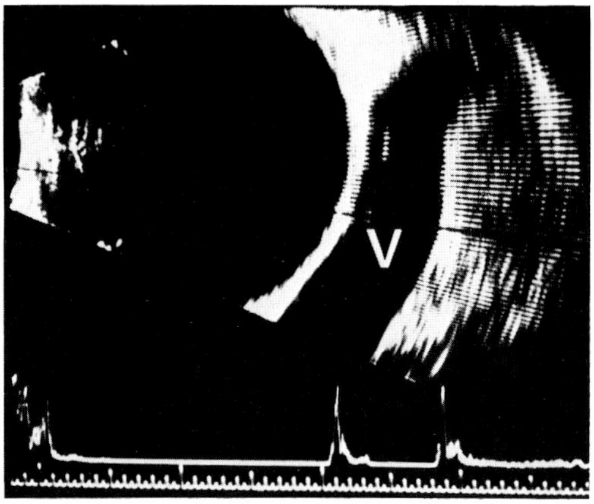

b

Fig. 6.**22a, b** Clinical picture and echographic findings in a case of traumatic cavernous sinus fistula
**a** Marked chemosis after acute deterioration of a traumatic fistula which had been present for years; the picture shows the patient after numerous attempts to close the fistula by embolization
**b** Widening of the ophthalmic vein to about 8 mm (V); upon pressure there is a collapse of the vessel synchronously with the pulse.

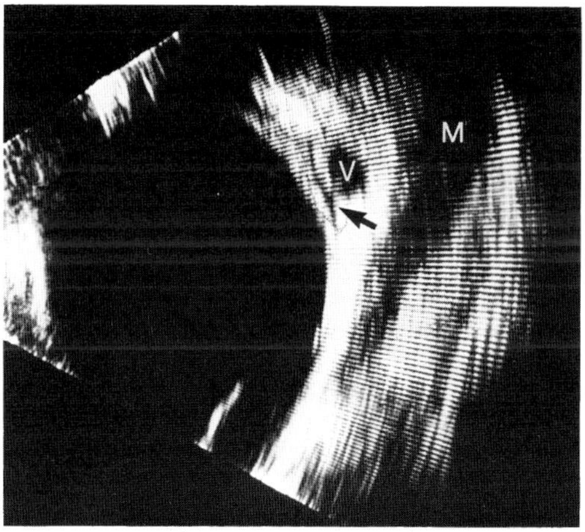

a

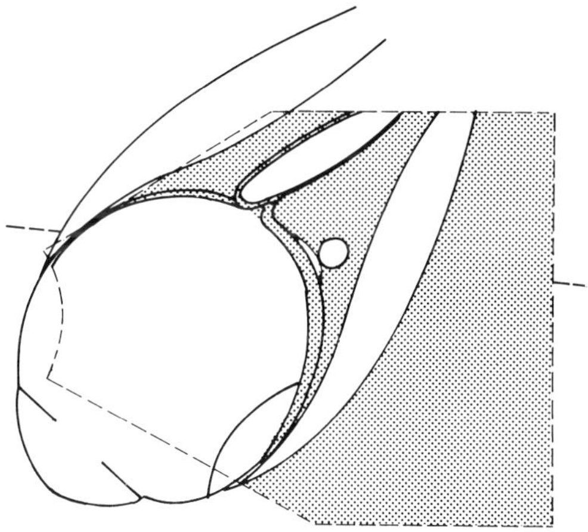
c

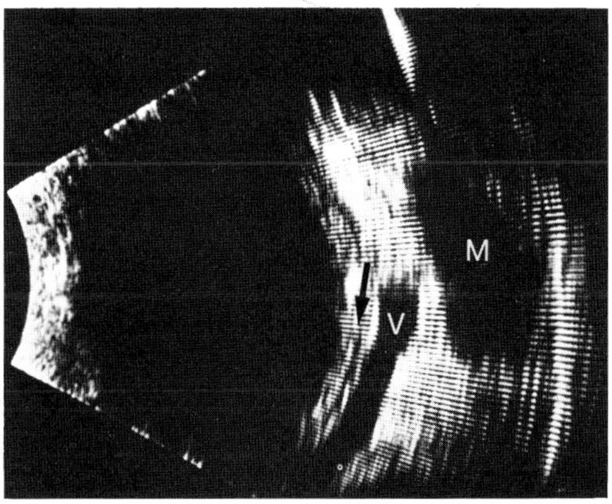

b

Fig. 6.**23a–c** Spontaneous arteriovenous fistula of the cavernous sinus in an 83-year-old woman. Increasing unilateral dilatation of the episcleral veins for the preceding four weeks. Progressive nonspecific decreased ocular motility
**a** Horizontal cross sectional echogram through the nasal part of the orbit
**b** Frontal cross sectional echogram. The overload on the venous vascular system has not only dilated the vein, but has also led to a circumscribed edema in Tenon's space, a widening of the recti muscles (here of the medial rectus), and a peripheral choroidal detachment
**c** Schematic drawing

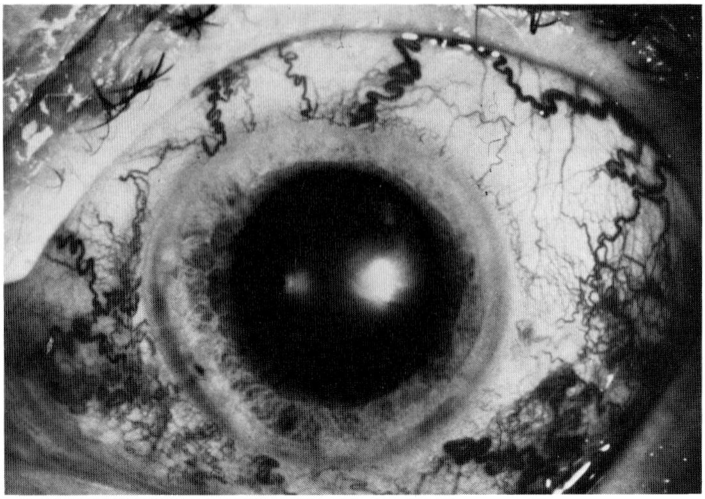

a

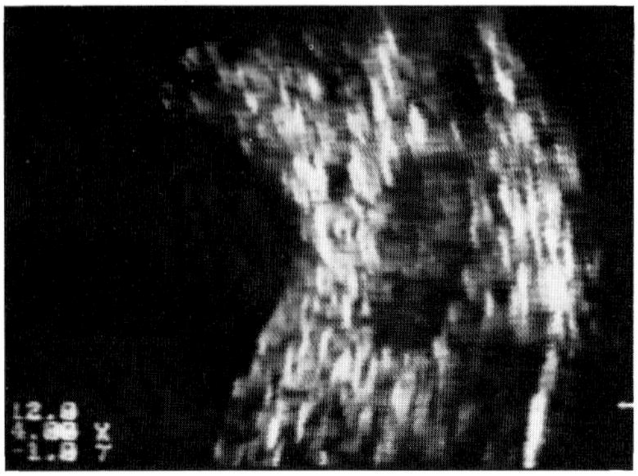


b

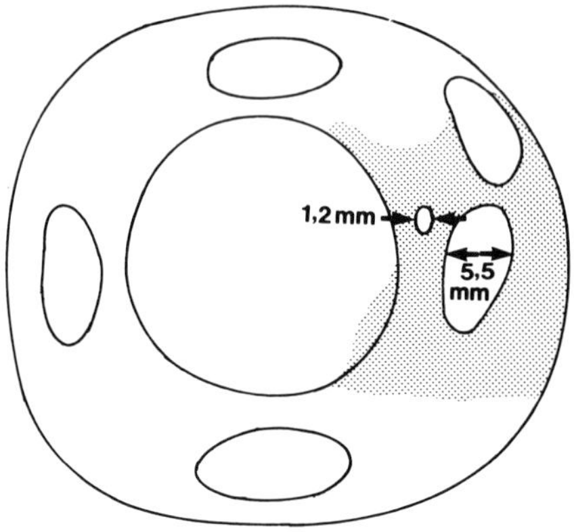


c

Fig. 6.**24a–c** Spontaneous dura-cavernous sinus fistula with small shunt volume
**a** There is moderate conjunctival and episcleral hyperemia and a difference in the intraocular pressure between right and left eyes (intraocular pressure in the affected eye is 8 mmHg higher than in the fellow eye); nonspecific decreased ocular motility of minor degree
**b** The internal diameter of the imaged vessel is about 1.2 mm; anterior diameter of the medial rectus muscle is about 5.5 mm
**c** Schematic drawing
**d, e** See color plates

arterialized veins by compressing the orbit manually. The previously easily identifiable vessel collapses synchronously with the pulse and disappears for a short time from the screen. In our experience, a vessel diameter of about 2 mm suffices to demonstrate this phenomenon (Fig. 6.**24**). The summation of image points on the B-mode echogram seems to be superior to the A-mode, and is preferred by most authors examining this disease entity.

In order to diagnose an arteriovenous fistula, we not only have to demonstrate the vessel, but also prove that pulsation occurs on pressure. This has been corroborated by individual observations on patients with expanding *thrombosis of the orbital veins* or with an inflammatory pseudotumor in which the cavernous sinus is also involved (Tolosa-Hunt syndrome). It is relatively easy to find the ophthalmic vein, but even marked up to pain-producing pressure will not make the vessel disappear on the echogram.

Using color-coded Doppler sonography facilitates the diagnosis and treatment control of orbital arteriovenous fistulas (Fig. 6.**24d, e**). A final evaluation cannot be made at the present time.

Table 6.6 **Referral diagnosis of patients with spontaneous cavernous sinus fistula** (n = 21)

| | |
|---|---|
| Orbital myositis | 6 |
| Orbital pseudotumor | 3 |
| Cavernous sinus fistula | 3 |
| Graves' orbitopathy | 2 |
| Retrobulbar tumor | 2 |
| Conjunctivitis | 2 |
| Angle closure glaucoma | 2 |
| Central vein thrombosis | 1 |

All disturbances of orbital circulation which impede venous outflow will lead to a widening of the extraocular muscles. This *widening of the muscles* can nearly always be found in patients with carotid-cavernous sinus fistula and is therefore an important differential diagnostic point of any myogenous exophthalmus. Table 6.**6** lists the referral diagnoses of 21 patients with spontaneous carotid-cavernous sinus fistula.

Occasionally, orbital veins can be demonstrated in cases of Graves' orbitopathy or in idiopathic myositis, but they disappear on moderate pressure without showing any pulsation. It is reasonable to assume that these veins, while exiting from the muscle cone, are being compressed by the markedly widened muscle bellies.

### Orbital Varices

*Orbital varix* can usually be diagnosed by the intermittent exophthalmus and the enophthalmus which occurs in between. Occasionally, we may be able to demonstrate echographically a widening of the veins during a Valsalva maneuver (Fig. 6.**25**).

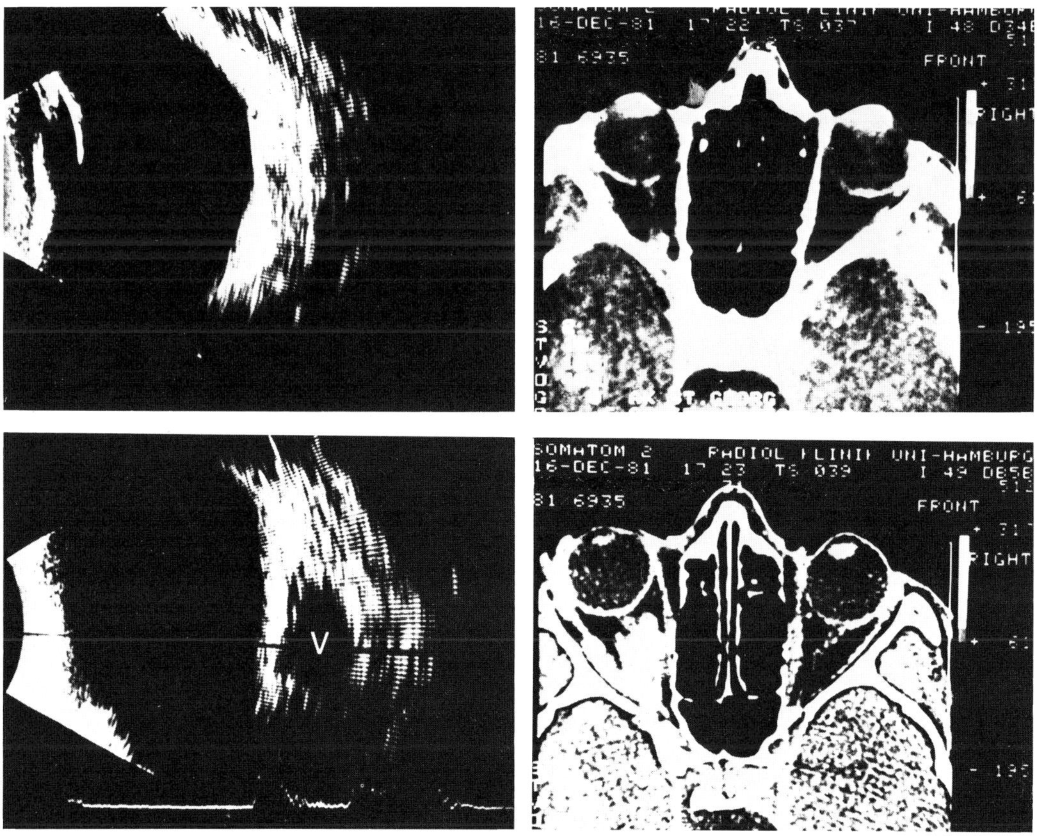


a b

Fig. 6.**25 a, b** Orbital varix in a 19-year-old woman
**a** During a Valsalva maneuver, we see an echo-free area in the central part of the orbit. This could be interpreted as the completely filled varix
**b** The same phenomenon can be demonstrated on CT scan

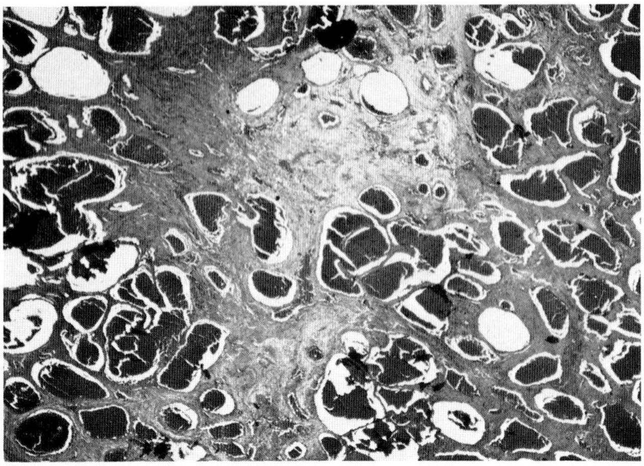

Fig. 6.**26** Histologic section of a cavernous orbital hemangioma. The septa are at a distance of 0.5–1 mm and therefore represent ideal acoustic interfaces for ultrasound. The regular structure of the lesion produces a nearly pathognomonic echogram

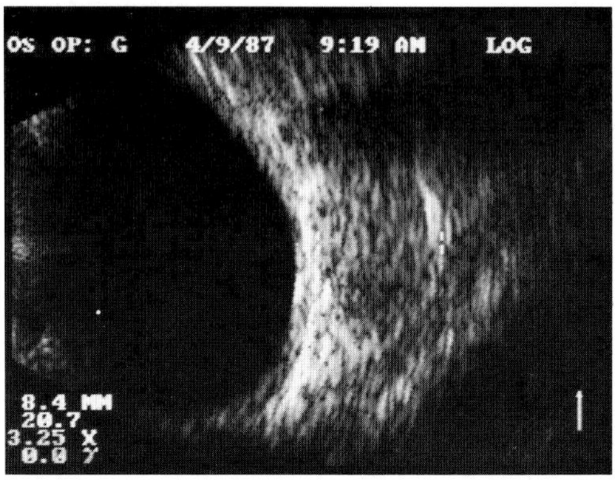


a

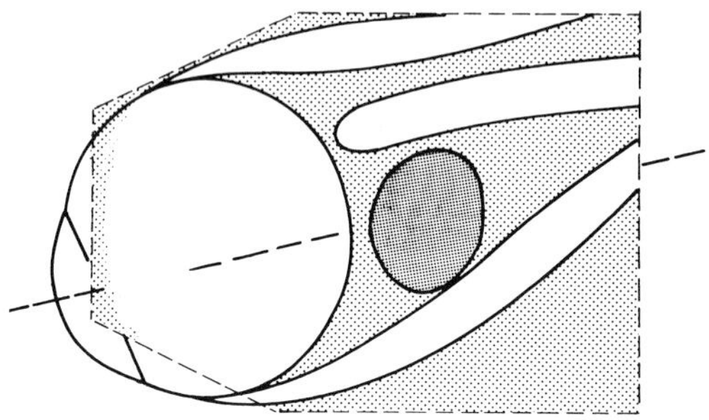

c

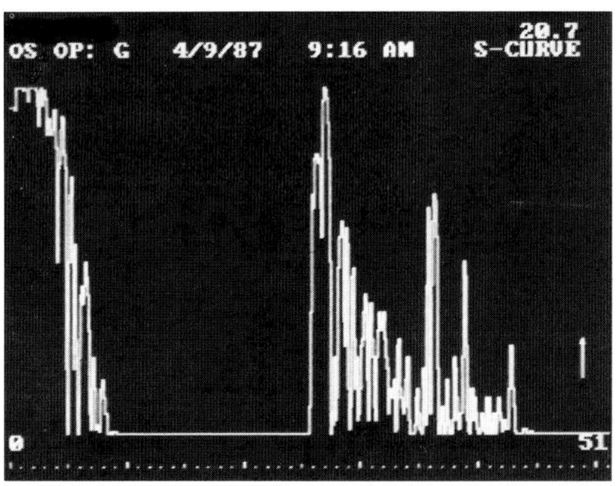


b

Fig. 6.**27 a–c** Small cavernous hemangioma in the muscle cone
**a** A suitable gray scale with logarithmic representation delineates the tumor clearly from the surroundings also on B-mode
**b** The diagnosis is corroborated by the characteristic sound attenuation with linearly decreasing internal echoes when the S-mode amplification is used for A-mode
**c** Schematic drawing

**Cavernous Hemangioma**

The *cavernous hemangioma* is one of the most common orbital tumors in adults (Hauff 1980, Henderson 1980). The tumor usually lies in the muscle cone and is encapsulated. It has a uniform histologic structure: blood-filled cavities are separated by septa. The lumen of the cavities is around 1 mm wide (Fig. 6.**26**). This framework of acoustic interfaces produces a strong acoustic reflectivity on

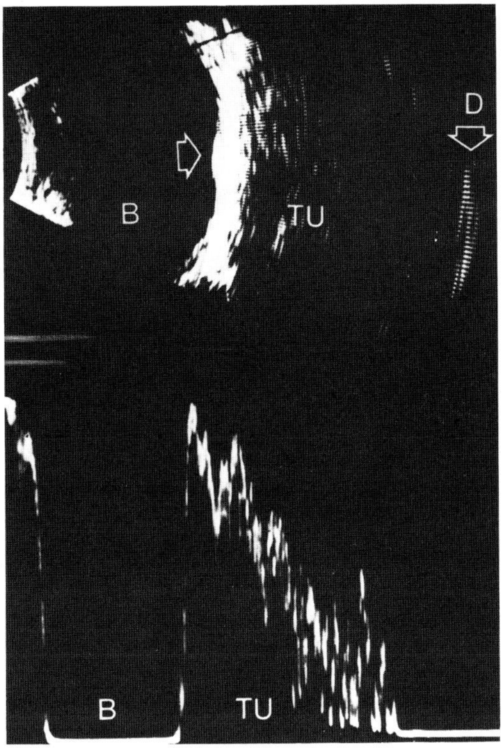


a

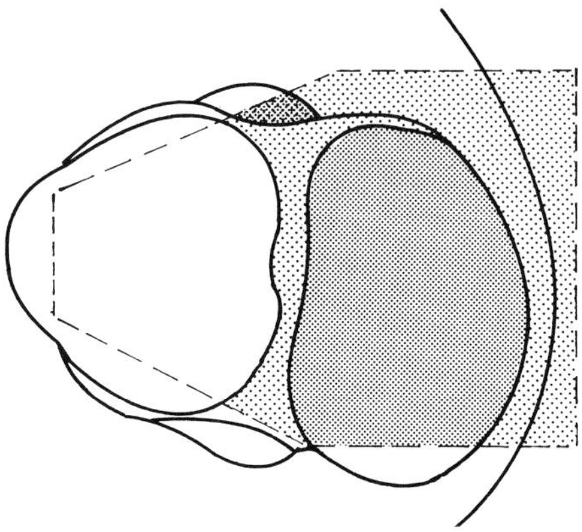

b

Fig. 6.**28a–c** Large cavernous orbital hemangioma pressing on the globe. The tumor has been present for many years and has caused complete optic atrophy. Vision is reduced to 0.05. Once the diagnosis has been ascertained, even small tumors should be excised early
**a** Standardized A-mode provides a nearly pathognomonic pattern. B = globe, arrow = pressure on the globe, TU = tumor, D = orbital roof
**b** Schematic drawing
**c** On CT scan the lesion is characterized by a round, sharply delineated space-occupying lesion in the muscle cone

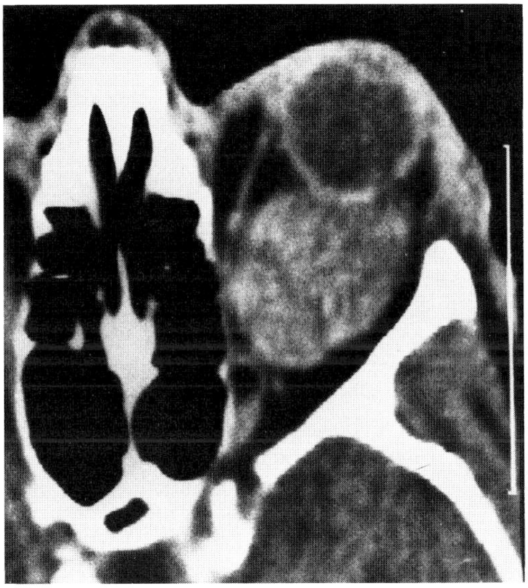

c

the usual ophthalmic ultrasound instruments, with a sound attenuation that extends into the tumor (Fig. 6.**27**). Using an S-shaped amplification with a well-calibrated apparatus, the A-mode echogram is nearly pathognomonic (Ossoinig et al. 1975) (Fig. 6.**28**).

#### Lymphangioma

*Lymphangiomas* are usually diagnosed by their typical clinical picture. They grow expansively and occasionally, the central orbital space is also involved. These are cystoid cavities of different size with a relatively high tendency to bleed, even after minor trauma (Fig. 6.**29**) (Jones 1959, Krohel et al. 1979, Wright 1974).

#### Metastatic Tumors

*Metastases* may develop anywhere in the orbit. Preferred sites are vascularized areas, extraocular muscles and the muscle cone. According to the literature (Shammas 1984) occasionally necroses develop centrally in the lesion, leading to typical A-mode patterns.

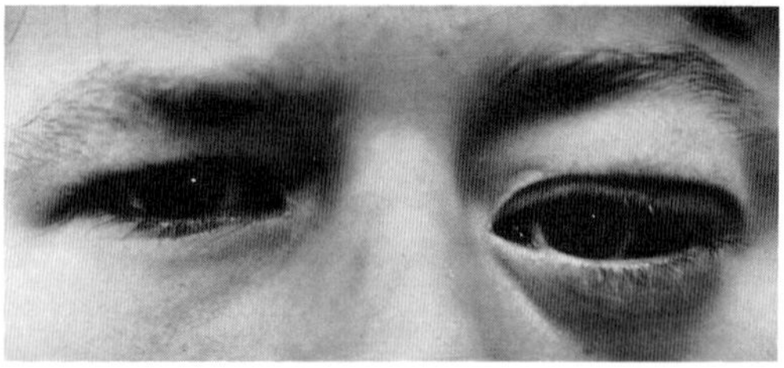
a

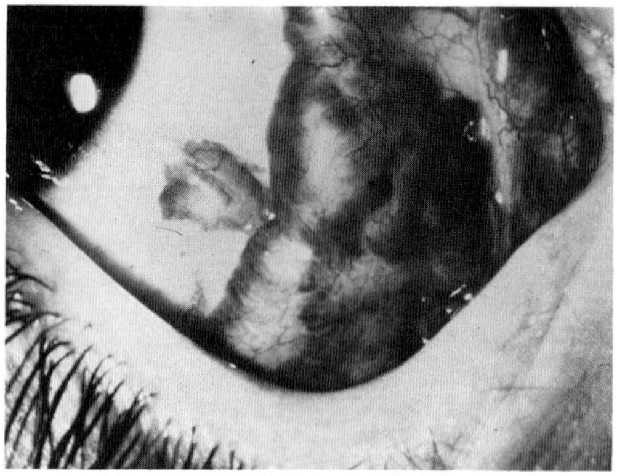
b

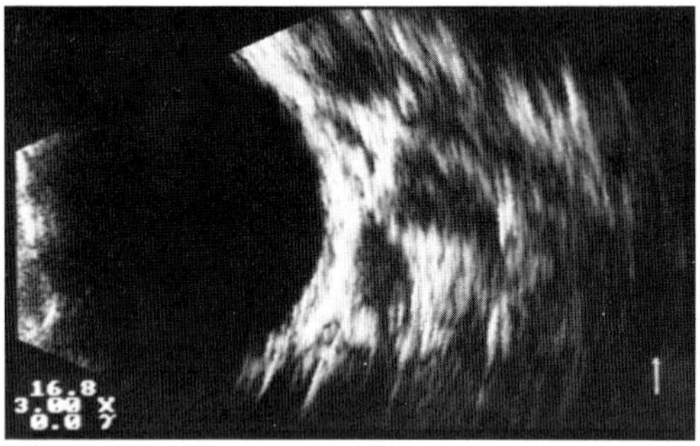
c

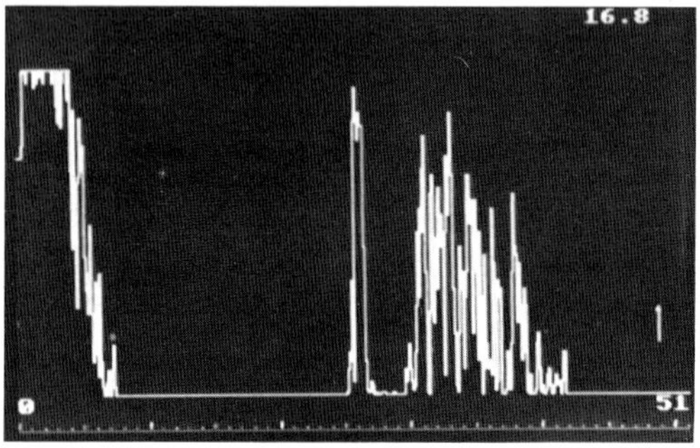

d

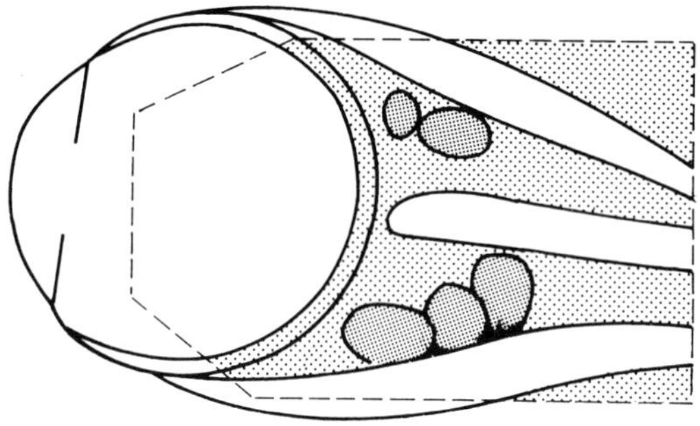
e

Fig. 6.**29 a–e** Lymphangioma in the anterior orbit, involving the subconjunctival space

**a, b** Clinically, the lesion is characterized by dilated, fluid-filled lymph spaces in the area of the bulbar conjunctiva; spontaneous hemorrhages into these cavities may occur
**c, d** On echography we see an extension of the lesion into the muscle cone. In spite of the tendency for the lesion to bleed, surgical treatment is only exceptionally indicated. The infiltrative character makes a total excision nearly impossible
**e** Schematic drawing

## 6.6 The Optic Nerve

Table 6.7 **Diseases with an echographically demonstrable widening of the dural diameter**

| |
|---|
| Optic neuritis |
| Retrobulbar neuritis |
| Papillitis |
| Disturbed circulation of the cerebrospinal fluid with or without papilledema |
| Optic nerve meningioma |
| Optic nerve glioma |
| Metastatic carcinoma of the meninges |

### Optic Neuritis

Already in the middle of the 19th century Cruveilhier established a correlation between visual loss and changes in the optic nerve on the basis of his pathologic anatomical investigations. In 1860 von Graefe published his paper on optic neuritis, and in 1885 Uhthoff wrote his study establishing a relationship between optic neuritis as defined by Graefe and multiple sclerosis. Echography was the first method with which it was possible to evaluate structural changes of the optic nerve, and within limits, to measure them. Abramson (1975) and

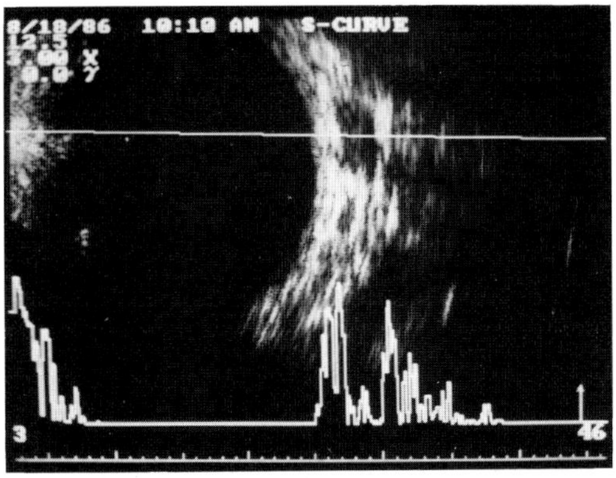

a

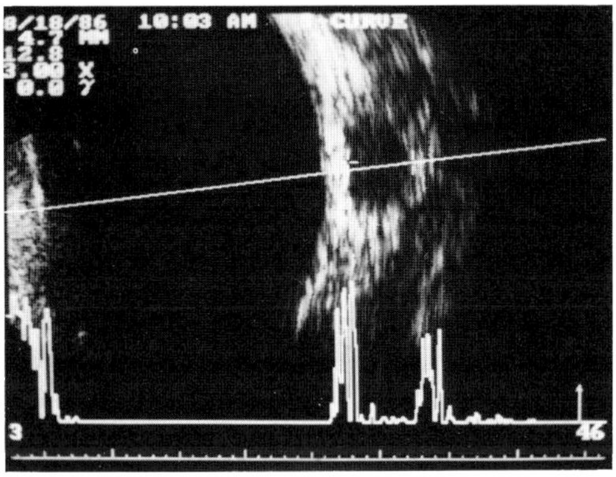

b

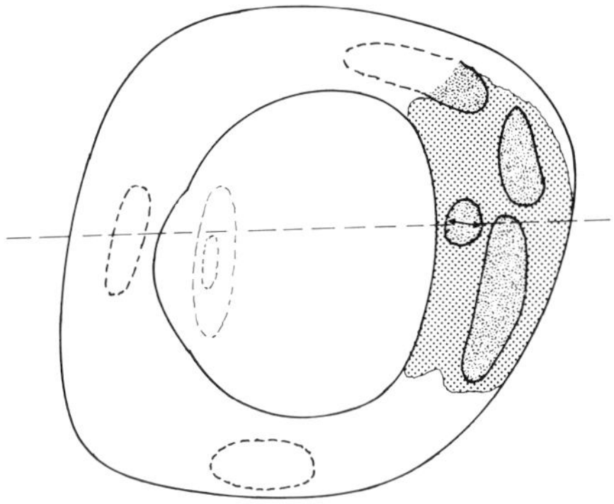

c

Fig. 6.**30a–c**
**a, b** Comparison of the A- and B-echograms of the orbits in a patient with acute retrobulbar neuritis. The dural diameter of the involved optic nerve is 4.7 mm. On the uninvolved side the diameter is 2.8 mm on the available cross section. Upon temporal examination with maximal abduction of the globe, the ultrasound encounters the optic nerve nearly vertically
**c** Schematic drawing

Coleman et al. (1972) reported for the first time on changes of horizontal sectional echograms in various optic nerve diseases. Schroeder (1976) and Ossoinig et al. (1977) published results of their measurements of the optic nerve diameter. Both autors listed characteristics according to which echograms could be evaluated in relation to the clinical picture. According to these studies, in about two-thirds of patients with retrobulbar neuritis we can expect a widening of the optic nerve diameter measured from the inner surface of the dura (dural diameter) (see Sect. 5.3).

In our experience, the most reliable results will be obtained if we measure when the globe is abducted and place the transistor on the temporal part of the lid fissure. If the optic neuritis is associated with papilledema (papillitis), we can expect a widening of the anterior part of the optic nerve in nearly 100% of the cases (Fig. 6.**30**). Schroeder (1976) points out that only two-thirds of patients with retrobulbar neuritis will show a pathologic echogram. He attributes this to the difficulties of the technique and to the fact that some of these inflammatory foci may lie close to the apex, where they cannot be demonstrated echographically. In the course of the disease the diameter of the optic nerve becomes normal again; if this was the first attack of optic neuritis, such a regression will usually be associated with an improvement of vision (Schroeder 1976).

### Disturbances of Cerebrospinal Fluid Circulation

A rise of intracranial pressure will, if it can extend into the subarachnoidal space of the orbital optic nerve, lead to swelling of the optic nerve head. This is due to a damming of axoplasmic flow, which develops in the area of the optic nerve head when the pressure in the subarachnoidal space of the optic nerve exceeds the intraocular pressure by a certain amount (Hayreh 1977). Echographically we can document a widening of the subarachnoidal space as an enlargement of the dural diameter. This can be achieved by A- and B-mode echography (Fig. 6.**31**). According to Ossoinig et al. (1977) and Skalka (1977, 1981), it is possible to use the

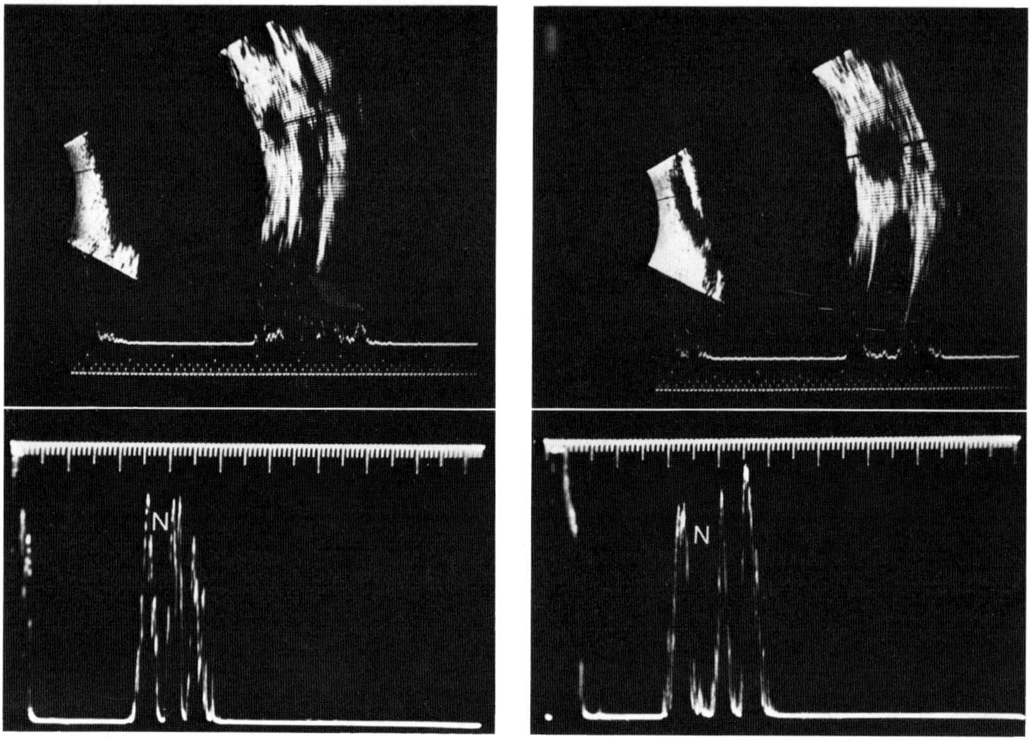


a b

Fig. 6.**31 a, b** Marked widening of the subarachnoidal space in chronic papilledema. If the optic nerve head has become atrophic, a dilated dural diameter represents an important proof that the intracranial pressure is still elevated

**a** Normal dural diameter (5.0 μs corresponds to 4.0 mm)
**b** Markedly dilated dural diameter (7.0 μs corresponds to 5.6 mm)

widened subarachnoidal space for differential diagnostic interpretations. We found in experiments on tissue models (Schroeder et al. 1969) that such a differentiation is questionable and the interpretation may be difficult, even when the echogram has been obtained under ideal conditions.

It is easy to learn the examination technique for determining the dural diameter in patients with increased intracranial pressure, because we know from experience that widened optic nerve sheaths are much more easily imaged by echography than a normal optic nerve. In cases of chronic papilledema with beginning optic atrophy, the widened dural diameter may be a sensitive indicator for a persisting, increased intracranial pressure, even without measuring the cerebrospinal fluid pressure (Guthoff et al. 1983).

### Papilledema of Orbital Etiology

Pressure by space-occupying lesions on the anterior visual pathway will lead to local ischemia and corresponding visual loss. There is usually papilledema, indicating impeded axoplasmic flow, when the compression involves the intraorbital or the intracanalicular part of the optic nerve. The changes at the optic nerve head are, according to Tso (1976), Wirtschafter et al. (1977) and Hayreh (1977), an expression of disturbed axoplasmic flow which will become visible at the cribriform plate as we see it with increased intracranial pressure. The orbital part of the optic nerve may be compressed not only by tumors, but also by enlarged extraocular muscles. The intracranial part of the nerve is most frequently compromised by sphenoidal meningiomas, more rarely by carotid aneurysms. This disturbed axonal transport may occasionally manifest itself by a widening of the optic nerve diameter before the disk edema itself develops (Guthoff 1987). This may lead to optic atrophy without a papilledema ever developing (Wright et al. 1989). The condition of the subarachnoidal space in such patients is debatable. Occasionally, the space around the optic nerve generates slight echos, but is not free of acoustic reflectivity. It is therefore possible that the arachnoid is edematous and there is no freely movable subarachnoidal fluid (Fig. 6.**32**). It is possible that this condition will be clarified by magnetic resonance imaging (MRI) examinations (Guthoff 1987).

### Optic Nerve Meningioma

Meningiomas of the optic nerve are rare tumors. They develop from arachnoidal endothelial cells and infiltrate the subarachnoidal space, thereby compressing the optic nerve. More frequently, we find extensions of meningiomas in the middle cerebral fossa, especially around the sphenoidal bone, extending through the optic canal or the superior orbital fissure to the orbital part of the optic nerve. This will characteristically lead to an early and progressive loss of vision associated with slight exophthalmus (Walsh 1970, Wright 1977, Wright et al. 1980). An initial disk edema may soon be followed by an early atrophy; in these cases the widening of the dural diameter is an important indication that there is a space-occupying lesion in the intradural space. A CT scan is always indicated to appreciate the extension of the lesion. In tumors close to the chiasm, an MRI examination should be performed. The combination of optic atrophy with the formation of opticociliary shunt vessels (Fig. 6.**33**) and an echographically appreciable enlargement of the dural diameter can be regarded as pathognomonic for an optic nerve meningioma.

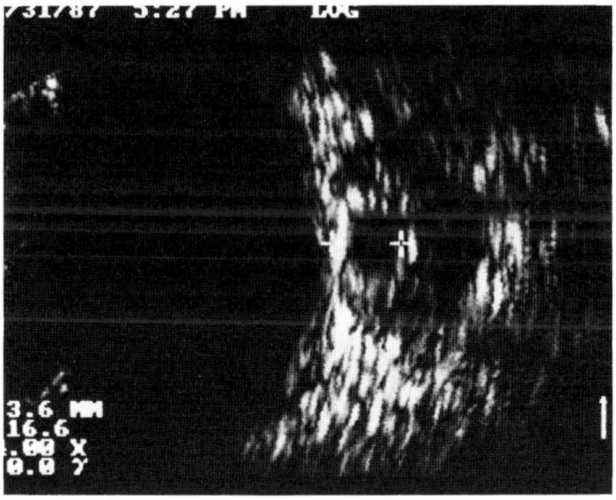


a

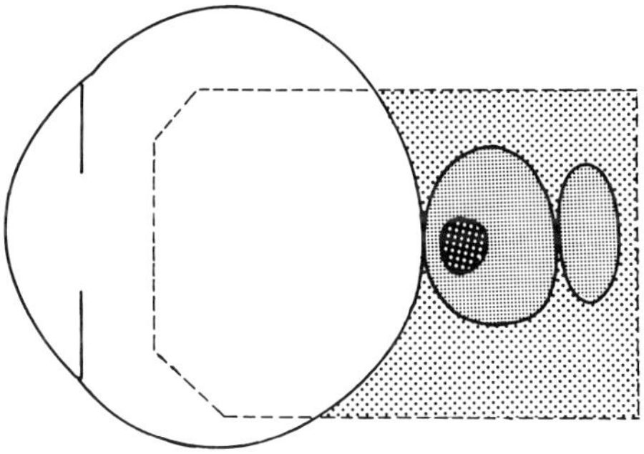

c

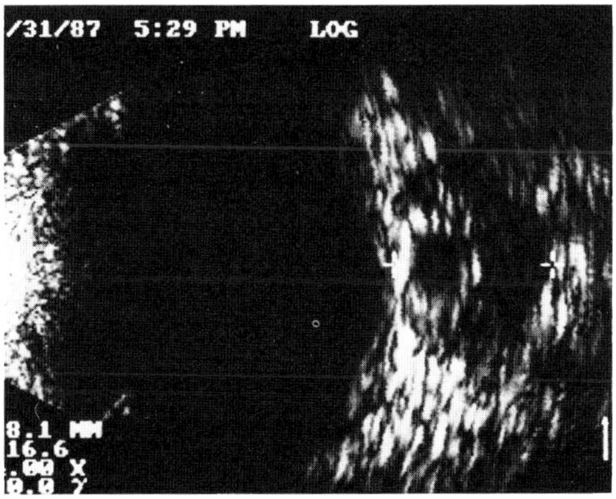


b

Fig. 6.**32 a–c**
**a, b** Cross sectional echogram through the nasal part of the orbit in Graves' orbitopathy. The diameter of the optic nerve is 3.6 mm and is therefore at the upper range of normal values. The dural diameter is 8.1 mm and therefore markedly enlarged. The medial rectus is only faintly visible on the cross sectional echograms lying between the nasal orbital wall and the optic nerve
**c** Schematic drawing

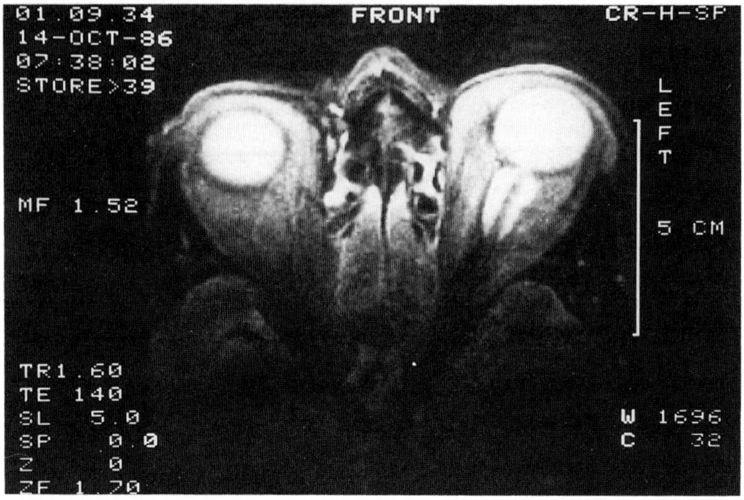


d

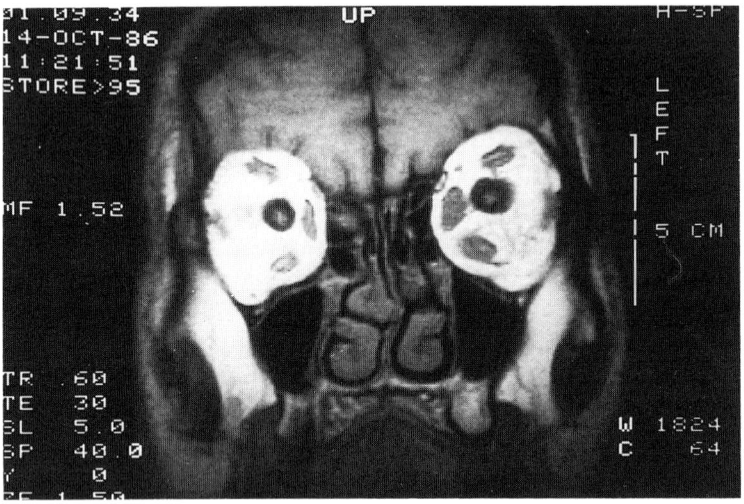


e

Fig. 6.**32d** In a T2-weighted axial magnetic resonance image, the thickening of the anterior perineural space, as suspected on echography, can be proven
**e** Magnetic resonance imaging in a coronary section. The T2-weighted image shows moderately dilated extraocular muscles. The dural space is dilated in both orbits and, within it, the optic nerve can be recognized as a concentric circle
The pathogenesis of the widening of the perineural space in Graves' orbitopathy is unknown. In the above-described patient, vision was 0.8 and there was no deficit of ocular motility. The optic nerve head was normal (from R. Guthoff: Zur Differentialdiagnose der endokrinen Orbitopathie. Fortschr. Ophthalmol., 1988)

### Optic Nerve Glioma

Gliomas of the optic nerve are seen mainly in children and young adults. They cause unilateral exophthalmus and early loss of vision. In about 60% of children with such a neoplasm, we find other stigmata of systemic neurofibromatosis (Wright 1980). The tumors usually have the character of a hamartoma. They originate in the optic nerve and may infiltrate the chiasm. There is nearly always an enlargement of the optic canal which can be proven radiologically (Lloyd 1975). Echographically, we usually find the optic nerve enlarged and spindle-shaped. This can be documented reliably only on B-mode echography (Fig. 6.**34**). On the A-mode echogram we find, depending upon the direction of the sound beam, a widening of the dural diameter.

### Metastatic Carcinoma of the Optic Nerve Sheaths

Infiltrations of the optic nerve sheaths can be seen in leukemic or carcinomatous meningeal involvement. They lead to a widening of the dural diameter. Echography does not provide any specific signs.

### Drusen of the Optic Nerve Head

The diagnosis is not difficult when the drusen lie superficially in the optic nerve head and are visible

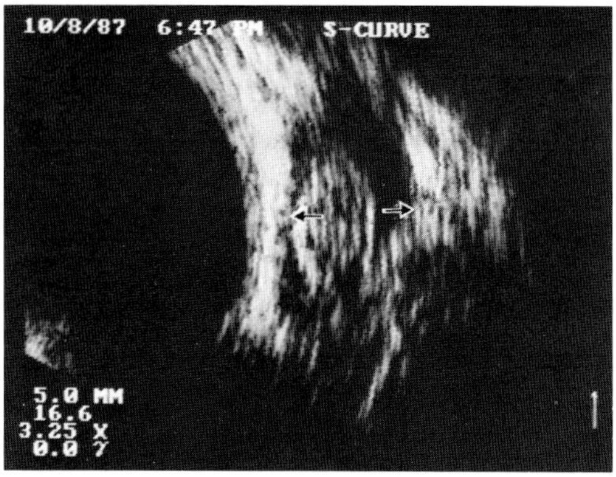


a

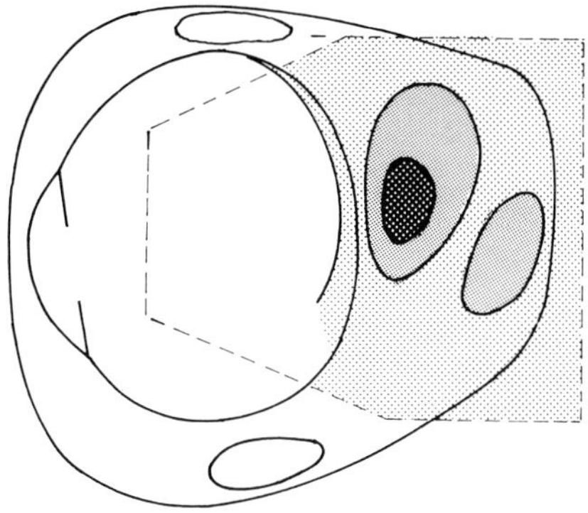

c

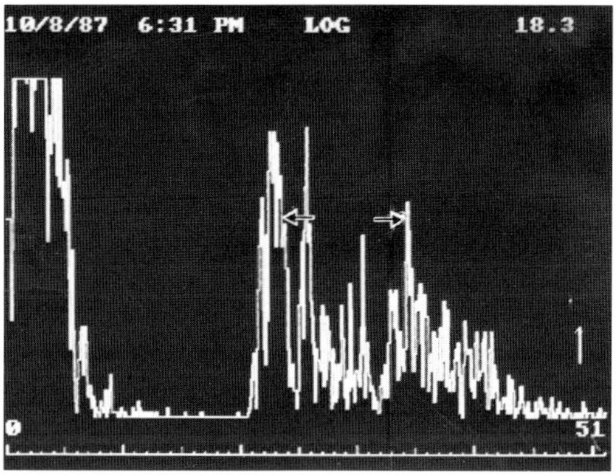


b

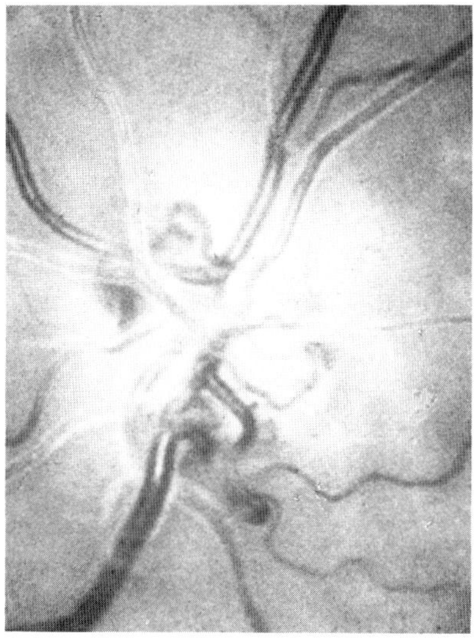

d

Fig. 6.**33a–d** Meningioma of the optic nerve sheath. Echographically, the dural diameter is widened to about 10 mm, both on A- and B-echography (arrows). The optic nerve is surrounded by a tumor envelope which shows low acoustic reflectivity. Cilioretinal shunt vessels on the optic nerve head associated with an echographically increased dural diameter can be regarded as pathognomonic for a meningioma of the optic nerve sheaths

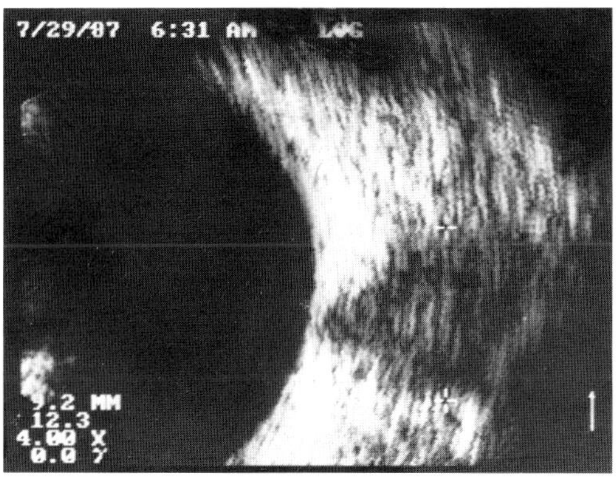


a

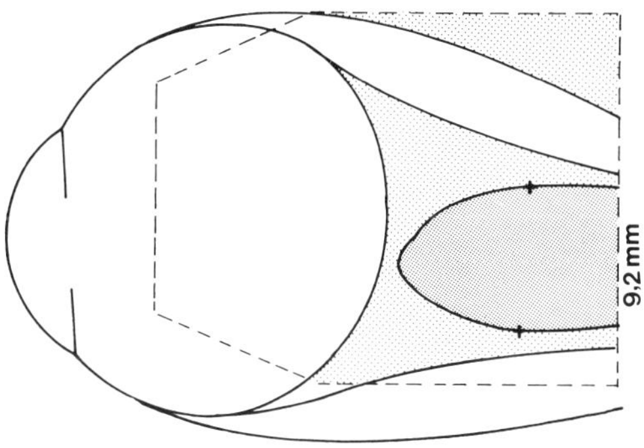


b

Fig. 6.**34a, b**
**a** Optic nerve glioma. Spindle-shaped dilatation of the optic nerve near the globe in a 22-year-old patient with von Recklinghausen disease. The orbital apex can not be evaluated echographically
**b** Schematic drawing

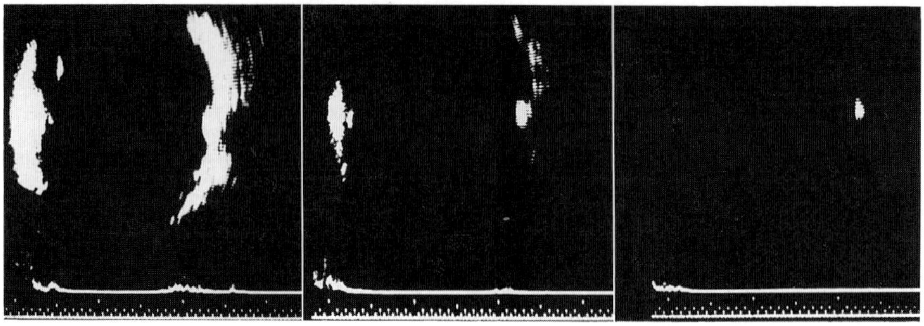

Fig. 6.**35 a–c** B-echogram of an eye with deep drusen. The sound intensity decreases from left to right in three steps, each one representing 10 db. High reflectivity in the area of the optic nerve head compared to the adjacent structures indicates drusen. With decreased sound intensity, only the druse remains visible in addition to the emission echo

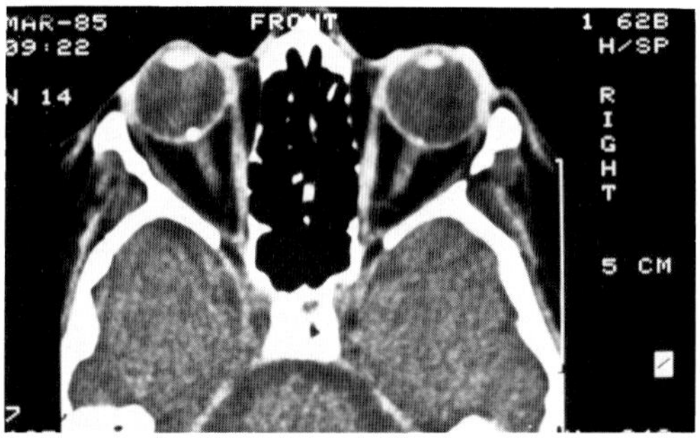


Fig. 6.**36** CT scan of a patient with bilateral drusen of the optic nerve. On the left, the drusen lie in the cross section; on the right, they are barely visible because they are only partly encompassed

a

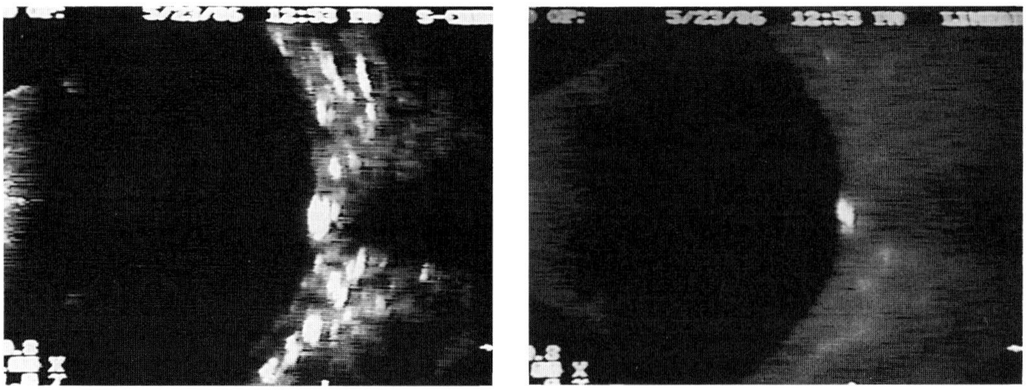

b

Fig. 6.**37 a, b** The high reflectivity of the drusen compared to the adjacent tissue and the sclera can be emphasized by appropriate amplification modes

**a** Optic nerve drusen seen with S-shaped amplification pattern. The optic nerve head is characterized by high reflectivity and traces of repeat echoes

**b** Linear amplifications will reduce small and average signals. High reflecting structures are therefore imaged nearly as isolated dots as glassy spheres (Mustonen et al. 1982; Friedman et al. 1977). They possess a strong autofluoresscence (Mustonen et al. 1982). There may be circumscribed or extensive nerve fiber bundle defects in the visual field (Friedman et al. 1975). Prognosis for vision is good, though occasionally, progressive visual loss or disk hemorrhages may develop (Brodrick 1973, Boyce et al. 1978, Mustonen et al. 1982).

Much more difficult is the situation when the drusen lie deep in the optic nerve head, causing blurred disk margins. The diagnosis cannot be established with the ophthalmoscope alone. This situation arises mainly in children and adolescents. Echography has proven especially useful here. On B-mode echograms, the drusen appear as spherical, sharply delineated structures with high acoustic reflectivity, lying close to the disk (Friedman et al. 1975). Figure 6.**35** shows the disk area with deep drusen. From left to right, the pictures show a decrease of sound intensity by 10 dB. The A-mode echogram shows, as expected, a normal dural diameter of the optic nerve (Schroeder 1979).

Calcified drusen can be diagnosed unequivocally by a CT scan (Fig. 6.**36**), but calcified deposits are necessary for imaging, and we find these only rarely in children. There are no reports comparing CT scan and echographic findings in such patients. Ossoinig maintains that the spherical shape of these hyaline bodies will produce a typical echogram even before they are calcified.

The recognition of these drusen can be facilitated by using various modes of amplification. A linear amplification may not be of much help for routine examinations, but it may occasionally be helpful for diagnosing deep drusen (Fig. 6.**37a, b**).

# 7 Echography within the Framework of Ophthalmologic Differential Diagnosis – Reviews and Tables

We shall attempt in this chapter to present a brief discussion on the role of echography within routine clinical practice. We shall only exceptionally mention those disease entities for which echography is not of diagnostic help.

## 7.1 The Red Eye

The conjunctival vessels can easily be examined with the biomicroscope because they lie superficially in the tissue, and the conjunctiva is only slightly pigmented. The degree of blood flow is regulated by arteriovenous anastomoses, which can be influenced by locally synthesized inflammatory mediators (Grasslin et al. 1953). This clinically produces the picture of a circumscribed hyperemia in which all vessels, which are otherwise only transiently open, will be filled with blood. This produces an intensive red discoloration which may be confined to the bulbar conjunctiva or may involve the entire conjunctival sac. On the other hand, passive hyperemia, as it is caused by a cavernous sinus fistule, will dilate the vascular network, in which, after a prolonged course, the blood vessels become rarified (Fig. 6.**23**).

Frequently, the clinical picture or history alone will not suffice for a differentiation between the *active hyperemia* produced by inflammatory mediators from a purely *mechanical orbital congestion*. Echography can give us important clues concerning the differential diagnosis (Hasenfratz 1986). In Table 7.**1** the final diagnoses of 93 patients are listed. Their main sign was a dilatation of the conjunctival and episcleral vessels, and echography was useful in establishing the correct diagnosis.

A spontaneous carotid cavernous sinus fistule will most often lead to a circular dilatation of the episcleral vessels. In patients with orbital pseudotumor, a sectorial vascular dilatation usually points toward an involvement of extraocular muscles. If all other etiologic factors can be excluded, these patients with unilateral increased intraocular pressure may suffer from an idiopathic dilatation of the episcleral veins (Radius et al. 1978, Ruprecht et al. 1984, Jörgensen et al. 1985).

Table 7.1 **Diseases with dilatation of the episcleral vessels** (n = 93)

| | |
|---|---|
| Spontaneous cavernous sinus fistula | 26 |
| Traumatic cavernous sinus fistula | 9 |
| Orbital pseudotumor ± involvement of extraocular muscles | 21 |
| Episcleritis | 5 |
| Brawny scleritis | 3 |
| Graves' orbitopathy | 5 |
| Aseptic thrombosis of orbital veins | 4 |
| Idiopathic dilatation of episcleral veins | 5 |
| Conjunctival nevus | 2 |
| Ciliary body melanoma | 3 |
| Metastatic bronchial carcinoma to the ciliary body | 1 |
| Tolosa-Hunt syndrome | 2 |
| Osler disease | 1 |
| Sturge-Weber syndrome | 4 |
| Arteriovenous anomaly of the orbit | 1 |

A massive circular vascular dilatation is the principal sign of a brawny scleritis. The differential diagnosis is especially important here because the intraocular elevation can clinically, echographically and by P32 test not be differentiated from a choroidal melanoma (von Domarus 1979, Feldon et al. 1978). Unfortunately, neither A- nor B-mode echography provides reliable differential diagnostic points, so that this disease, even today, may occasionally lead to an unnecessary enucleation because a melanoma had been suspected. A pseudotumor of the anterior orbit may lead to less conspicuous and partly sectorial vascular dilatations. In myositis a few or individual extraocular muscles are affected and the conjunctival hyperemia is sectorially limited to the area of their insertions. The ensuing motility deficits are discussed in Sect. 7.8. Table 7.**2** compares diagnoses and typical echographic findings for the main sign "red eye".

Episcleral vascular dilatations which present diagnostic difficulties are mainly (in a ratio of 3:1) due to congestion. Table 7.**1** summarizes the etiologic possibilities of congestive hyperemia; the numbers behind the diagnosis refer to the location of the lesion as discussed in the subsequent paragraph.

Most numerous are spontaneous cavernous sinus fistules (1), which can only exceptionally be diagnosed before their first radiologic or echographic examination. An obstacle for outflow may lie in the superior orbital fissure (2) and will usually be produced by a tumor or pseudotumor. According to the reports published so far, the impedance for outflow in idiopathic episcleral venous stasis lies in the extraocular muscles (3). From a theoretical point of view and also according to the published literature, a thoracic stasis, as it exists in the superior vena cava syndrome, may cause similar signs and symptoms (4). Conspicuous arteriovenous shunts, as we see them in traumatic cavernous sinus fistules (5), can usually be diagnosed by history and the clinical picture.

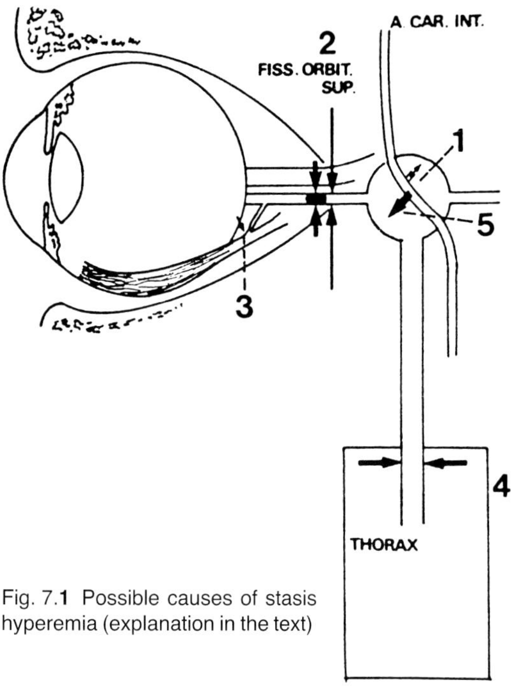


Fig. 7.**1** Possible causes of stasis hyperemia (explanation in the text)

Table 7.**2** **The red eye**. Echographic findings

| **Sectorial Vascular Dilatation** | |
|---|---|
| Diagnosis | Echographic Finding |
| Ciliary body melanoma | Evident tumor |
| Metastatic tumor to the ciliary body | Evident tumor |
| Scleritis | Widening of sclera and of Tenon's space |
| Episcleritis | Widening of Tenon's space |
| Myositis | Widening of the muscle, also at the insertion. Low acoustic reflectivity of the muscle belly |
| **Circular Vascular Dilatation** | |
| Diagnosis | Echographic Finding |
| Uveitis | Vitreous opacities |
| Secondary glaucoma due to intraocular tumor | Evident tumor |
| Orbital pseudotumor | Widening of various orbital structures with low acoustic reflectivity |
| Orbital cellulitis | Widening of serveral orbital structures with low acoustic reflectivity, ± detachment of periosteum, sound propagation into perinasal sinuses |
| Thrombosis of orbital veins | The ophthalmic vein or its branches can be echographically demonstrated, not compressible, not pulsating |
| Spontaneous cavernous sinus fistula (Red eye shunt syndrome) traumatic cavernous sinus fistula | Ophthalmic vein or its branches demonstrable, on pressure pulsation, muscles widened |
| Graves' orbitopathy | Widening of muscles, high acoustic reflectivity of muscle belly |
| Idiopathic dilatation of episcleral veins | No pathologic findings |

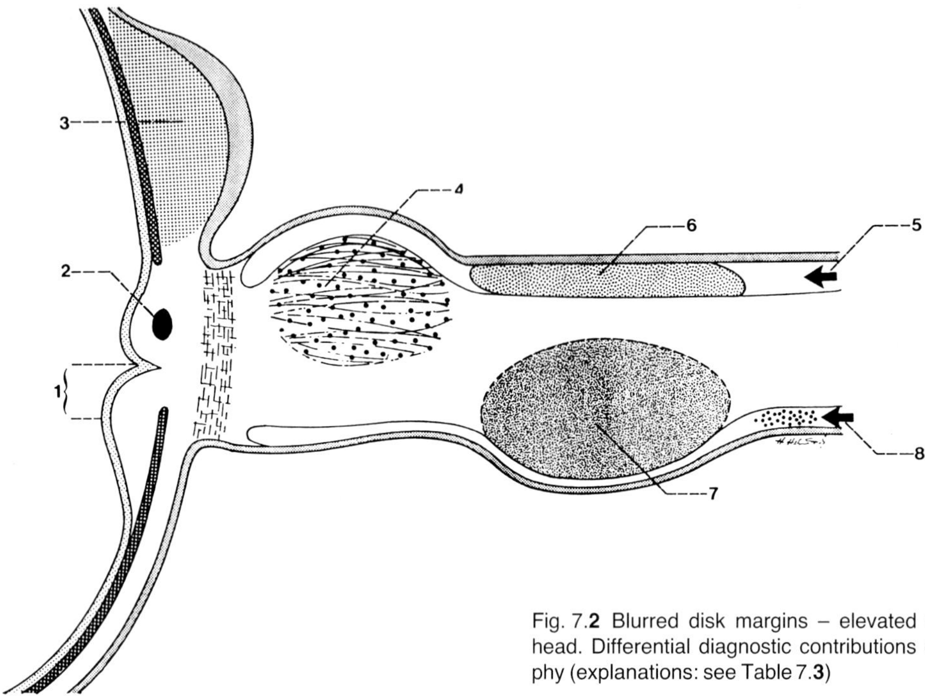


Fig. 7.**2** Blurred disk margins – elevated optic nerve head. Differential diagnostic contributions of echography (explanations: see Table 7.**3**)

Table 7.**3** **Blurred disk margins – elevated optic nerve head.** Echographic contributions to the differential diagnosis (numbers behind the diagnosis refer to the location of a lesion in Fig. 7.**2**)

| Diagnosis | Echographic Finding |
|---|---|
| Pseudopapilledema in hyperopia (1) | Short axial length, widened ocular wall |
| Disc drusen (2) | Structures of high acoustic reflectivity in the area of the optic nerve head (independent from the degree of calcification) |
| Ocular hypotony | Widening of ocular coats, occasionally with choroidal detachment |
| Posterior scleritis (3) | Widening of ocular coats, Tenon's space demonstrable |
| Optic neuritis (4) | Widening of dural diameter (always found in diskedema, present in 70% of eyes with retrobulbar neuritis) |
| Optic disk edema (5) | Widening of dural diameter |
| – Due to increased intracranial pressure | |
| – Due to compression of the orbital part of the optic nerve | |
| Optic nerve tumors | |
| – Meningioma (6) | Widening of dural diameter (opticociliary shunt vessels!) |
| – Glioma (7) | Widening of dural diameter, occasionally spindle-shaped thickening of optic nerve |
| – Metastatic carcinoma (8) | Widening of dural diameter |
| Blurred disk margins without echographically demonstrable changes | |
| – Congenital disk anomalies | |
| – Central vein occlusion | |
| – Anterior ischemic optic neuropathy | |

Mixtures between active and passive hyperemia may develop, especially in patients with an inflammatory orbital pseudotumor.

## 7.2 Blurred Disk Margins – Elevation of the Optic Nerve Head

We frequently cannot decide with certainty whether a disk with blurred margins and slight elevation represents a pathologic condition or not. If unequivocal pathologic findings are lacking, it is up to the examiner to decide how far the diagnostic procedures should be carried. It may be necessary to obtain neurologic consultation and to perform neuroradiologic investigations, including an MRI. On the other hand, after weighing the cost-benefit ratio and the risk of some side effects, the investigator may rely on his clinical acumen and decide that the condition only represents a variant of the norm.

Echographic examinations make it possible to support the clinical impression to a certain extent and to delineate somewhat the diagnosis of blurred disk margins. Figure 7.**2** in association with Table 7.**3** facilitate in a schematic form the correlation between clinical and echographic findings.

## 7.3 Choroidal Folds

In the older literature choroidal folds were always interpreted as a sign of an orbital space-occupying lesion (Vedel-Jensen 1959, Wolter 1974). They are typically horizontal folds and rarely extend beyond the equator. Fluorescein angiography allows an exact differentiation between retinal and choroidal folds (Norton 1969, Winning 1973). Newell (1973) was the first to express some critical comments on the above interpretation. Reports appeared in the literature (Hyvärien et al. 1970 Bird et al. 1973, Cappaert et al. 1977) describing intraocular diseases or scleritis, producing a comparable ophthalmoscopic picture. Our own examinations (Singh et al. 1986) show that during a long-term follow up, the pathologic ophthalmoscopic findings may disappear and the associated refractive errors may return to normal values. Verbeek (1981) summarized, on the basis of a literature review complemented by his own findings, the importance of echography for the differential diagnosis. Analyzing 167 patients, he found an ocular cause in 46 of them; in 26, an orbital lesion, and in 17, an atypical papilledema was diagnosed. No definite diagnosis could be established in 11 patients (Tables 7.**4**, 7.**5** and 7.**6**; Fig. 7.**3**).

## 7.4 Leukokoria

Whenever we diagnose leukokoria, a retinoblastoma has to be excluded. Figure 7.**4** and Table 7.**7** illustrate and list the differential diagnostic help given by echography.

## 7.5 Vitreous Hemorrhage

An acute vitreous hemorrhage will nearly always lead the patient to the ophthalmologist. As discussed in Sect. 3.21, echography is the method of choice to evaluate the situation and to estimate the prognosis. Entoptic functional tests can complement the echographic findings. Figure 7.**5** and Table 7.**8** summarize the most important differential diagnoses.

Table 7.**4** **Choroidal folds.** Orbital causes (after Verbeek)

| Diagnosis | Number of Patients |
|---|---|
| Graves' orbitopathy | 11 |
| Sinusitis | 5 |
| Mucocele | 2 |
| Hemangioma | 6 |
| Orbital pseudotumor | 5 |
| Various orbital tumors | 8 |
| Unexplained | 6 |
| Total | 43 |

Table 7.**5** **Choroidal folds.** Ocular causes

| Diagnosis | Number of Patients |
|---|---|
| Hyperopic eye | 17 |
| Macular degeneration | 12 |
| Ocular hypotony | 12 |
| Posterior scleritis | 9 |
| Buckling operation | 9 |
| Trauma | 6 |
| Intraocular tumor | 3 |
| Miscellaneous | 10 |
| Total | 78 |

Table 7.**6** **Choroidal folds.** Echographic findings

| Diagnosis | Echographic Findings |
|---|---|
| Myositis, Graves' orbitopathy (1) | Thickened extraocular muscles |
| Periorbital spaceoccupying lesion (2) | Change in the relief of the orbital wall, sound propagation into the perinasal sinuses |
| Orbital neoplasms (3) | Directly evident (it may be difficult to demonstrate a small cavernous hemangioma because of its high acoustic reflectivity) |
| Inflammatory orbital pseudotumor (4) | Widening of normal orbital structures, low acoustic reflectivity, Tenon's space may be demonstrable |
| Disk edema (5) | Widened dural diameter of the optic nerve |
| Axial hyperopia (6) | Axis length below 22 mm, ocular coats concentrically thickened |
| Ocular hypotony (7) | Ocular coats concentrically thickened |
| Macular degeneration | Thickening of the ocular coats in the area of the macula, high acoustic reflectivity |
| Scleritis (8) | Circumscribed widening of the ocular coats, Tenon's space demonstrable |

Table 7.**7** **Leukokoria.** Echographic findings helpful for differential diagnosis (numbers behind the diagnosis refer to the location of the lesion in Fig. 7.**4**)

| **The Axial Length Normal for Patient's Age** | |
|---|---|
| Diagnosis | Echographic Findings |
| Retinoblastoma (1) | Widening of the ocular coats, extremely high acoustic reflectivity, shadowing effect, atypical findings possible! |
| Congenital cataract (2) | Increased reflectivity from the posterior lens surface, vitreous space empty, ocular coats normal |
| **Shortened Axial Length** | |
| Diagnosis | Echographic Findings |
| Retinopathy of prematurity (3) | In stages IV and V, beginning or complete traction detachment (normal echographic findings in stages I-III) |
| Persistent hyperplastic primary vitreous (PHPV) (4) | Dense strand of tissue between optic nerve head and posterior lens pole; formes frustes may occur (posterior or anterior PHPV) |
| Retinal anomalies | Membranes in the vitreous, atypical detachment, which in part appears solid (no typical echogram) |
| Fundus coloboma (5) | Directly demonstrable protrusion of ocular coats, sometimes with orbital cyst! (microphthalmus with cyst) |
| Coats' disease (6) | Floating crystals in the vitreous and subretinal space (fast flickering spikes on A-mode) |

## 7.6 Examination before a Vitrectomy

Up to a few years ago echography was the decisive examination to determine the indications for vitreous surgery. Further development of surgical methods, especially the advances in illumination technique, prove that the surgeon may not need a detailed knowledge of the conditions within the vitreous body. A few findings which can only be obtained echographically are still important to estimate prognosis and risks of an operation. Figure 7.**6** and Table 7.**9** list some of the possible echographic information and the subsequent conclusions as far as the operative plan is concerned.

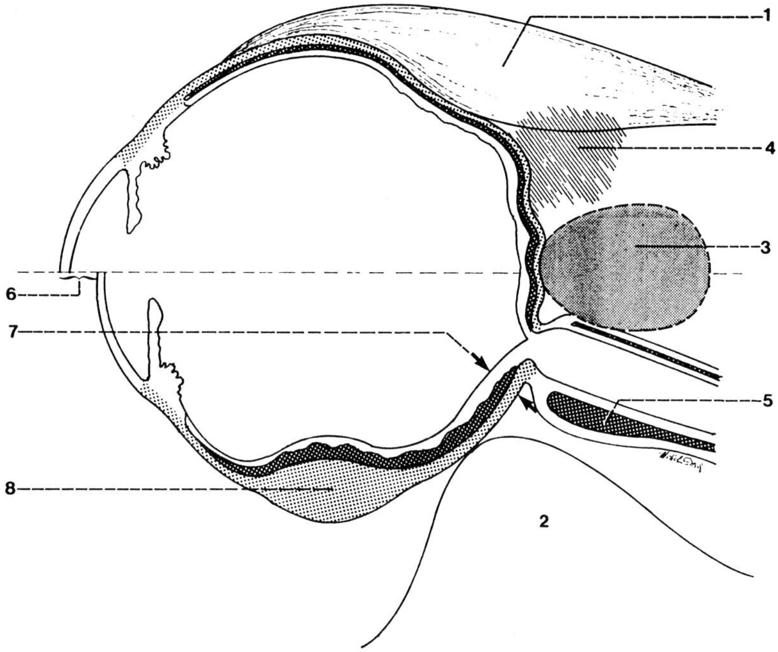


Fig. 7.**3** Choroidal folds – echographic contributions to the differential diagnosis (explanation: see Table 7.**6**)

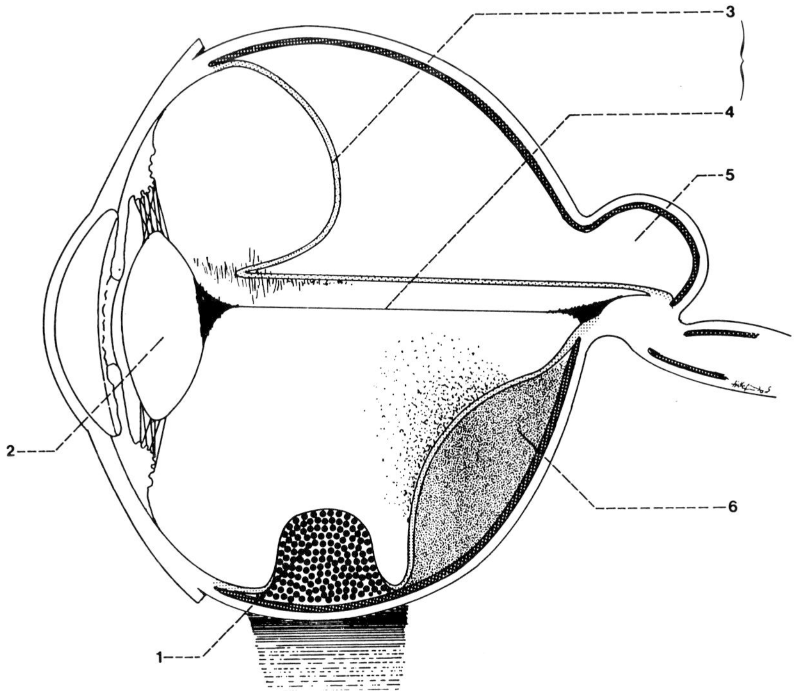


Fig. 7.**4** Leukokoria – echographic contributions to the differential diagnosis (explanation: see Table 7.**7**)

Table 7.**8** **Vitreous hemorrhage.** Echographic findings helpful for establishing the etiology (numbers behind the diagnosis refer to the location of the lesion in Fig. 7.**5**)

| Diagnosis | Echographic Findings |
|---|---|
| Symptomatic posterior vitreous detachment (1) | Thickened detached posterior hyaloid membrane, occasionally beginning retinal detachment |
| Recently formed retinal break with torn vessel (2) | Blood-covered vitreous strands converge toward the retinal break; occasionally a high floating operculum may be detected |
| Proliferative retinopathy (3) | Strands or membranes extending from the optic nerve head or the posterior pole, high acoustic reflectivity |
| Terson syndrome (vitreous hemorrhage after subarachnoidal bleeding) (4) | Vitreous opacities in front of the optic nerve head or behind the detached vitreous |
| Disciform macular degeneration (5) | Widening of the ocular coats in the macular area, high acoustic reflectivity, vitreous strands extending from the macula |
| Choroidal melanoma (6) | Biconvex thickening of the ocular wall, low acoustic rereflectivity, sometimes mushroom-shaped. Accompanying retinal detachment distant from the tumor |

Table 7.**9** **Examination before a vitrectomy**. Echographic findings helpful for planning the operation (numbers behind the questions refer to the location of the lesion in Fig. 7.**6**)

| **Questions on the Echographic Examination** | **Consequences for Planning the Operation** |
|---|---|
| Choroidal detachment including the pars plana? (1) | Avoiding this area when inserting the ports |
| Post-traumatic vitreous hemorrhage, retina attached? | If retina detached, strong indication for vitrectomy |
| Intraocular foreign body demonstrable? Location in regard to ocular coats (2) | Choice of surgical approach; magnet extraction possible? |
| **Estimating the Prognosis** | |
| Choroidal detachment caused by blood (3) | Extremely poor prognosis; perhaps even abandon the operation |
| Free-floating retinal detachment (4) | Reattachment probable, can be achieved without tamponade from the inside |
| Rigid retinal detachment? Thickened retina? (5) | Removal of preretinal membranes necessary |
| Vitreous strands with traction effect demonstrable? (6) | Cutting the strands |
| Retinal parts behind the lens? (7) | Special care indicated when entering the vitreous space |
| Thickened ocular coats in the macula (disciform degeneration?) (8) | Poor prognosis for central vision |
| Indications of a secondary, e.g., solid, retinal detachment? (9) | Additional diagnostic examinations; enucleation may be necessary |
| Attached retina with minimal remaining vision? | Reconsider indication for operation; prognosis for vision extremely poor |

## 7.7 Exophthalmus

Before CT was introduced, echography was the only diagnostic method which enabled us to examine soft tissue pathology in the orbit. Ossoinig and Till, in particular, contributed to the value of echography for the preoperative differential diagnosis of orbital lesions. However, it seems dubious whether it is reasonable to delineate – as some authors have attempted to do – 80 different pathologic processes involving the orbit by echographic findings. When a malignant space-occupying lesion is suspected, a histologic examination will be necessary in all doubtful cases in order to ascertain a correct diagnosis. Speculations about the benign or malignant nature of a lesion on the basis of echographic findings are of little help.

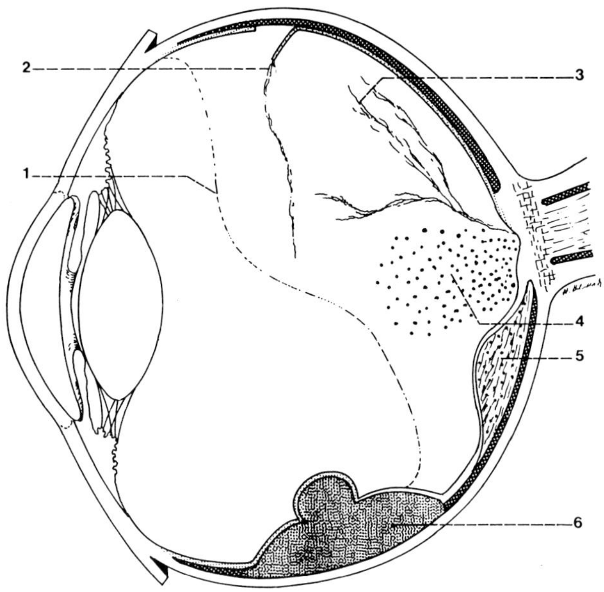


Fig. 7.**5** Vitreous hemorrhage – echographic contributions to determine the pathogenesis (explanation: see Table 7.**8**)

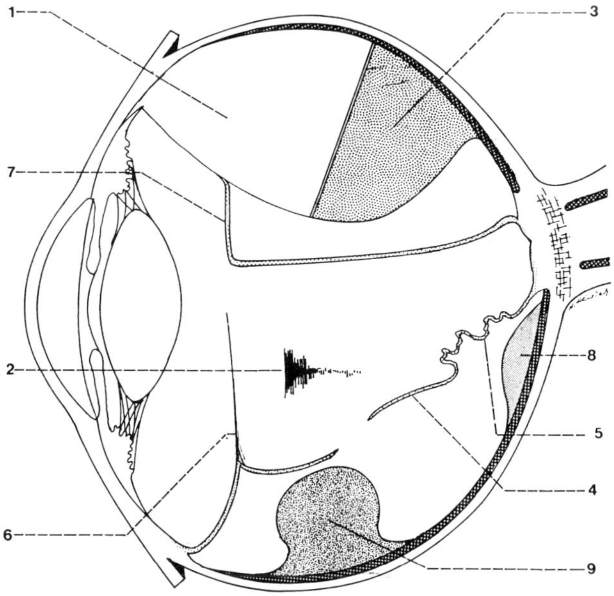


Fig. 7.**6** Examination before a vitrectomy – echographic contributions to the planning of the operation (explanation: see Table 7.**9**)

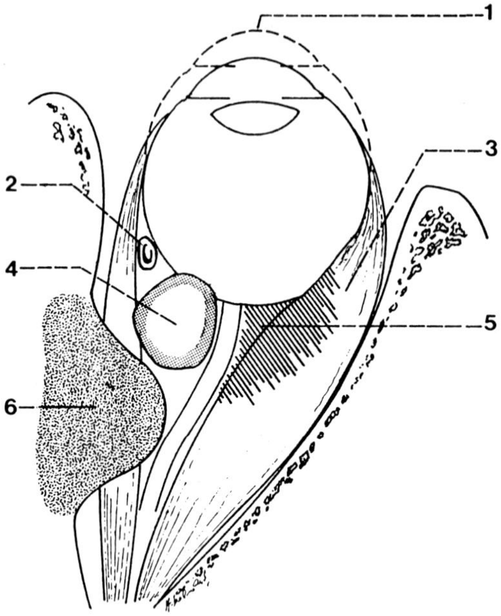


Fig. 7.**7** Exophthalmus – echographic contributions to differential diagnosis (explanation: see Table 7.**10**)

We attempt here to present a classification which enables the examiner to use the echographic diagnosis as a filter to separate those disease processes in which the echographic examination can ascertain the diagnosis from pathologic processes in which other diagnostic examinations, usually by other medical specialists, will be necessary. Figure 7.**7** and Table 7.**10** correlate the most frequent causes of exophthalmus with the echographic findings (the numbers behind the diagnoses indicate the location of the lesion as shown in Fig. 7.**7**).

Patients with *pseudoexophthalmus* may be diagnosed by measuring the refractive error of the affected eye, but they can be definitely recognized echographically.

The various types of *vascular exophthalmus* can be echographically differentiated up to a certain degree. In our experience, the entity of "red eye shunt syndrome", the spontaneous dura cavernous sinus fistule, has so far been diagnosed too sparingly. The diagnosis can be regarded as certain if we find a combination of a slightly elevated intraocular pressure, a red eye and veins that pulsate on pressure. The condition occurs mainly in older patients and has, with few exception, a good prognosis with a good chance of spontaneous healing (Phelps et al. 1982, Guthoff et al. 1987). In the individual patient we have to consider whether angiography would not constitute an unjustifiably high risk.

The differential diagnostic conditions of a *myogenic exophtalmus* are listed in Table 7.**10**. The clinical picture including laboratory work-up, will usually allow a definite diagnosis. A CT scan is often unnecessary.

*Cysts*, especially those associated with microphthalmus, are usually congenital and need no further diagnostic test or treatment if they cause no signs or symptoms.

*Dermoids* do not always appear echographically as true cysts because the varying components have

Table 7.**10** **Exophthalmus**. Echographic findings helpful for differential diagnosis

| Diagnosis | Echographic Findings |
|---|---|
| Pseudoexophthalmus (1) | Myopic globe, flat orbit |
| Vascular exophthalmus (2) | Branches of the ophthalmic vein demonstrable |
| ● Spontaneous or traumatic cavernous sinus fistula | Venous branches pulsate on pressure |
| ● Thrombosis of orbital veins | Noncompressible venous branches demonstrable |
| Myogenic exophthalmus (3) | Widening of the recti muscles (differential diagnosis: Graves' orbitopathy, myositis, lymphoma, metastatic carcinoma, carotid-cavernous sinus fistules) |
| Neoplasms (4) | Space-occupying lesion separated from orbital fat, varying acoustic reflectivity |
| Inflammatory infiltration (5) | Widening of pre-existing orbital structures, homogeneous acoustic properties. Tenon's space demonstrable |
| Exophthalmus caused by spaceoccupying lesion extending from the surroundings (6) | Changes in the contour of the orbital walls, detachment of periosteum, sound propagation into the perinasal sinuses |

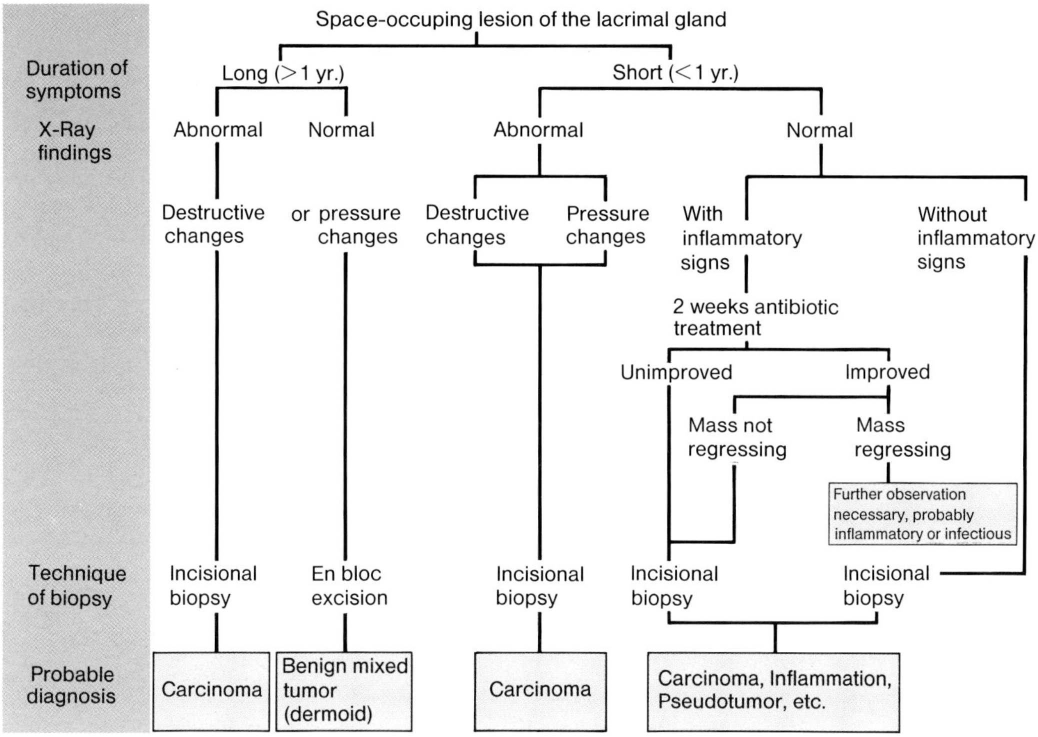


Fig. 7.**8** Space-occupying lesions of the lacrimal gland (from Spalton and Wright: The Orbit and Lacrimal System. In: Spalton, D. J., R. A. Hitchings and P. A. Hunter, Atlas of Clinical Ophthalmology, Lippincott, Philadelphia 1984)

different acoustic reflectivities. In case of doubt, a CT scan will help to characterize and diagnose these space-occupying lesions because of their fat content.

Echography alone will not suffice if there is an involvement of *periorbital structures*. In these cases, we need other methods to image soft tissues for diagnostic purposes in order to evaluate the pathologic process affecting adjacent structures. The treatment is often provided by nonophthalmologists.

The *inflammatory exophthalmus* usually presents a differential diagnostic problem. We first have to exclude a propagation of the inflammation from the perinasal sinuses by using other diagnostic procedures. It then has to be decided individually whether a working diagnosis of orbital pseudotumor is justified and whether such a diagnosis can be ascertained by a trial run of systemic treatment with corticosteroids. In case of doubt, a histologic clarification will be necessary.

A CT scan is indispensable when an *orbital neoplasm* needing as surgical intervention is suspected. With the exception of the cavernous hemangioma, which, due to its internal structure, provides a nearly pathognomonic echogram, the ultrasonic differential diagnosis remains speculative.

Space-occupying lesions of the *lacrimal fossa* need, independent from the echographic findings, a therapeutic approach which is mainly guided by clinical and radiological parameters. Wright (1984) has published a schematic orientation for this purpose (Fig. 7.**8**).

## 7.8 Deficits in Ocular Motility

Deficits in ocular motility can be analyzed by diagnostic methods revealing the soft tissue of the orbit whenever the cause of the deficit lies in the orbit itself. Neurogenic lesions cannot be imaged echographically. In our experience, which differs in this aspect from that of other authors (Rochels et al. 1986), echographic examinations are only of lim-

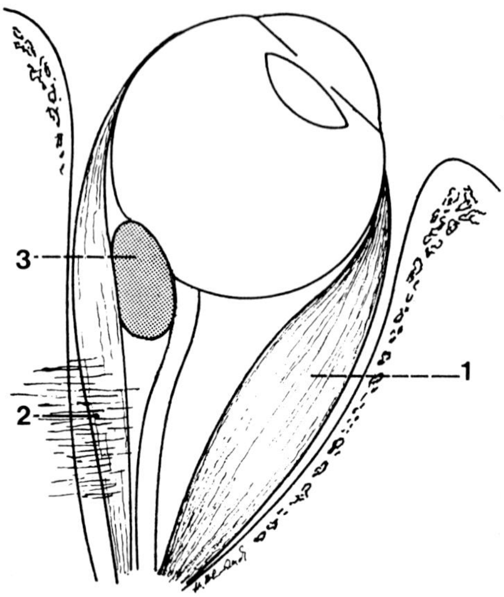


Fig. 7.**9** Orbital causes of disturbed ocular motility – echographic contributions to the differential diagnosis (explanation: see Table 7.**11**)

Table 7.**12** **Widened extraocular muscles.** Correlation between etiology and expected motility defect

| Diagnosis | Motility Defect | |
|---|---|---|
| | Decreased Stretchability | Decreased Contractility |
| Graves' orbitopathy | + | (+) in late stages |
| Idiopathic myositis | + | (+) |
| Metastatic carcinoma | + | (+) |
| Lymphomatous infiltration | (+) | + |
| Muscle involvement in orbital cellulitis | (+) | + |
| Muscle edema in circulatory disorders | (+) | (+) |

ited help when evaluating posttraumatic motility deficits. We are, however, capable of differentiating between lesions within and outside of the muscle. Figure 7.**9** and Table 7.**11** list the most frequent echographically demonstrable etiologic factors.

#### Myogenic Deficits of Ocular Motility

If an enlarged muscle has been found, we have to decide whether loss of effective contraction or loss of stretchability is the cause of reduced activity of the involved muscle. If only one muscle is affected, the answer to the question is simple. In doubtful cases, we have to consider the concept of common visual axes between the two eyes. Whenever one muscle cannot be normally stretched, contraction of the antagonist will press on the globe and therefore increase the intraocular pressure, depending on the direction of gaze. Table 7.**12** lists the correlation between possible muscle widening and the expected ocular motility deficits. Unequivocal statements can only be made about *Graves' orbitopathy*: whenever there is a motility deficit in this disease, we always find a loss of stretchability of the involved muscle. In late stages the contraction capability of the muscle is further decreased by the atrophy of normal muscle fibers which are replaced by connective or adipose tissue.

In the literature (Esslen et al. 1961) *idiopathic myositis* is nearly exclusively associated with de-

Table 7.**11** Orbital causes of decreased ocular motility. Echographic findings helpful for the differential diagnosis (numbers behind the diagnosis refer to the location of the lesion in Fig. 7.9)

| Diagnosis | Echographic Findings |
|---|---|
| Widened extraocular muscle (1) | Myositis: Low acoustic reflectivity of muscle belly; insertion also widened |
| | Graves' orbitopathy: Muscle belly with strong acoustic reflectivity; in protracted course muscle can barely be differentiated from orbital fat |
| | Metastatic carcinoma |
| | Lymphoma |
| | Cavernous sinus fistula |
| Extension of a pathologic process (2) | Purulent sinusitis, tumor invasion |
| Expanding orbital process (3) | E.g., hemangioma, neurinoma |

creased contractility. According to our examinations (Guthoff et al. 1988), this narrow correlation does not exist. In more than 50% of such patients there is primarily a loss of stretchability of the affected muscles. If the area of the cavernous sinus is also involved (Tolosa-Hunt syndrome), we primarily find neurogenic deficits.

*Metastatic tumors to the muscles* may produce both kinds of motility deficits. In our experience a loss of stretchability is more frequently seen.

In cases of **bacterial infection** the contractility of the muscle will be decreased, even if the muscle itself is only slightly enlarged.

**Circulatory disorders**, e.g., cavernous sinus fistules or thrombosis of the orbital veins, will usually produce a mixed picture with reduced contractility and stretchability.

**Expanding space-occupying lesions** may have a mechanical effect on ocular motility without directly invading the muscle. This applies especially to intraconal lesions. In these cases the intraocular pressure will nearly always increase in certain directions of gaze. If this sign is absent, we should consider a neurogenic component of the decreased motility.

## 7.9 Ultrasound Biometry for Intraocular Lens Implantation

There are a number of ways to correct the refractive error of aphakia. Two possibilities have to be stressed:

1. a correction which leads to emmetropia, i.e., sharp distance vision, without a visual aid;
2. a correction which leads to isokonia between the two eyes.

The second solution is only exceptionally met by the implantation of an intraocular lens which produces emmetropia. From a clinical point of view, we have to consider the error margins when measuring the optical components.

**1. Corneal curvature**

When calculating the refractive power of the cornea, we have to measure corneal curvature in mm. Various devices allow us to read the corneal refractive power in diopters. These are measurements already derived which, in individual instruments, are calculated by different methods. Errors in measuring the radius of curvature will have a considerable influence on calculating refractive power. An error of 0.1 mm corresponds to a difference in corneal refractivity of 0.5 diopter. Under these circumstances, a spectacle correction of 0.5 diopter would be necessary. With precise instruments, we can measure the corneal diameter with an average error of 0.03 mm. Therefore, the measuring error in keratometry can, under optimal conditions, be reduced to 0.1–0.2 diopters.

**2. Axial length determination by ultrasound**

The systematic error of ultrasound biometry is about 0.1 mm. The actual error depends upon the instrument and the examiner, but should not exceed 0.3 mm. An error in axial length of 0.1 mm corresponds to a refractive correction by spectacles of 0.3 diopters.

**3. Anterior chamber depth**

The third uncertainty factor in measurements is the postoperative location of the intraocular lens within the optical system of the eye. The size of this error cannot be decreased ad lib. The correlation is similar to the difference of refractive power of a cataract lens, depending upon its position. A change in the calculated position of the intraocular lens by 0.1 mm changes the optical power by 0.2 diopters. The surgeon will, of course, base his decision on his own experience. The depth of the anterior chamber in an eye with a posterior chamber lens is assumed to be 3.8–5.4 mm; in an eye with an anterior chamber lens it is 2.2 mm. Other surgeons recommend also considering the preoperative depth of the anterior chamber, and advise subtracting 1.2 mm from this value to calculate the postoperative position of an anterior chamber lens, and adding 0.5 mm for the location of a posterior chamber lens which lies in the capsular sac. In addition, there are a number of imponderable factors, such as the individual surgical technique. It is therefore highly recommended that personal statistics be used in order to calculate these corrections.

### The Various Equations to Calculate the Refractive Power of an Intraocular Lens

Various calculations have been devised in order to use these biometric data. There is a principal difference in the concepts of deriving such calculations:

1. The equations are based on the principles of physiologic optics in which, in the individual case, the empirically determined correction factors are considered (equations of Gernet, Binkhorst and Colenbrander).

2. Without using any assumptions of physiologic optics, regression formulas have been calculated on the basis of statistical analysis using a large number of pre- and postoperative refraction data, e.g., SRK formula, Daxecker formula.

If we now compare the expected results with the various methods of calculation, we find only insignificant deviations. For extreme cases of refractive error, correction factors have been suggested.

The goal of any lens implantation should be to provide the patient with comfortable binocular vision. This requires exact isokonia programs as they have been supplied by a few manufacturers or as they could be laboriously calculated from sets of formulas (Gernet et al. 1973). In general, we aim to achieve a slight postoperative myopia (at the most 3 diopters) with a tolerable anisokonia (at the most 6–8%).

# References

## Textbooks and Overviews


Berges OM, Torrent M. Echographie de l'oeil et de l'orbite. Paris: Vigot, 1986.

Bronson NR, Fisher YL, Pickering NC, Trayner EM. Ophthalmic contact-B-scan ultrasonography. Westport, CT: Intercontinental, 1976.

Buschmann W. Ophthalmologische Ultraschalldiagnostik. In: Velhagen K, ed. Der Augenarzt, vol 2. Leipzig: VEB Thieme, 1972:391.

Buschmann W, Trier HG. Ophthalmologische Ultraschalldiagnostik, mit Atlas, Standardisierung und Einordnung in den ophthalmologischen Untersuchungsbefund. Berlin: Springer, 1989.

Coleman DJ, Lizzi SL, Jack RL. Ultrasonography of the eye and orbit. Philadelphia: Lea and Febiger, 1977.

Gernet H, Ostholt H, Werner H. Intraokulare Optik in Klinik und Praxis. Munich: Rothacker, 1978.

Guthoff R. Die Stellung der Kontakt-B-Bild-Echographie im Rahmen der Orbitadiagnostik dissertation. University of Hamburg, 1985.

Guthoff R. Ultraschall in der opthalmologischen Diagnostik. Ein Leitfaden für die Praxis. Stuttgart: Enke, 1988.

Ossoinig KC. Clinical echo-ophthalmography. In: Blodi FC, ed. Current concepts in ophthalmology, vol 19. St.Louis: Mosby, 1972:127.

Poujol J, Iris M, Armand J. Correlation entre la reflectivit et l'attenuation ultrasonore des tumeurs intraoculaires et leur structures histologiques. Bibl Ophthalmol 1975;83:172.

Rochels R. Ultraschalldiagnostik in der Augenheilkunde. Lehrbuch und Atlas. Munich: Ecomed, 1986.

Sampaolesi R. Ultrasonidos en oftalmologia. Buenos Aires: Panamericana, 1984.

Shammas HJ. Atlas of ophthalmic ultrasonography and biometry. St.Louis: Mosby, 1984.

Stefani FH, Hasenfratz G. Macroscopic ocular pathology: an atlas including correlation with standardized echography. Heidelberg: Springer, 1987.


## General


Abramson DH, Coleman DJ, Franzen LA. Ultrasonography of optic nerve lesions. Bibl Ophthalmol 1975;83:231.

Ashton N, Morgan G. Discrete carcinomatous metastases in the extraocular muscles. Br J Ophthalmol 1974;58:112.

Basedow KA von. Exophthalmus durch Hypertrophie des Zellgewebes in der Augenhöhle. Kaspars Wochenschr Ges Heilkd 1840;1314:220.

Baum G. Use of ultrasonography in the differential diagnosis of ocular tumors. In: Boniuk M, ed. Ocular and adnexal tumors. St.Louis: Mosby, 1964:308.

Baum G. Ultrasonic characteristics of malignant melanoma. Arch Ophthalmol 1967;78:12.

Baum G, Greenwood J. The application of ultrasonic locating techniques to ophthalmology, part 1. Am J Ophthalmol 1958;46:319.

Bedford PD, Daniel PM. Discrete carcinomatous metastases in the extrinsic extraocular muscles. Am J Ophthalmol 1960;49:723.

Berger RW, Guthoff R, Helmke K, Winkler B, Draeger J. Dopplersonographische Befunde der Arteria und Vena centralis retinae. Fortschr Ophthalmol 1988;:85:

Berges OM, Torrent M. Echographie de l'oeil et de l'orbite. Paris: Vigot, 1986.

Best W, Rentsch F. Über das Pseudogliom bei der Incontinentia pigmenti. Klin Monatsbl Augenheilkd 1974;164:19.

Bigar F. Die echographische Differentialdiagnose der Leukokorie. Klin Monatsbl Augenheilkd 1986;188:385.

Bird AC, Sanders MD. Choroidal folds in association with papilloedema. Br J Ophthalmol 1973;57:89.

Bloch RS, Gartner S. The incidence of ocular metastatic carcinoma. Arch Ophthalmol 1971;85:673.

Blodi FC. Eine Aderhautblutung, ein Melanom vortäuschend. Klin Monatsbl Augenheilkd 1972;160:46.

Blodi FC. Ein Tuberkulom der Aderhaut, ein Melanom vortäuschend. Klin Monatsbl Augenheilkd 1977;170:845.

Blodi FC, Gass JDM. Inflammatory pseudotumor of the orbit. Br J Ophthalmol 1968;52:79.

Bluth K. Ultrasonic biometry in congenital glaucoma. In: Hillmann JS, Le May MM, eds. Ophthalmic ultrasonography. The Hague: Junk, 1983:267.

Bluth K, Planitzer J. Comparison of echographic and computer-tomographic examinations in orbital diseases. Doc Ophthalmol Proc Ser 1981;29:293.

Boyce SW, Platia EV, Green WR. Drusen of the optic nerve head. Ann Ophthalmol 1978;10:659.

Brockhurst RJ. Vortex vein decompression for nanophthalmic uveal effusion. Arch Ophthalmol 1980;98:1987.

Brodrick JD. Drusen of the disc and retinal hemorrhages. Br J Ophthalmol 1973;57:299.

Bronson NR. Development of a simple B-scan ultrasonoscope. Trans Am Ophthalmol Soc 1972;70:365.

Bronson NR, Fisher YL, Pickering NC, Trayner EM. Ophthalmic contact-B-scan ultrasonography. Westport, CT: Intercontinental, 1976.

Brunner R, Meyer-Schwickerath R, Schmidel R, Sickel W, Wiedemann P. Uveales Effusions-Syndrom. Eine Verlaufsdokumentation. Paper presented at the 84th meeting of the German Ophthalmologic Society, Aachen, 1986.
Bujara K, Domarus D von, Guthoff R. Nekrotisches malignes Melanom der Aderhaut mit ungewöhnlichem klinischen Verlauf. Ophthalmologica 1980;180:222.
Buschmann W. Ultrasonic examinations of arteries and veins. In: Goldberg R, Sarin L, eds. Ultrasound in ophthalmology. Philadelphia: Saunders, 1967:183.
Buschmann W. Ophthalmologische Ultraschalldiagnostik. In: Velhagen K, ed. Der Augenarzt, vol 2. Leipzig: VEB Thieme, 1972.
Buschmann W, Bluth K. Regelmässige echographische Messung der Achsenlänge des Auges zur Kontrolle der Druckregulierung bei Hydrophthalmie. Klin Monatsbl Augenheilkd 1974;165:878.
Buschmann W, Haigis W. Influence of equipment parameters on results in ophthalmic ultrasonography. Doc Ophthalmol Proc Ser 1981;29:487.
Buschmann W, Haigis W. Measurement-based ophthalmic ultrasonography. Ultrasound Med Biol 1989;15:161.
Buschmann W, Staudt J. Fundaments of echographic differential diagnosis. In: Böck J, Ossoinig K, eds. Ultrasonographia medica (SIDUO III). Vienna: Wiener Medizin-Akademie, 1971:395.
Bustos B de, Augsburger JJ, Shields JA, Shakin EP, Pryor CC. Intraocular metastasis from cutaneous malignant melanoma. Arch Ophthalmol 1985;103:937.
Canning CR, Restori M. Doppler ultrasound studies of the ophthalmic artery. Eye 1988;2:92.
Cappaert WE, Purnell EW, Frank KE. Use of B-scan ultrasound in the diagnosis of benign choroidal folds. Am J Ophthalmol 1977;84:375.
Cennamo G, Loffredo A, Sammartino A, de Lellis A. A comparative echographic and biochemical study of the subretinal fluid in idiopathic retinal detachment. Doc Ophthalmol Proc Ser 1981;29:249.
Chappell JJ. Pseudotumor cerebri following an atrial septal defect repair in a child. Ann Ophthalmol 1969;14:1127.
Clemens S, Kroll P, Busse H. Echographie der Hinterkapsel vor Implantation einer Kunstlinse. Klin Monatsbl Augenheilkd 1987;191:110.
Coleman DJ. Measurement of choroidal pulsation with M-scan ultrasound. Am J Ophthalmol 1971;71:363.
Coleman DJ, Caroll FD. Evaluation of optic neuropathy with B-scan ultrasonography. Am J Ophthalmol 1972;74:281.
Coleman DJ, Franzen LA. Vitreous surgery: preoperative evaluation and prognostic value of ultrasonic display of vitreous hemorrhage. Arch Ophthalmol 1974;92:375.
Coleman DJ, Jack RL, Franzen LA. B-scan ultrasonography of orbital lymphangiomas. Br J Ophthalmol 1973;57:193.
Coleman DJ, Abramson DH, Jack RL, Franzen LA. Ultrasonic diagnosis of tumors of the choroid. Arch Ophthalmol 1974;91:344.
Coleman DJ, Lizzi SL, Jack RL. Ultrasonography of the eye and orbit. Philadelphia: Lea and Febiger, 1977.
Daiker D. Das gewebliche Substrat der verdickten äusseren Augenmuskeln bei der endokrinen Orbitopathie. Klin Monatsbl Augenheilkd 1979;174:843.
Darnley-Fisch DD, Frazier-Byrne S, Hughes JR, Parrish RK, Feuer BJ. Contact B-scan echography in the assessment of optic nerve cupping. Am J Ophtalmol 1990;109:55.
Diamond JG, Keffring SL, Ossoinig KC. Echography and vitrectomy. In: White B, Brown RE, eds. Ultrasound in medicine, vol 3a. New York: Plenum Press, 1977:971.
Domarus D von. Sulzige Skleritis. Heidelberg: 7. Ophthalopathologisches Kolloquium, 1979.
Draeger J. Pseudoglaukom bei endokrinem Exophthalmus. Berichte Dtsch Ophthalmol Ges 1960;63:148.
Draeger J, Schneider C. Ein Beitrag zur Differenzierung der Verlaufsform der endokrinen Orbitopathie. Klin Monatsbl Augenheilkd 1963;143:104.
Edwards MK, Buncic JR, Harwood-Nash DC. Case report: optic disc drusen. J Cataract Refract Surg 1982;6:383.
Eichler C, Hertel PK, Lommatzsch P, Fuhrmann K. Echographische Befunde vor und nach Betabestrahlung. Ru-106 Rh von Aderhautmelanomen. Klin Monatsbl Augenheilkd 1987;190:17.
Esslen E, Papst W. Die Bedeutung der Elektromyographie für die Analyse von Motilitätsstörungen der Augen. Bibl Ophthalmol 1961;57:168.
Feke G, Tagawa H, Deupree DM, Goger DG, Sebag J, Weiter JJ. Bloodflow in the normal human retina. Invest Ophthalmol Vis Sci 1989;30:58.
Feldon SE, Sigelman J, Albert DM, Smith TR. Clinical manifestations of brawny scleritis. Am J Ophthalmol 1978;85:781.
Ferry AP. Lesions mistaken for malignant melanoma of the posterior uvea. Am J Ophthalmol 1964;72:463.
Ferry AP, Font RL. Carcinoma metastatic to the eye and the orbit, 1: a clinicopathological study of 227 cases. Arch Ophthalmol 1974;92:276.
Fledelius H. Orbital malignancies in infancy and childhood in Denmark: recommendations for diagnosis and therapy. Acta Ophthalmol 1976;54:704.
Flocks M, Gerende JH, Zimmerman LE. The size and shape of malignant melanomas of the choroid and ciliary body in relation to prognosis and histologic characteristics. Trans Am Acad Ophthalmol Otolaryngol 1955;59:740.
Font RL, Ferry AP. The phacomatoses. Int Ophthalmol Clin 1972;12:1.
Francois J, Goes F. Ultrasonography in pediatric ophthalmology. J Pediatr Ophthalmol 1971;8:221.
Francois J, Goes F. Ocular biometry: introductory lecture. Doc Ophthalmol Proc Ser 1981;29:135.
Francois J, Goes F, Yobbagyi P. Etude biomtrique d'une ectasie sclrale pripapillaire congnitale (staphylome postrieur vrai). Ophthalmologica 1967;154:446.
Freyler H. Beginnende Bulbusatrophie. Eine echographisch-histologische Vergleichsstudie. Graefes Arch Klin Exp Ophthalmol 1975a;197:203.
Freyler H. Ultraschalldiagnostik des Pseudotumors der Macula. Graefes Arch Klin Exp Ophthalmol 1975b;194:283.
Freyler H, Arnsfelder H. Relation between histological structure and ultrasonogram in malignant melanoblastoma of the choroid. Bibl Ophthalmol 1975;83:163.

Freyler H, Weiss H. Echographie bei experimentellen Glaskörpermembranen. Versuch einer Standardisierung. Graefes Arch Klin Exp Ophthalmol 1974;191:315.

Fried M, Foerster MH, Wessing A, Meyer-Schwickerath G. Echographische Grössenbestimmung von Tumor und Lageüberprüfung des Applikators in der Ruthenium-Therapie beim Aderhautmelanom. Fortschr Ophthalmol 1982;79:193.

Friedman AH, Gartner S, Modi SS. Drusen of the optic disc: a retrospective study in cadaver eyes. Br J Ophthalmol 1975;59:413.

Frisen L, Schöldström G, Svendsen P. Drusen in the optic nerve head: verification by computerized tomography. Arch Ophthalmol 1978;96:1611.

Gass JDM. New observations concerning choroidal osteomas. Int Ophthalmol 1979;1:71.

Gass JDM, Guerry RK, Jack RL, Harris G. Choroidal osteoma. Arch Ophthalmol 1978;96:428.

Gerke E. Dimensionen des Bulbus bei Ablatio retinae. Berichte Dtsch Ophthalmol Ges 1979;76:549.

Gernet H. Biometrische Befunde bei Rissamotio im kurzsichtigen Auge. Beitrag zur Pathogenese. Ophthalmologica 1965;150:386.

Gernet H, Hollwich F. Oculometrie des kindlichen Glaukoms. Berichte Dtsch Ophthalmol Ges 1969;69:341.

Gernet H, Worst JGF. Klinische Okulometrie und Linseneinpflanzung nach Binkhorst. In: Massin M, Poujol J, eds. Diagnostica ultrasonica in ophthalmologica. Paris: Centre Nationale Ophtalmologique Quinze-Vingt, 1973:247.

Gernet H, Ostholt H, Werner H. Intraokulare Optik in Klinik und Praxis. Munich: Rothacker, 1978.

Gonvers M, Zografos L, Gailloud CL. Tumeurs malignes de la chorode: confrontation anatomo-ultrasonographique. Klin Monatsbl Augenheilkd 1979;174:934.

Graefe A von, Saemisch T. Handbuch der gesamten Augenheilkunde, vol 9.1. 2nd ed. Berlin:, 19071930.

Grasslin HL, Bagley EH. Studies of peripheral blood vascular beds. Bull Johns Hopkins Hosp 1953;92:47.

Graves RJ. Clinical lectures, 12. Lond Med Surg J 1835;7:516.

Griffin DR. Listening in the dark. New Haven: , 1958.

Guerry RK, Lawton-Smith J. Paranasal sinus carcinoma causing orbital mucocele. Am J Ophthalmol 1975;80:943.

Guthoff R. Die Differentialdiagnostische Bedeutung des Tenonschen Raums. Fortschr Ophthalmol 1974;81:388.

Guthoff R. Modellmessungen zur Volumenbestimmung des malignen Aderhautmelanoms. Graefes Arch Klin Exp Ophthalmol 1980;214:139.

Guthoff R. Techniques in ocular biometry: influences of intraocular pressure and probe contact pressure. In: Thissen JM, Hillman JS, Galenga PE, Cennamo G, eds. Proceedings, SIDUO XI. Dordrecht: Kluwer, 1988:309.

Guthoff R. Ruthenium plaque therapy on malignant melanomas of the choroid: analysis of failures due to unsatisfactory placement of the applicator. In: Olah Z, ed. Proceedings of the symposium on intraocular tumors. Bratislava: Slovak Medical Society, 1989:.

Guthoff R. Zur Diagnose der endokrinen Orbitopathie. Fortschr Ophthalmol (in press).

Guthoff R, Abramo F. Osteome der Bulbuswand. Erscheinungsformen in Abhängigkeit von Lage und Ausdehnung. Klin Monatsbl Augenheilkd (in press).

Guthoff R, Hamann KU. Ophthalmologische Probleme des Pseudotumor cerebri. Fortschr Ophthalmol 1983;80:94.

Guthoff R, Jörgensen J. Long-term follow-up in patients with spontanous AV fistulas affecting the orbit. Orbit 1987;6:229.

Guthoff R, Schroeder W. Korrelation von pathologisch-anatomisch und schnittbildechographischen Befunden. In: Gernet H, ed. Proceedings, SIDUO VII. Münster: Remy, 1979.

Guthoff R, Schroeder W. Swollen extraocular muscles: ultrasonographic findings and clinical appearances. Doc Ophthalmol Proc Ser 1981;29:337.

Guthoff R, Singh G. Posterior scleritis: the role of ultrasonography in the follow-up of the disease. In: Hillmann JS, Le May MM, eds. Ophthalmic ultrasonography. The Hague: Junk, 1983:169.

Guthoff R, Schroeder W, Hallermann D. Echographische Befunde nach Ruthenium-Bestrahlung intraokularer Tumoren. Berichte Dtsch Ophthalmol Ges 1977;74:723.

Guthoff R, Domarus D von, Schroeder W. Gegenüberstellung klinischer, echographischer und histologischer Befunde beim malignen Melanom der Aderhaut. Klin Monatsbl Augenheilkd 1981;179:330.

Guthoff R, Hagemann J, Heller M. Möglichkeiten der computertomographischen Fremdkörperlokalisation. Graefes Arch Klin Exp Ophthalmol 1982;218:307.

Guthoff R, Domarus D von, Steinhorst U, Hallermann D. Ruthenium-106/Rhodium-106-Behandlung des malignen Melanoms der Aderhaut. Klin Monatsbl Augenheilkd 1986;188:576.

Guthoff R, Berger R, Draeger J. Ultrasonographic measurements of the posterior coats of the eye and their relation to axial length. Graefes Arch Klin Exp Ophthalmol 1987a;225:374.

Guthoff R, Terwey B, Burk R, Domarus D von. Versuch einer präoperativen Differenzierung des malignen Melanoms der Aderhaut. Klin Monatsbl Augenheilkd 1987b;191:45.

Guthoff R, Berger RW, Helmke K, Winkler B. Dopplersonographische Befunde bei intraokularen Tumoren. Fortschr Ophthalmol 1989;86:239.

Guthoff R, Abramo F, Jörgensen JS. Die okuläre Myositis Morphologie und Funktion. Langzeitbeobachtungen bei 15 Patienten. Klin Monatsbl Augenheilkd (in press).

Gutjahr E, Lederka LD, Müller-Hermeling HK, Nover A. Klinik und Morphologie kindlicher Rhabdomyosarkome der Orbita. Graefes Arch Klin Exp Ophthalmol 1975;196:113.

Gärtner J, Löpping G. Über Glaskörperveränderungen im Verlauf des Alters. Untersuchungen mit Ultraschall. Graefes Arch Klin Exp Ophthalmol 1967;173:283.

Gärtner J, Löpping G. Der Glaskörper bei systemischen Bindegewebsveränderungen. Untersuchungen mit Ultraschall. In: Jaeger J, ed. Berichte, 68. Zusammenkunft der Deutschen Ophthalmologischen Gesellschaft. Munich: Bergmann, 1968:40.

Haigis W, Buschmann W. Die Benutzung von Testreflektoren zur schnellen klinischen Überprüfung von Geräten für die ophthalmologische Ultraschalldiagnostik. Proc Ges Biomed Technik Berlin 1980a;:53.

Haigis W, Buschmann W. Klinisch anwendbare Methoden zur Überprüfung von diagnostisch relevanten Geräteparametern von Impulsechogeräten. In: , ed. Ultraschall in der Medizin. Stuttgart: Thieme, 1980b:.

Hallermann D, Guthoff R. Regression of choroidal melanoma after beta-irradiation with ruthenium-106: contribution to the International Symposium. In: Lommatzsch PK, Blodi FC, eds. Intraocular tumors. Berlin: Akademie, 1983:307. (Fortschritte in der Onkologie, 9).

Harris EJ. Subperiostal abscess of the orbit. Arch Ophthalmol 1983;101:751.

Hasenfratz G. Echographische Befunde orbitaler Gefässanomalien bei conjunctivaler Kongestion als Leitsymptom. Fortschr Ophthalmol 1986;83:275.

Hasenfratz G. Echographische Befunde mit standardisierter Echographie bei akuter Endophthalmitis. Fortschr Ophthalmol 1987;84:255.

Hasenfratz G, Ossoinig KC. The diagnosis of orbital mucoceles and pyoceles with standardized echography. In: Hillmann JS, Le May MM, eds. Ophthalmic ultrasonography. The Hague: Junk, 1983:407.

Hasenfratz G, Riedel KG, Markl A, Stefani FH. Echographische Befunde bei Metastasierung in einem äusseren Augenmuskel. Klin Monatsbl Augenheilkd 1987;191:229.

Hauff W, Till P. Malignes Melanom oder Aderhautmetastase? Eine echographische Differentialdiagnose. Klin Monatsbl Augenheilkd 1980;176:341.

Hayreh SS. Optic disc edema in raised intracranial pressure. Arch Ophthalmol 1977;95:1553.

Hedges TR, Pozzi-Mucelli R, Char DH, Newton TH. Computed tomographic demonstration of ocular calcification: correlations with clinical and pathological findings. Neuroradiology 1982;23:15.

Henderson JW. Orbital tumors. 2nd ed. New York: Stratton-Thieme, 1980:497.

Hinzpeter EN, Naumann GOH. Cornea and sclera. In: Naumann GOH, Apple DJ, eds. Pathology of the eye. New York: Springer, 1985:317.

Horn DL van, Aalberg TM, Machemer R, Fenzl R. Glial cell proliferation in human retinal detachment with massive periretinal proliferation. Am J Ophthalmol 1977;84:383.

Horst W. Methoden und Ergebnisse des Radiojodstoffwechselstudiums zur Diagnostik thyreoidaler und extrathyreoidaler Erkrankungen. Klin Wochenschr 1952;30:439.

Howard GM, Ellsworth RM. Differential diagnosis of retinoblastoma: a statistical survey of 500 children, 2: factors relating to the diagnosis of retinoblastoma. Am J Ophthalmol 1965;60:618.

Hoyt WF, Pont ME. Pseudopapilledema: anomalous elevation of optic disk. Pitfalls in diagnosis and management. J Am Med Assoc 1962;181:191.

Hyvärien L, Walsh FB. Benign chorioretinal folds. Am J Ophthalmol 1970;70:14.

Iejima Y, Asanagi K. A new B-scan ultrasonographic technique for observing ciliary body detachment. Am J Ophthalmol 1983;95:498.

Jacobs L, Weissberg LA, Kinkel WR. Computerized tomography of the orbit and the sella turcica. New York: Raven Press, 1980.

Jaeger W. Tiefenmessung der menschlichen Vorderkammer mit planparallelen Platten (Zusatzgerät zur Spaltlampe). Graefes Arch Klin Exp Ophthalmol 1952;153:120.

Jaffe NS. The vitreous in clinical ophthalmology. St.Louis: Mosby, 1969.

Jaffe NS, Jaffe GF, Jaffe MS. A randomized prospective evaluation of planned extracapsular cataract extraction versus phacoemulsification with posterior chamber lenses. In: , ed. Proceedings of the 5th Congress of the European Intraocular Implant Council, Jerusalem 1987 (in press).

Jansson F. Measurements of intraocular distances by ultrasound. Acta Ophthalmol Suppl (Copenh) 1963;74:1.

Jansson F, Kock E. Determination of the velocity of ultrasound in the human lens and vitreous. Acta Ophthalmol (Copenh) 1962;40:420.

Jansson F, Sundmark E. Determination of the velocity of ultrasound in ocular tissues at different temperatures. Acta Ophthalmol (Copenh) 1961;39:899.

Jensen SF. Endocrine ophthalmoplegia: is it due to myopathy or to mechanical immobilisation? Acta Ophthalmol (Copenh) 1971;49: 679.

Jones IS. Lymphangiomas of the ocular adnexa: an analysis of 62 cases. Trans Am Ophthalmol Soc 1959;57:602.

Jörgensen JS, Guthoff R. 24 cases of carotid cavernous fistulas: frequency, symptoms, diagnosis and treatment. Arch Ophthalmol Suppl (Copenh) 1985;173:67.

Jörgensen JS, Guthoff R. Sturge-Weber-Syndrom: Glaukom mit erhöhtem episkleralen Venendruck. Klin Monatsbl Augenheilkd 1987;191:275.

Kalina RE, Mills RP. Acquired hyperopia with choroidal folds. Ophthalmology 1980;87:44.

Kamin DF, Hepler RS, Foos RY. Optic nerve drusen. Arch Ophthalmol 1973;89:359.

Khan SG, Frenkel M. Intravitreal hemorrhage associated with rapid increase of intracranial pressure (Terson's syndrome). Am J Ophthalmol 1975;80:37.

Kline LE, Skalka HW, Davidson JD, Wilmes FJ. Bilateral choroidal osteomas associated with fatal systemic illness. Am J Ophthalmol 1982;93:192.

Koch A, Gerke E, Höpping W. Echography in retinoblastoma. Graefes Arch Klin Exp Ophthalmol 1983;221:27.

Kolozsvary L. Diagnostic ultrasound in cases of experimental vitreous hemorrhage. Doc Ophthalmol Proc Ser 1984;38:175.

Koorneeff L. Orbital septa: anatomy and function. Ophthalmology 1971;91:303.

Koorneeff L. Sectional anatomy of the orbit: a 20-slide atlas of histological sections of human orbits. Amsterdam: Aelus Press, 1980.

Kramer KKM, Lapiana LF. Quantification of intraocular malignant melanoma volume: a preliminary report. Ann Ophthalmol 1976;8:781.

Krohel GB, Wright JE. Orbital hemorrhage. Am J Ophthalmol 1979;88:254.

Krohel GB, Steward WB, Chavis RM. Orbital disease: a practical approach. New York: Grune and Stratton, 1981.

Langenbruch K. Die Computertomographie der Orbita bei der endokrinen Orbitopathie. RöFo 1981;135:29.

Laqua H, Machemer R. Sternfalten bei Netzhautablösung. Graefes Arch Klin Exp Ophthalmol 1974;191:273.

Le May M. B-scan ultrasonography of the anterior segment of the eye. Br J Ophthalmol 1978;62:651.

Lepper RD. Ultraschallmessungen an der Rückwand des lebenden menschlichen Auges dissertation. University of Bonn, 1978.

Lepper RD, Trier HG. Computer-aided ultrasonic measurements of the corneal thickness. Ophthalmol Res 1984;16:163.

Lepper RD, Trier HG, Reuter R. Neuartige Ultraschallbiometrie. Klin Monatsbl Augenheilkd 1980;177:101.

Lieb W Jr, Cohen SM, Mitchell D, Merton D, Shields J. Darstellung von intraokularen und orbitalen Gefässen mittels Angiodynographie. Paper presented at the 87th meeting of the German Ophthalmologic Society, Heidelberg, 1989.

Lloyd GAS. The radiological investigation of proptosis. Br J Radiol 1970;43:1.

Lloyd GAS. Radiology of the orbit. London: Saunders, 1975:30.

Lloyd GAS. Primary orbital meningioma: review of 41 patients investigated radiologically. Clin Radiol 1982;33:181.

Lopez JFV, Alvarez JC. Atypical echographic forms of retinoblastoma. J Pediatr Ophthalmol Strabismus 1983;20:230.

Machemer R, Aalberg TM. Glaskörperchirurgie, Vitrektomie. Indikationen und Technik. Berne: Huber, 1981.

McLeod D chair. Round table discussion on vitreous pathology. Doc Ophthalmol Proc Ser 1981;29:547.

McLeod D, Restori M. Real time B-scanning of the vitreous. Trans Ophthalmol Soc UK 1977;97:547.

McNutt L, Kaeffring SL, Ossoinig KC. Echographic measurements of extraocular muscles. In: White D, Brown RE, eds. Ultrasound in medicine, vol 3a. New York: Plenum Press, 1977:927.

McRae A. Prognosis in malignant melanoma of the choroid and ciliary body. Trans Ophthalmol Soc UK 1953;73:3.

Makabe R. Echographische Untersuchungen bei exzentrischen hinteren Skleraektasien. Klin Monatsbl Augenheilkd 1975;167:97.

Manschot WA. The relation between histopathology and ultrasonography in intraocular tumors. Doc Ophthalmol Proc Ser 1981;29:71.

Marushak D. Uveal effusion attending scleritis posterior: a case report with A- and B-scan echograms. Acta Ophthalmol 1982;16:773.

Mazzeo VL, Ravalli L, Spettoli M, Rossi A. Is it possible to differentiate histological types of choroidal malignant melanoma with Kretz technique 7200 MA scans? Doc Ophthalmol Proc Ser 1988;48:357.

Mornix R, Fournier G, Berthezenne F. Ophthalmic Graves' disease. Mod Probl Ophthalmol 1975;14:426.

Mottow-Lippa L, Jacobiec FA, Smith M. Idiopathic inflammatory pseudotumor in childhood, 2: results of diagnostic tests and biopsies. Ophthalmologica 1981;88:565.

Mundt GH, Hughes WS. Ultrasonics in ocular diagnosis. Am J Ophthalmol 1956;41:488.

Mustonen E, Nieminen H. Optic disc drusen a photographic study, 1: autofluorescence pictures and fluorescein angiography. Acta Ophthalmol (Copenh) 1982a;60:849.

Mustonen E, Nieminen H. Optic disc drusen a photographic study, 2: retinal nerve fibre layer photography. Acta Ophthalmol (Copenh) 1982;60b:859.

Nasr AM, Ipektchi A. The diagnosis of an aerocele with standardized echography. Orbit 1984;3:275.

Naumann GOH, Apple DJ. Pathology of the eye. New York: Springer, 1985.

Naumann GOH, Portwich E. Ätiologie und akuter klinischer Anlass zu 1000 Enukleationen. Eine klinische ophthalmo-pathologische Studie. Klin Monatsbl Augenheilkd 1976;168:622.

Newell FW. Choroidal folds. Am J Ophthalmol 1973;75:930.

Newton TH. Radiology in lacrimal gland tumors. Radiation 1962;79:598.

Norton EW. A characteristic fluorescein angiography pattern in choroidal folds. Proc Roy Soc Med 1969;62:119.

Nover A, Glanschneider D. Ultraschalldiagnostik intraokularer Tumoren. Fortschr Med 1965a;83:433.

Nover A, Glanschneider D. Die Untersuchungen über die Fortpflanzungsgeschwindigkeit und Absorption des Ultraschalls im Gewebe. Experimentelle Beiträge zur Ultraschalldiagnostik intraokularer Tumoren. Graefes Arch Klin Exp Ophthalmol 1965b;168:304.

Nover A, Grote W. Untersuchungen über die Reflexion des Ultraschalls an Netzhaut, Aderhaut und Sklera, das sogenannte "Rückwandecho". Graefes Arch Klin Exp Ophthalmol 1965;168:388.

Nover A, Rochels R. Echographische Differentialdiagnostik posttraumatischer Motilitätsstörungen des Auges. Klin Monatsbl Augenheilkd 1986;189:206.

Nover A, Rochels R, Queckenstedt U, Wende S. Vergleich echographischer, computertomographischer und histologischer Befunde bei Orbitatumoren. Fortschr Ophthalmol 1982;79:22.

Oksala A. Echogram in melanoma of the choroid. Br J Ophthalmol 1959;43:408.

Oksala A. Melanoma of the choroid examined with an acoustic biomicroscope. Br J Ophthalmol 1961;45:218.

Oksala A. Ultrasonic diagnosis in melanoma and retinoblastoma. Arch Ophthalmol Suppl (Copenh) 1974;123:136.

Oksala A. Ultrasonic findings in vitreous bodies at different ages and in patients with detachment of the retina. Graefes Arch Klin Exp Ophthalmol 1975;197:83.

Oksala A. Ultrasonic findings in the vitreous body. In: Gernet H, ed. Proceedings, SIDUO VII. Münster: Remy, 1979:85.

Oksala A, Kause GR. On the differential diagnosis of retinitis proliferans intraocular tumor by ultrasound. In: , ed. Ultrasonics in ophthalmology, vol 19. Basel: Karger, 1967:143.

Ossoinig KC. Über die Beurteilung der kinetischen Eigenschaften von Echogrammen. In: , ed. Ultrasonics in ophthalmology, vol 19. Basel: Karger, 1967:88.

Ossoinig KC. Grundlagen der klinischen Echo-Ophthalmologie. Vienna: Wiener Medizin-Akademie, 1971.

Ossoinig KC. Clinical echo-ophthalmography. In: Blodi FC, ed. Current concepts in ophthalmology, vol . St. Louis: Mosby, 1972:101.

Ossoinig KC. Preoperative differential diagnosis of tumors with echography, 4: diagnosis of orbital tumors. In: Blodi FC, ed. Current concepts in ophthalmology, vol 4. St. Louis: Mosby, 1974:313.

Ossoinig KC. Echography of the eye. In: Arger PH, ed. Regiology of the Orbit. New York: Wiley, 1976:.

Ossoinig KC. Spezielle echographische Methoden zur Beurteilung okularer Fremdkörper. In: Neubauer H, Rüssmann W, Kilp H, eds. Intraokulare Fremdkörper und Metallose. Munich: Bergmann, 1977:247.

Ossoinig KC. Standardized echography: basic principles, clinical applications and results. In: Int Ophthalmol Clin 1979;19(4):127.

Ossoinig KC. Ein neues Merkmal zur verlässlichen Differentialdiagnostik des endokrinen Exophthalmus. Klin Monatsbl Augenheilkd 1982;180:198.

Ossoinig KC. Advances in diagnostic ultrasound. In: Henkind P, ed. Acta, 14th International Congress of Ophthalmology. Philadelphia: Lippincott, 1983:89.

Ossoinig KC. Echographic detection and classification of posterior hyphaemas. Ophthalmologica 1984;189:2.

Ossoinig KC, Blodi FC. Preoperative differential diagnosis of tumors with echography, 3: diagnosis of intraocular tumors. In: Blodi FC, ed. Current concepts in ophthalmology, vol 4. St. Louis: Mosby, 1974:296.

Ossoinig KC, Seher K. Einige Erkenntnisse über das histologische Substrat der Echogramme. In: , ed. Ultrasonics in ophthalmology, vol . Basel: Karger, 1967:103.

Ossoinig KC, Seher K. Ultrasonic diagnosis of intraocular foreign bodies. In: Gitter KA, Keeney AH, Sahin LK, eds. Proceedings of the 4th International Congress of Ultrasonography in Ophthalmology, Philadelphia 1968. St. Louis: Mosby, 1969:311.

Ossoinig KC, Till P. Methods and results of ultrasonography in diagnosing intraocular tumors. St. Louis: Mosby, 1969.

Ossoinig KC, Till P. 10 years' study on clinical echography in orbital disease. Bibl Ophthalmol 1975;83:200.

Ossoinig KC, Keenan TP, Bigar F. Cavernous hemangioma of the orbit: a differential diagnosis in clinical echography. Bibl Ophthalmol 1975;83:236.

Ossoinig KC, Kaefring SL, McNutt L, Weinstock SJ. Echographic measurement of the optic nerve. In: White D, Brown RE, eds. Ultrasound in medicine, vol 3. New York: Plenum Press, 1977:.

Ossoinig KC, Reshef DS, Harries RP, Hasenfratz GC. Acoustic tissue differentiation with standardized echography in reference to melanomas and pseudomelanomas. Doc Ophthalmol Proc Ser 1988;48:363.

Pallikaris I, Gruber H. Determination of sound velocity in different forms of cataracts. Doc Ophthalmol Proc Ser 1981;29:165.

Paulmann H, Heimann K. Das uveale Effusions-Syndrom. Berichte Dtsch Ophthalmol Ges 1977;74:545.

Pavlin CJ, Sherar MD, Foster FS. Subsurface ultrasound microscopic imaging of the intact eye. Ophthalmology 1990;97:244.

Pavlin CJ, Sherar MD, Foster FS. Ultrasound biomicroscopy: research in clinical application [paper presented at the 13th Biennial Congress of the Intraocular Society of Ophthalmic Ultrasound, Vienna, July 1–5 1990].

Peeters FLM, Kröger R. Dural and direct cavernous sinus fistulas. Am J Radiol 1979;132:599.

Phelps CD, Thompson HF, Ossoinig KC. The diagnosis and prognosis of atypical carotid cavernous fistula (red-eye shunt syndrome). Am J Ophthalmol 1982;93:423.

Poujol J. Echographie en Ophtalmologie. Paris: Masson, 1981.

Poujol J, Iris M, Armand J. Corrlation entre la rflectivit et l'attnuation ultrasonores des tumeurs intraoculaires et leur structures histologiques. Bibl Ophthalmol 1975;83:172.

Radius LA, Maumenee AE. Dilated episcleral vessels and open angle glaucoma. Am J Ophthalmol 1978;86:31.

Ramirez H, Blatt ES, Hibri NS. Computed tomographic identification of calcified optic nerve drusen. Radiation 1983;148:137.

Rentsch F. The ultrastructure of preretinal macular fibrosis. Graefes Arch Klin Exp Ophthalmol 1977;203:321.

Restori M, McLeod D. Ultrasonic examination of the vitreous. Doc Ophthalmol Proc Ser 1981;29:47.

Riva CE, Grunwald JE, Sinclair SH, Petrig BL. Blood velocity and volumetric flow rate in human retinal vessels. Invest Ophthalmol Vis Sci 1985;26:1024.

Rochels R, Nover A. Echographische Differentialdiagnose der Leukokorie im Kindesalter. Ophthalmologica 1979;178:215.

Rochels R, Nover A. Echography of paranasal tumors invading the orbit. Orbit (in press).

Rochels R, Reis G. Echographische Befunde bei traumatischer Linsenluxation. In: Berneaud-Kötz G, ed. Sitzungsbericht der 139. Versammlung des Vereins der Rheinisch-Westfälischer Augenärzte. Balve: Zimmermann, 1980a:69.

Rochels R, Reis G. Echographie bei orbitalen Rhabdomyosarkomen im Kindesalter. Ophthalmologica 1980b;180:274.

Rochels R, Nover A, Neuhann TH, Adam F. Echographic examination of 110 histologically proven intraocular melanomas. In: Lommatzsch PK, Blodi FC, eds. Intraocular tumors. Berlin: Akademie, 1983:176.

Rochels R, Geyer G, Wleier R. Echographische Diagnostik bei orbitaler Mucocele. Laryn Rhinol Otol 1985;64:181.

Rochels R, Nover A, Hackelbusch R. Echographische Befunde und Differentialdiagnostik. Klin Monatsbl Augenheilkd 1986;188:101.

Rootmann J, Quenville N, Owen D. Recent advances in pathology as applied to orbital biopsy. Ophthalmology 1984;91:708.

Roth A. Les myosites orbitaires aigues et chroniques. Klin Monatsbl Augenheilkd 1985;186:450.

Ruchmann MC, Flanagan J. Cavernous hemangioma of the orbit. Ophthalmology 1983;90:1328.

Ruprecht KW, Naumann GOH. Einseitiges sekundäres Offenwinkelglaukom bei idiopathisch dilatierten episkleralen Gefässen. Klin Monatsbl Augenheilkd 1984;184:23.

Rüssmann W, Bös W, Neubauer H. Klinische Ultraschalldiagnostik bei intraokularen Fremdkörpern. Bibl Ophthalmol 1975;83:96.

Sampaolesi R. La pression oculaire et le sinus camrulaire chez l'enfant normal et dans le glaucome congnitale au-dessous de l'age de cinq ans. Doc Ophthalmol Proc Ser 1969;26:497.

Sampaolesi R. Ocular echometry in the diagnosis of congenital glaucoma. Doc Ophthalmol Proc Ser 1981;29:177.

Schelenz J, Stodollick H, Kammann J. Der Einfluss unterschiedlicher Messverfahren auf die Berechnung der Brechkraft intraokularer Linsen. In: Jacobi KW, Schott K, Gloor B, eds. DGII-Berichte. Heidelberg: Springer, 1988:39.

Scherer U, Osterheld B. Echographische Befunde bei Zyklitis anularis pseudotumorosa und Ringmelanom des Ziliarkörpers. Klin Monatsbl Augenheilkd 1985;187:455.
Scherer U, Rochels R. Artefakte im A- und B-Bild-Echogramm nach Implantation von Kunstlinsen. Ophthalmologica 1983;187:192.
Schmidt B, Trojan HJ. Augenhintergrundsbefunde und histologische Untersuchungen bei Pachymeningitis haemorrhagica interna des Kindes. Klin Monatsbl Augenheilkd 1970;157:239.
Schnaudigel OE. Intraokulare Knochenbildung. Klin Monatsbl Augenheilkd 1989;195:232.
Schroeder W. Nutzen der A-Bild-Echographie in der Diagnostik des persistierenden hyperplastischen primären Glaskörpers. Klin Monatsbl Augenheilkd 1976a;168:210.
Schroeder W. Ergebnisse der A-Bild-Echographie bei einseitigen Sehnervenerkrankungen. Klin Monatsbl Augenheilkd 1976;169b:30.
Schroeder W. Schallaufzeitmessung im distalen Sehnervquerschnitt. Klin Monatsbl Augenheilkd 1976c;169:743.
Schroeder W. Topographische Orbitadiagnostik mit der Kontakt-B-Bild-Echographie. Klin Monatsbl Augenheilkd 1978;172:12.
Schroeder W. Ultraschalldiagnostik des Sehnerven. Dissertation. University of Hamburg, 1979.
Schroeder W, Guthoff R. Modellversuche zur Messung des Sehnerven. In: Gernet H, ed. Proceedings, SIDUO VII. Münster: Remy, 1979:3.
Schwab B, Nover A. Ergebnisse der Orbita-Echographie im A-Bild-Verfahren. Klin Monatsbl Augenheilkd 1975;166:758.
Shammas HJ. Atlas of ophthalmic ultrasonography and biometry. St. Louis: Mosby, 1984a.
Shammas HJ. A comparison of immersion and contact techniques for axial length measurements. Am Intraocular Implant Soc J 1984b;10:444.
Shammas HJ, Blodi FC. Prognostic factors in choroidal and ciliary body melanomas. Arch Ophthalmol 1977;95:63.
Shammas HJ, Minckler DS, Owden C. Ultrasound in early thyroid orbitopathy. Arch Ophthalmol 1980;98:277.
Shapiro DR, Stone RD. Ultrasonic characteristics of retinopathy of prematurity presenting with leukokoria. Arch Ophthalmol 1985;103:1690.
Shibata H, Misuyama Y, Mishimoto Y, Savada A. Echography in orbital myositis. Doc Ophthalmol Proc Ser 1981;29:343.
Shields CL, McDonald RP. Improvements in the diagnosis of posterior uveal melanomas. Arch Ophthalmol 1974;91:259.
Shields CL, Shields JA, Augsburger JJ. Update on choroidal osteomas. In: , ed. Proceedings of the 2nd International Meeting on the Diagnosis and Treatment of Intraocular Tumors, Lyons 1987 (in press).
Shields JA, Joffe L, Giubor P. Choroidal melanoma clinically simulating a retinal angioma. Am J Ophthalmol 1978;85:67.
Singh G, Guthoff R, Foster S. Observations on long-term follow-up of posterior scleritis. Am J Ophthalmol 1986;101:570.
Skalka HW. Quantitative ultrasonographic examination of perineuralorbital optic nerve cerebrospinal fluid. In: White D, Brown RE, eds. Ultrasound in medicine, vol 3. New York: Plenum Press, 1977:.
Skalka HW. The use of ultrasonography in the diagnosis of endocrine orbitopathy. Neuro-Ophthalmol 1980;1:109.
Skalka HW. Ultrasonography of the optic nerve. Neuro-Ophthalmol 1981;1:261.
Spallanzani IL. Opere, ed. Fabroni VA. :, 1825:.
Spalton DJ, Hitchings RA, Hunter PA. Atlas of clinical ophthalmology. Philadelphia: Lippincott, 1984.
Stewart WB, Krohel GB, Wright JE. Lacrimal gland and fossal lesions: an approach to diagnosis and management. Ophthalmology 1979;86:886.
Strobel J, Jacobi KW. Zur Brechkraft der Intraokularen Linsen. Berichte Dtsch Ophthalmol Ges 1978;75:603.
Susal AL, Walker JT. In vivo measurements of vitreous and retinal acceleration. In: Hillmann JS, Le May MM, eds. Ophthalmic ultrasonography. The Hague: Junk, 1983:163.
Takahashi T, Oda Y, Isayama Y. Leukemic opticoneuropathy. Ophthalmologica 1982;185:37.
Takeuchi S. Ultrasonic diagnosis of massive periretinal proliferation. Doc Ophthalmol Proc Ser 1981;29:13.
Tane S, Komatsu A. Ultrasonic characteristics of ocular trauma, especially diagnostic application of ophthalmic ultrasonic high-speed electronic scanning display. In: Hillmann JS, Le May MM, eds. Ophthalmic ultrasonography. The Hague: Junk, 1983:127.
Thijssen JM. Echo ophthalmography: physical principles and diagnostic value. Doc Ophthalmol Proc Ser 1973;3:273.
Thomas JW, Green BA, Maumenee AE. Small choroidal melanomas: a long-term follow-up study. Arch Ophthalmol 1979;97:861.
Till P. Echography in intraocular tumors. In: Gernet H, ed. Proceedings, SIDUO VII. Münster: Remy, 1979:144.
Till P, Hauff W. Echographic findings in orbital mucoceles. In: Gernet H, ed. Proceedings, SIDUO VII. Münster: Remy, 1979:151.
Till P, Hauff W. Differential diagnostic results of clinical echography in intraocular tumors. Doc Ophthalmol Proc Ser 1981;29:91.
Till P, Ossoinig KC. Echographie des Retinoblastoms. In: Jaeger W, ed. Berichte der 69. Zusammenkunft der Deutschen Ophthalmologischen Gesellschaft. Munich: Bergmann, 1969:203.
Till P, Ossoinig KC. Echographische Befunde bei Retinopathia proliferans. Klin Monatsbl Augenheilkd 1972;161:297.
Till P, Ossoinig KC. 10 years' study on clinical echography in intraocular disease. Bibl Ophthalmol 1975;83:49.
Till P, Steinkogler JF, Hauff W. Die Bedeutung der echographischen Gewebsdifferenzierung für die Orbitachirurgie. Klin Monatsbl Augenheilkd 1985;186:296.
Trier HG. Gewebsdifferenzierung mit Ultraschall. Bibl Ophthalmol 1977;86:92.
Trier HG, Böhm HW. B-Bild bei inverser Papille mit hinterem Staphylom. In: , ed. Diagnostica Ultrasonica. Brno: , 1968:263.

Trokel SL, Hilal SK. Recognition and differential diagnosis of enlarged extraocular muscles in computed tomography. Am J Ophthalmol 1979;87:503.
Trokel SL, Jacobiec FA. Correlation of CT-scanning and pathologic features of ophthalmic Graves' disease. Ophthalmology 1981;88:553.
Tso MOM, Fine BS. Electron-microscopic study of human papilledema. Am J Ophthalmol 1976;82:424.
Tso MOM, Shih CY. Disruption of bloodretinal barrier in ocular hypotony: preliminary report. Exp Eye Res 1976;23:209.
Ullerich K, Fischedick O. Spezialuntersuchungen, insbes. nuklearmedizinische Methoden zum Nachweis einer endokrinen Orbitopathie. In: , ed. . Stuttgart: Enke, 1976:.
Ulrich WD, Ulrich C. Okulo-oszillo-Dynamographie. Ein neues Verfahren zur Bestimmung des Ophthalmica-Blutdrucks und zur okulären Pulskurvenanalyse. Klin Monatsbl Augenheilkd 1985;186:385.
Unsöld R, Newton TH, de Grot J. CT evaluations of extraocular muscles: anatomicCT correlations. Graefes Arch Klin Exp Ophthalmol 1980a;214:155.
Unsöld R, Ostertag CH, Newton TH. Zur Differentialdiagnose der endokrinen Orbitopathie und entzündlicher Pseudotumoren der Orbita. Computertomographie-Befunde. Klin Monatsbl Augenheilkd 1980b;177:31.
Unsöld R, Ostertag CH, de Groot J. Computer reformations of the brain and skull base: anatomy and clinical applications. Berlin: Springer, 1982.
Vedel-Jensen N. Retinal grooves caused by pressure on the globe. Acta Ophthalmol 1959;37:279.
Verbeek AM. Retinal tear on B-scanning. Doc Ophthalmol Proc Ser 1981a;29:269.
Verbeek AM. A choroidal oat cell carcinoma metastasis mimicking a choroidal melanoma. Doc Ophthalmol Proc Ser 1981b;29:367.
Verbeek AM. Echographic findings in 36 patients with choroidal folds. Doc Ophthalmol Proc Ser 1981c;29:.
Walsh FB. Meningioma primary within the orbit and optic canal. In: Smith JL, ed. Neuro-ophthalmological Symposium, University of Miami and Bascon Parmer Eye Institute, vol 5. St. Louis: Mosby, 1970:240.
Watson PG, Hayreh SS. Scleritis and episcleritis. Br J Ophthalmol 1976;60:163.
Wende S, Aulich A, Nover A, et al. Computer tomography of orbital lesions: a cooperative study of 210 cases. Neuroradiology 1978;13:123.
Werner SC. Euthyroid patients with early signs of Graves' disease. Am J Med 1955;18:608.
Wing GL, Schepens CL, Trempe CL, Weiter JJ. Serous choroidal detachment and the thickened choroid sign detected by ultrasonography. Am J Ophthalmol 1982;94:499.
Winning CHOM. Fluorography of choroidal folds. In: , ed. 165th Netherlands Opthalmogolic Society Meeting, The Hague 1973. :, :167:436.
Wirtschafter JD, Slagel DE, Fox WJ, Rizzo FJ. Intraocular axonal swelling produced by partial immediately retrobulbar ligature of the optic nerve. Invest Ophthalmol Vis Sci 1977;16:537.
Witold J, Orlowski-Szczypinski J. Ultrasonography of the subretinal space in rhegmatogenous retinal detachment. Z Mod Probl Ophthalmol 1976;18:40.
Witschel H, Font RL. Hemangioma of the choroid: a clinico-pathologic study of 71 cases and a review of the literature. Surv Ophthalmol 1976;20:415.
Wolf S, Bertram B, Jung F, Kiesewetter H, Teping C, Reim M. Videofluoreszenzangiographische Verlaufsbeobachtungen bei Patienten mit retinalem Stasesyndrom. Klin Monatsbl Augenheilkd 1988;193:39.
Wolter JR. Parallel horizontal choroidal folds secondary to an orbital tumor. Am J Ophthalmol 1974;77:669.
Wolter JR, Shut AL, Martonyi CL. Hemangioma-like clinical appearance of a collar-button melanoma caused by the strangulation effect of Bruch's membrane. Am J Ophthalmol 1973;76:730.
Wright JE. Orbital vascular anomalies. Trans Am Acad Ophthalmol Otolaryngol 1974;78:78.
Wright JE. Primary optic nerve sheath meningioma: clinical presentation and management. Br J Ophthalmol 1989;73:960.
Wright JE, Steward WB, Krohel GB. Clinical presentation and management of lacrimal gland tumors. Br J Ophthalmol 1979;63:600.
Wright JE, McDonald IW, Call MB. Management of optic nerve gliomas. Br J Ophthalmol 1980;64:545.
Wright JE, Wong D, Guthoff R. The management of severe Graves' ophthalmopathy. Br J Ophthalmol (in press).
Zakow ZN, Berlin LA, Gutman FA. Ultrasonographic mapping of vitreoretinal abnormalities. Am J Ophthalmol 1963;96:622.
Zakow ZN, Berlin LA, Meyers AM, Zachary IG. Atypical choroidal osteomas. In: , ed. Proceedings of the 2nd International Meeting on the Diagnosis and Treatment of Intraocular Tumors, Lyons 1987 (in press).
Zimmerman LE, Naumann G. Pathology of retinoschisis. In: McPherson A, ed. New and controversal aspects of retinal detachment. New York: Harper and Row, 1968:.

# Index